AF680039

Causes, Diagnosis and Treatment of Tuberculosis

Causes, Diagnosis and Treatment of Tuberculosis

Editor: Morris Beckler

AMERICAN
MEDICAL PUBLISHERS
www.americanmedicalpublishers.com

AMERICAN
MEDICAL PUBLISHERS
www.americanmedicalpublishers.com

Cataloging-in-publication Data

Causes, diagnosis and treatment of tuberculosis / edited by Morris Beckler.
p. cm.
Includes bibliographical references and index.
ISBN 979-8-88740-538-4
1. Tuberculosis. 2. Tuberculosis--Etiology. 3. Tuberculosis--Diagnosis. 4. Tuberculosis--Treatment.
5. Mycobacterium tuberculosis. 6. Mycobacterial diseases. I. Beckler, Morris.
RC311 .C38 2023
616.995--dc23

© American Medical Publishers, 2023

American Medical Publishers,
41 Flatbush Avenue,
1st Floor, New York,
NY 11217, USA

ISBN 979-8-88740-538-4 (Hardback)

This book contains information obtained from authentic and highly regarded sources. Copyright for all individual chapters remain with the respective authors as indicated. All chapters are published with permission under the Creative Commons Attribution License or equivalent. A wide variety of references are listed. Permission and sources are indicated; for detailed attributions, please refer to the permissions page and list of contributors. Reasonable efforts have been made to publish reliable data and information, but the authors, editors and publisher cannot assume any responsibility for the validity of all materials or the consequences of their use.

Trademark Notice: Registered trademark of products or corporate names are used only for explanation and identification without intent to infringe.

Contents

Preface

Tuberculosis (TB) is an infectious disease caused by the bacteria Mycobacterium tuberculosis (MTB). It is disseminated through air when persons with active tuberculosis in their lungs cough, spit, speak or sneeze. Tuberculosis affects the lungs in most cases, but it can also affect other parts of the body such as brain, lymphatic system or bones. In the majority of infections, there are no visible symptoms, known as latent tuberculosis. Chronic cough with bloody mucus, fever, night sweats and weight loss are all common symptoms of active tuberculosis. It is diagnosed by chest X-rays and culture of bodily fluids. The tuberculin skin test (TST) or blood tests are used for the diagnosis of latent tuberculosis. Multiple antibiotics must be used over a long period of time to treat this infection. Antibiotic resistance is becoming a problem as the number of people with multidrug-resistant tuberculosis (MDR-TB) is rising. This book contains some of the path-breaking studies related to tuberculosis. It includes some of the vital pieces of work being conducted across the world on the diagnosis, causes and treatment of this disease. This book will serve as a reference to a broad spectrum of readers.

Various studies have approached the subject by analyzing it with a single perspective, but the present book provides diverse methodologies and techniques to address this field. This book contains theories and applications needed for understanding the subject from different perspectives. The aim is to keep the readers informed about the progresses in the field; therefore, the contributions were carefully examined to compile novel researches by specialists from across the globe.

Indeed, the job of the editor is the most crucial and challenging in compiling all chapters into a single book. In the end, I would extend my sincere thanks to the chapter authors for their profound work. I am also thankful for the support provided by my family and colleagues during the compilation of this book.

Editor

1

Tuberculosis Vaccine Development — Its History and Future Directions

Elizabeth M. MacDonald and Angelo A. Izzo

1. Introduction

Mycobacterium tuberculosis is the world's most successful pathogen, having survived over 70,000 years and currently infecting nearly 2 billion people worldwide [1]. With around 9 million new cases of tuberculosis (TB) each year, almost one third of the population is at risk for developing active disease [2]. In 2012 alone, an estimated 3,500 people *per day* died of TB and, in fact, human immunodeficiency virus (HIV) is the only other infectious disease responsible for more deaths each year than *M. tuberculosis* [1, 3]. Because of these deadly statistics, the World Health Organization (WHO), the Centers for Disease Control (CDC), and the Bill and Melinda Gates foundation, among many others, have committed to eradicating *M. tuberculosis* by the year 2050. A combined strategy of drug treatment, better diagnostics, and prevention (i.e. vaccine development) is the only way to reach this goal [4].

While finding a cure and treating the disease is an essential aspect of medicine, of equal importance are prevention measures to stop contracting the disease in the first place. Because extreme and totally drug resistant strains of *M. tuberculosis* are appearing with increasing frequency, it is essential that we block the spread of this pathogen by developing a vaccine that provides protection against infection.

1.1. Vaccine development

The hallmark of an effective vaccine is one that can be given to a young population, with no adverse side effects, and which will provide lifelong immunity against a particular pathogen. The basis of a functional vaccine is dependent on the immune system's ability to 'remember' an encounter with a foreign pathogen. Typically, immunological memory is established upon the first encounter with a pathogen by the creation of memory T cells. These memory T cells are specific to a particular antigen and will reside in tissues and lymph nodes until they recognize their specific pathogen and become activated. Upon activation by a second exposure, the memory T cells will quickly and efficiently initiate a response to eliminate the pathogen and prevent disease. The creation of memory T cells and life-long immunity can be obtained either by primary exposure to the pathogen followed by disease and eventual recovery, or by being given a vaccine. Vaccines act to prime the immune system by exposing a person to a non-lethal, milder version of the pathogen's antigens so that those memory T cells can be created without causing disease in the individual. Ideally, a vaccine is made of pathogen-derived components that are critical for induction of protective immunity and consequently, are often composed of either an attenuated (non-virulent) or killed version of the bacteria, inactivated bacterial toxins, or subunits of the pathogen. The vaccines will have antigens similar to the virulent version of the pathogen but would lack factors necessary for disease. Thereafter, if a vaccinated individual is exposed to that particular set of antigens a second time, the immune system will quickly eliminate the pathogen and prevent disease. The immune system is therefore required to respond in a proper manner both to vaccination and to subsequent challenges with the pathogen.

In the case of *M. tuberculosis* infection, however, the immune response initiated upon exposure does not result in memory and instead, infection follows a more complex pathogenesis route. The main route of transmission for *M. tuberculosis* is via aerosolization of liquid droplets containing bacilli that are then breathed in by an individual. After inhalation, organisms are carried into the deep lung where it is phagocytosed by antigen presenting cells (APCs), such as macrophages or dendritic cells, which then travel to the draining lymph nodes and initiate an immune response [1, 5]. *M. tuberculosis* specific T cells then migrate to the lungs and are required for the formation of a granuloma around the site of infection [1]. In an immunocompetent individual, this granuloma will contain the infection in the lungs and prevent active disease [6] [1].

CD4+T cells are the hallmark of the immune response to *M. tuberculosis* infection and, together with CD8+T cells play significant roles in the various stages of infection and disease [6, 7]. Interferon (IFN)-γ and tumor necrosis factor (TNF)-α are essential cytokines for the induction of immunity to infection [6, 7]. Our understanding of the network of immune cells and cytokines required by the host to contain the infection, generate granulomas, and limit the extent of tissue involvement is increasing and will provide a better understanding of the requirements for generating vaccine mediated immunity.

This chapter will focus on the varied and unique aspects of *M. tuberculosis* that have made the development of a vaccine a challenging prospect. We will discuss the only vaccine currently on the market, BCG, its history, and why it has failed to prevent the spread of this pathogen. We will also discuss the various animal models and methodologies that are used by researchers to study the immune response to *M. tuberculosis* in the hopes of developing a more effective vaccine. We will also discuss a few of the vaccines that have already been developed and are being tested in clinical trials. Additionally, we will briefly discuss the various regulatory approval processes that are required to test a vaccine before it can finally be approved for release on the market.

2. The BCG vaccine

Bacillus Calmette-Guérin (BCG) is the most widely used vaccine having been delivered to nearly 3 billion people [8-10]. Despite its widespread use, BCG delivers only minimal protection and has failed to eradicate or reduce the disease burden of TB. The mechanisms by which BCG works to provide its marginal protection are incompletely understood. Even though BCG provides an imperfect defense against *M. tuberculosis* infection, it is still the best vaccine available. In this section of the chapter we will discuss the history of BCG and some possible reasons why it has failed to stem the tide of deaths due to *M. tuberculosis* infection.

2.1. History

Albert Calmette and Camille Guérin developed BCG at the beginning of the 20th century. Developed from a virulent strain of *Mycobacterium bovis,* the BCG vaccine was attenuated by serially passing the strains on potato slices supplemented with glycerol over a period of 13 years until a non-virulent strain was obtained [8-10]. Trials of the newly developed vaccine were performed in cows, monkeys, and African apes and proved to be efficacious [11] [12]. The strain was first used as a vaccine in humans in 1921 with few adverse side effects observed in the patients who received it [8, 9]. The non-virulence of this strain was then established before it was sent out to several laboratories throughout the world and used as a vaccine. The vaccine was then propagated in the various countries in different ways with varying passage numbers, resulting in the emergence of different variants of the BCG vaccine [8, 10].

2.2. World use

BCG is very cheap to produce and at only $2-3USD per dose, it is one of the most cost effective ways to provide at least partial protection against *M. tuberculosis* to millions of children worldwide [13]. Most of the BCG given in the world is supplied by UNICEF – obtained from three major sources; producers in Denmark, Japan, and Russia [8, 9]. Most countries around the world require that the BCG vaccine be given during childhood. The US, Canada, and Italy are some of the very few countries that have never required that children be given BCG. Most of Europe and Australia did at some point in their history require BCG to be given to children, but have since changed their policies. All of Africa, Asia, and most of South America currently require BCG to be given in early childhood [14].

2.3. Safety and efficacy

A huge reason for the widespread use of BCG is that it is considered to be one of the safest vaccines on the market [15]. Side effects of BCG are very rare with the most common complication being swelling around the injection site [15]. The most significant issue to arise from BCG vaccination is in HIV infected and other immunocompromised individuals. The increased risk of dissemination in HIV infected children lead the WHO to change its policy and recommend that they not be given BCG [15, 16]. Even so, BCG is still part of the WHO's expanded program of vaccination [8].

Studies into the efficacy of BCG have revealed wide-ranging results from vaccination programs with some reports suggesting 80% efficacy and others showing no protection at all [15, 17]. BCG is thought to convey protection against dissemination of the mycobacteria to other organs during childhood, an event that is highly fatal if left untreated. BCG does not, however, provide protection against adult pulmonary disease, which is the main route by which *M. tuberculosis* is transmitted [16].

2.4. Variability in efficacy

There are several possible reasons behind the huge variability in the reported efficacy of BCG; we will discuss some of these reasons in this section. It is important to keep in mind that some of the issues surrounding BCG efficacy variability are also issues which apply to the new *M. tuberculosis* vaccines currently being developed.

2.4.1. Variation in the strain of BCG that is used for vaccination

There are at least 11 different types of BCG vaccines currently available throughout the world [8]. A major reason for the different types of BCG and the genetic variability between the strains is mainly a product of the time period when the vaccine was developed. When Calmette and Guérin first developed BCG, they sent it out to several other laboratories around the word. Those laboratories cultured, grew, and stored BCG, each in their own way. It must be remembered that this occurred in the early part of the 20th century, before the advent of current molecular techniques and storage methods that can maintain parent strain homogeneity. Instead, as BCG was grown and cultured in these various laboratories, it accumulated a series of independent mutations that continued to build upon themselves [8]. It was not until the 1960s, with the introduction of culture seed stocks that soon became the norm, that the standardization of these lines became possible. By that time, however, the various strains of BCG had diverged and modern analysis has demonstrated that there is significant variability in the genetic make-up of these strains [8, 10]. The genetic variation in BCG strains can lead to variation in how well they protect against infection due to difference in the cell surface proteins that would elicit an immunogenic response [10]. However, all of these BCG strains have remained non-virulent and a commonality among all of the strains is the loss of the ESX-1 excretion system. It is still not completely understood how the loss of the ESX-1 system blocks virulence since its re-addition to at least two separate BCG strains does not restore virulence back to wild type levels [10, 18]. Due to this variation in BCG strains, it is essential that accurate record keeping be in place when conducting efficacy studies for the vaccine [8].

2.4.2. The genetic diversity of the tested population

The genetic diversity of a population can affect the outcome of any clinical research study and this is an important factor to consider when examining vaccine efficacy. Various single nucleotide polymorphisms (SNPs) within a genome can affect a person's susceptibility to disease and how their immune system responds to a vaccine. The spectrum of immune system responses to a vaccine can vary from no response to complete activation and protection. Variations within a person's genome could prevent their immune system from properly responding to the vaccine and therefore it would not convey protection when the person is exposed to the pathogen. For instance, it has been found that mutations in the IFN-γ receptors leads to an increased risk of developing disseminated disease from BCG vaccination rather than protection from *M. tuberculosis* infection [19]. Individuals with mutations in these susceptibility genes are also more prone to infection by non-virulent, environmental mycobacteria as well [19] [19].

Therefore, it is essential when designing a vaccine study in humans to have a large population that is statistically powerful enough that some variability in immune response will not skew the data. Additionally, no matter where a study is being conducted, the genetic diversity of the population must be considered. An ethnically homogenous population is more desired for a research study since that population will be more likely to share SNPs, and therefore more likely to respond to a vaccine in a similar manner. It also follows that it may also be useful to test multiple ethnic groups; indeed, some studies have suggested that the reason some vaccine trails show high protection with BCG is because they were conducted within certain population groups [15].

2.4.3. *Pre-vaccination exposure to the pathogen*

Another issue that is of huge importance when conducting vaccine efficacy tests is whether or not an individual has been pre-exposed to the pathogen. The immune response of an individual who has already been exposed may be quite different than someone without prior exposure. Especially in areas where TB is endemic, it is likely that a child will have already been exposed to *M. tuberculosis* prior to vaccination [1]. A child could be exposed to both *M. tuberculosis* in the form of infected adults, or to environmental nontuberculous mycobacteria (NTM) – both of which could alter how that child responds to a vaccine. Some studies have also suggested that pre-exposure to NTM may provide some protection that cannot be improved upon by BCG delivery [9, 15, 20]. This may indeed be the case with BCG as it has been found that vaccine programs with the highest degree of efficacy are those with more rigorous screening to only include children who had not been previously exposed to the antigen [17].

2.4.4. *Inaccurate diagnostic methods*

Because of the complications that result from pre-exposure to the pathogen, it is essential to have accurate diagnostic methods available when deciding which individuals to include in a study. A non-homogeneous population (a mixture of non-and pre-exposed individuals) can produce misleading results that can hinder accurate interpretation of vaccine efficacy. In the case of *M. tuberculosis,* current diagnostic methods are often slow or inaccurate. One of the most common diagnostics for *M. tuberculosis* is the tuberculin skin test (TST), a delayed-type hypersensitivity reaction to protein purified from *M. tuberculosis* and injected just below the skin [21, 22]. It takes two to three days after injection of the purified protein derivative (PPD) before the results can be read; a delay that can result in loss of study participant compliance or even exposure. Additionally, the TST, as well as many new serological tests, cannot distinguish between exposure to environmental NTM and infectious *M. tuberculosis* [23]. Newer IFN-γ release assays (IGRAs) are, however, becoming more commonly used for research studies since they are selective for *M. tuberculosis* and are more sensitive than the TST [21, 22]. IGRAs are *in vitro* tests that stimulate T cells with *M. tuberculosis* specific antigens (such as ESAT-6), if the T cells have been previously exposed to these antigens, they will release IFN-γ [22].

3. Specific difficulties associated with M. tuberculosis vaccine development

The complications involved with studying *M. tuberculosis* in a laboratory are numerous and range from the practical to the scientific. Due to the complex nature of the pathogen, *M. tuberculosis* presents some very unique challenges for the researcher studying it. In this section we will go into more depth as to the specifics of these challenges and how they have delayed the development of a vaccine.

3.1. Biosafety considerations

When a researcher decides to investigate the development of a vaccine against *M. tuberculosis* one of the very first considerations that must be taken into account is the safety of those working with the pathogen. In the United States, the CDC provides a set of guidelines for the safety measures that need to be in place in order to work with various pathogenic organisms. These biosafety levels range from 1 (least likely to cause harm to an individual) to 4 (most harmful and infectious) [24]. The basis for these biosafety measures are derived from the WHO, which, in turn, base their recommendations upon the availability of effective preventive measures and treatment options [25]. As the biosafety level of a pathogen increases, it is necessary to increase the safety measures for a person working in these conditions. In the research laboratory setting, *M. tuberculosis* is considered a biosafety level 3 (BSL3) pathogen; a BSL3 pathogen is defined by the WHO as one that poses a high risk for an individual but a low risk for the community and can cause serious harm to an infected human. The various safety measures that must be put in place include laboratory practices, facility construction, security, and safety equipment. The exact nature of the measures put in place will vary slightly from facility to facility but in general, this includes separate rooms and equipment for work with the pathogen. Rooms in which the pathogen is manipulated must be under negative pressure so that airflow is directed from a clean room into a 'dirty' room to prevent it from spreading. All work done with the microbe needs to be conducted in a properly outfitted biosafety cabinet and special personal protective equipment (e.g. respirators) must be worn at all times.

These biosafety mechanisms can be a limiting factor when attempting to study *M. tuberculosis*, as they require full facility involvement and specialized equipment to be in place. Additionally, these biosafety measures, while necessary, can be relatively uncomfortable, and may therefore limit the time with which a person can work under them. While these are obviously not insurmountable obstacles, they should be taken into consideration before research of this nature is undertaken.

3.2. Slow growth of the pathogen

M. tuberculosis is a slow growing pathogen with a doubling time of approximately 24 hours [26]. Because it grows so slowly, it is necessary to let a significant amount of time pass after infection in order to resolve differences in vaccine treatments. If an unvaccinated mouse is given a low dose aerosol infection of virulent *M. tuberculosis*, it can take upwards of 3 to 4 weeks before visible granulomatous lesions will form in the lungs [6]. When conducting immunological research, mice are generally sacrificed 30 to 120 days after infection to examine short and long term immunity and determine if a vaccine has had any effect on the reduction in mycobacterial number. When the animal is sacrificed, the lungs must then be plated on selective agar media in order to enumerate the number of mycobacteria growing in the lungs. The time of plating the lungs until the formation of visible colonies is between 2-3 weeks. All told, experiments of this nature often require 6-9 months of work before any data is even collected. Therefore, when planning out experiments involving infected animals, researchers must consider the significant amount time it will take between the initiation of the experiment and the completion of the study.

3.3. Disease stages

As mentioned previously, infection with *M. tuberculosis* can be divided into distinct stages. In humans, infection with *M. tuberculosis* can be divided into four stages: infection, latency, reactivation, and transmission [5]. At each of these stages, the proteins expressed by the organism are thought to vary significantly and therefore protection in one stage may not protect in all. After primary infection, in an immunologically healthy individual, an infection will progress to a latent TB infection (LTBI). The persistence of infection despite no active disease in a clinically 'cured' individual, make end point goals difficult to define for a researcher developing a vaccine [16]. There is significant evidence that sterile clearance of *M. tuberculosis* is a rare occurrence and rather, it is the maintenance of an active immune system to contain the mycobacteria in the latent state that prevents active disease from forming [1, 27]. In most individuals, this is where the infection will remain unless there is an outside occurrence that reduces the functionality of their immune system [1]. A person with a LTBI will not have active disease, but will have developed memory cells against *M. tuberculosis* antigens. It is generally believed that when *M. tuberculosis* is in a latent stage it is slow growing or non-replicative and most likely expresses a different set of antigens than during the primary infection stage of the life cycle [1]. The exact immunological events that are required in order for the pathogen to progress from latency into an active state are incompletely understood.

The immune response that humans develop against *M. tuberculosis* infection appears to contain the bacteria and induce it into a latent stage, yet fails to sterilize the infection [5]. This leads to some interesting questions as to what types of antigens to target for vaccine development. When a person has a LTBI, their immune system is effectively containing the mycobacteria and they do not get sick. Do we therefore design vaccines to elicit an immune prolife similar to someone with a latent infection even though that profile is not sufficient to eliminate the pathogen? It is interesting to note that individuals that are infected with *M. tuberculosis* and progress on to latency are not protected from re-infection. However, because detection of *M.*

tuberculosis when it is in a latent stage is quite difficult with our current diagnostic methods, it is often challenging to distinguish between reactivation of the primary (latent) infection or re-infected from a new exposure [1, 16]. Since our understanding of the possibility of lung sterilization post-*M. tuberculosis* infection is incomplete, the comparison of persons with LTBI to those with active disease is limited in what it can tell us about protective immunity.

Ideally, the best vaccine would be one that provides protection from all stages of infection, i.e. a vaccine must be effective against primary infection, latency, reactivation, and reinfection [1, 2].

3.4. Vaccination in immunocompromised individuals

Of the estimated 1.3 million people who died of TB in 2013 around 25% of them were co-infected with HIV [3]. In fact, TB is the number one killer of HIV infected individuals [7, 28-30]. The resurgence of *M. tuberculosis* infections in the 1990s has largely been attributed to the advent of the HIV epidemic [30, 31]. The reasons behind the increased susceptibility of HIV infected individuals to *M. tuberculosis* infection are not completely understood. An infection with HIV leads to a reduction in CD4+T cells and this is believed to be the cause of greater susceptibility to *M. tuberculosis* by most individuals [28, 30, 32]. One hypothesis is that HIV disrupts the function of the granuloma and allows for the replication of the organism [28]. The immune system of an HIV infected individual is, therefore, not able to control or contain the *M. tuberculosis* infection, resulting in reactivation of the disease [28, 30]. HIV infection may also disrupt the function of macrophages and *M. tuberculosis* specific T-cells that prevents the killing of the pathogen [28]. An interesting aspect of the *M. tuberculosis*-HIV co-infection is that HIV infection leads to susceptibility to *M. tuberculosis* even after anti-retroviral therapy has commenced and CD4+T cell counts have been restored to normal [33] [30, 34]. It has also been found that HIV infected infants do not produce a robust T helper (Th)1 immune response when vaccinated with BCG [30]. Additionally, HIV positive infants are at a significantly increased risk of dissemination of BCG after vaccination [7, 15, 16].

Another group of immunocompromised individuals that must be considered are those with poor living conditions and poor nutrition. TB is a disease of the poor and mainly affects those who are already at a socioeconomic disadvantage. Poor nutrition and living conditions increases a person's susceptibility to disease and dampens their immune response to a challenge. These living conditions could impair the ability of the immune system to respond properly both to a vaccination and exposure to a pathogen. Other conditions, such as diabetes or vitamin D deficiency, can also impair the ability of the immune system to produce a robust response and indeed, both conditions have been associated with an increased risk for developing TB [35-37].

3.5. Vaccination post exposure to the pathogen

In the case of TB, it is important to consider if the vaccine is aimed at pre or post-exposure to the pathogen. As mentioned in the previous section, a person's immune system will respond differently to a vaccine if they have already been exposed to the pathogen. Since the immune system will have already been primed to respond to particular *M. tuberculosis* antigens that are not capable of protection, it is necessary to find a new method of immune activation. Because of the high prevalence of *M. tuberculosis* in endemic countries, it is likely that in order to eradicate TB, a vaccine will need to be effective post-exposure.

3.6. Laboratory strains versus clinical isolates

Mycobacteria from clinical isolates are often quite different than the strains commonly used in laboratory practice. Laboratories, by necessity for the repeatability of their experiments, must maintain an unchanging common lab strain. There are currently several strain types used in laboratories throughout the world (H37Rv, HN878, Erdman, CDC1551, etc.) that vary in their virulence and antigenic composition. Variation can also occur within a strain depending on how it is handled in the laboratory. Unfortunately, however, these strains can be significantly different than the mycobacteria isolated from infected patients. The mycobacteria found 'in the wild' is going to be constantly changing and mutating depending on various selection factors. The extent of the divergence between laboratory strains and clinical isolates will depend upon the strength of the selection factor. These selection factors can include incomplete drug treatments or the strength of a non-drug treated person's immune response to the pathogen. Additionally, there is a natural mutation rate for the genome of all organisms independent of selection factors due to DNA replication errors or un-repaired DNA damage. The selection factors and mutational changes observed in clinical isolates are most apparent with the emergence of multi, extreme, and totally drug resistant organisms. While it is hoped that there is enough similarity between laboratory strains and the clinical isolates that vaccination against one will provide protection from all forms of *M. tuberculosis*, the constant mutation of wild-type strains should be considered.

3.7. Intrinsic properties of *M. tuberculosis* which make it difficult to immunize against

Currently, almost all vaccines that have proven to be efficacious in humans against infectious pathogens convey protection through the production antibodies [1, 38]. These antibodies will coat a pathogen and signal to the immune cells that it should be removed from the system. *M. tuberculosis*, however, is intracellular, which means that the immune system must be able to recognize and then eliminate infected host cells without causing excessive damage to the host.

M. tuberculosis has established several methods by which it can evade recognition by the host immune system. Most of these mechanisms revolve around ways of keeping the pathogen in a quiescent state within the macrophage. For example, the recruitment of professional phagocytic cells to the site of infection provides an increased number of ideal environments for *M. tuberculosis* survival. Once phagocytic cells have taken up the organism, it can survive within macrophages by arresting and inhibiting the maturation of the phagosome to prevent its own clearance from the cell [37]. These blocks in phagosome maturation prevent fusion of the phagosome with the lysosome and acidification of the compartment and thus elimination from the cell [37]. This block in phagocytosis also prevents proper presentation of *M. tuberculosis* antigens [1]. Presentation of antigens is essential for recognition that an antigen is foreign and needs to be eliminated, as well as for the creation of immune memory. *M. tuberculosis* also evades removal by the ability to regulate both the necrotic and apoptotic death of host cells [5].

All of the elimination avoidance methods developed by *M. tuberculosis* serve to maintain the pathogen within the macrophages where it can live for decades as a latent infection [1, 37]. While *M. tuberculosis* infection does produce an immune response in the host, this response fails to result in protection or complete clearance of the pathogen [1, 5]. Therefore, when designing a vaccine, it is necessary to activate the immune system in such a way that the host can overcome these evasion methods and recognize that the pathogen infected cells should be destroyed.

4. Animal models used for vaccine development

In some cases where the pathogen is non-lethal or there are readily available treatment options (such as malaria or influenza), it is possible to test the efficacy of a vaccine in a human model. In these instances, a willing volunteer is vaccinated, and then exposed to the pathogen by the researcher in a controlled manner [16]. In the case of *M. tuberculosis* however, this course of experimentation is unethical as it is still controversial if sterilization of the lungs post-infection is even possible. It is therefore imperative that we use animal models for the development of vaccines. A vaccine is considered efficacious in an animal model if it is able to reduce the number of colony forming units (CFU) in the lung. Currently, the goal for new vaccines is to reduce the number of CFU in the lung better than BCG, which consistently provides around a 1 $\log_{10}$ CFU reduction in the mouse model of tuberculosis.

4.1. Mouse model

4.1.1. Advantages

Cost effectiveness and scalability. One of the biggest reasons for the use of mouse models in research is their cost effectiveness. With the exception of highly specialized knock-in or knock-out models, inbred mice can be purchased in large numbers at very low cost. Since mice can often be housed with multiple animals per cage, this further reduces the facilities cost by utilizing less space per animal. A researcher can therefore scale a study up to a magnitude that would be impossible with larger or more costly animals.

Inbred mouse strains and genetically modified models. Through the use of genetically identical inbred strains, researchers from all over the world have the ability to collaborate using the same set of tools and more effectively build upon previous studies. The ready availability of facilities like The Jackson Laboratories and Charles Rivers, which specifically maintain these inbred mouse strains are an invaluable resource for researchers. These facilities also make it easy to custom order genetically modified mouse models to test the importance of various proteins during vaccination or pathogen challenge. The availability of total or conditional knock-out mice, as well as knock-in models, allows researchers to effectively use *in vivo* system to ask questions that are unavailable by other methods.

Availability of immunological reagents. The use various molecular assays after completion of an animal experiment can provide vital information about the function of the immune system. An additional advantage to using the mouse model is that because it is so widely used, reagents are available for many types of immunological assays. In particular, antibodies for western blot, enzyme linked immunosorbent assays (ELISAs), flow cytometry, and many others, are commonly used on mouse models and are therefore relatively easy to optimize for a particular experiment.

Susceptibility of various strains. The strain of mouse that will be used for an experiment is of great importance when designing an experiment. There is significant variability between mouse strains as to their susceptibility to TB infection. This variance in susceptibility of a mouse strain can depend up on several important factors including the route of infection, the dosage, and the strain of *M. tuberculosis* [39]. While genetic modification is commonly done on a C57Bl/6 background, these mice are actually resistant to *M. tuberculosis* infection and aerosol infection does not reduce their lifespan [39]. Some strains such as CBA are very susceptible to infection, while others, such as the BALB/c, appear to be susceptible depending on the route of infection [39]. These last two strains, however, do have the disadvantage that there are fewer genetically modified strains available with this background. The immune systems of both the susceptible and resistant strains clearly respond differently to both vaccination and challenge infection and therefore, it is often useful for researchers to test a vaccine in more than one mouse model.

4.1.2. Disadvantages

A major disadvantage of the mouse model is that the immune system is not the same as that of a human. The underlying genomic inflammatory response to infection in a mouse has been shown to bear little correlation to what occurs in humans [40]. Many drugs that have been designed to modify inflammatory responses in mice, have failed human clinical trials [40]. While humanized mice (a mouse containing human genes, cells, or tissue) may allow for an immune response closer to that of a human, it is impossible to create an identical response. Additionally, unlike in humans, BCG vaccination of a mouse model does convey some protection from *M. tuberculosis* infection and reduces the number of CFU in the lungs. A better understanding of the critical cellular differences between the mouse and human immune system is needed before we can effectively translate studies from the bench to the clinic.

4.2. Guinea pig model

4.2.1. Advantages

Historically, the guinea pig was the first animal model used for tuberculosis research. Guinea pigs are considered the gold standard by which *M. tuberculosis* vaccines are tested before continuing to larger animal models or even humans. This is because guinea pigs have an immune response that more closely resembles that which is seen in susceptible humans. Guinea pigs are very susceptible to infection and demonstrate a tuberculosis disease progression that is similar to that seen in humans [41].

One aspect of guinea pig research that is both an advantage and a disadvantage is the lack of in-bred laboratory strains. There are only a handful of laboratory guinea pig strains available commercially and these are mostly out-bred stock that will not be genetically identical at every locus. This provides greater genetic diversity within an animal strain with which to tests vaccine efficacy. Obviously when vaccines move into human trials, genetic diversity will be unavoidable (as mentioned previously), and therefore the guinea pig provides a more realistic model of what will happen in humans. However, this does limit the exact repeatability of an experiment due to the lack of genetically identical animals.

4.2.2. Disadvantages

A disadvantage of the guinea pig model is that they are very susceptible to infection, but humans are relatively resistant. While the phenotype observed during disease progression does resemble that of humans with active disease, this represents only a small fraction of people infected with *M. tuberculosis*. It is believed that most humans are resistant to infection and will not go on to active disease unless an outside force reduces their immune response and ability to contain infection in a latent state [6, 7]. The exact mechanisms behind reactivation of latent *M. tuberculosis* are not completely understood, but it is a vital step in disease pathogenesis that is missed in the guinea pig model.

The guinea pig also has the disadvantage that, because it is a larger animal, housing costs tend to be much higher than for mice. Guinea pigs require larger cages with fewer animals per cage and thus facility space limitations may reduce the number of animals included in a study. Additionally, because they are not as commonly used as the mouse model, it is more difficult to find the facilities and veterinary expertise necessary to house and care for guinea pigs.

Of great importance is the lack of genetically modified guinea pig models for the researcher to use. This can severely limit the ability of the researcher to develop and improve upon vaccine models.

4.3. Other animal models

The mouse and guinea pig are the most commonly used animal models for research into *M. tuberculosis* vaccine development. However, there are several other animal models that are also sometimes utilized for this purpose including rabbit, cattle, non-human primates (NHP) and even zebrafish [42-44].

Macaques are an NHP that are a promising model to use for the development of a tuberculosis vaccine. The pathophysiology of TB infection in a macaque closely resembles that of what occurs in human populations, including latency – an aspect of infection that has been difficult to model in other animals [43, 45]. Due the size of the animals, their limited availability, the cost of housing and care, as well as ethical considerations, use of NHP, while highly informative, is extremely limited and generally only done after a vaccine has been tested in smaller animal models.

One of the biggest disadvantages to use of any of these non-mouse models is that there are very few reagents available for post-mortem tissue analysis. Few antibodies or other commonly used immunological reagents are available for the study of the immune response in many animal models. Sometimes there is enough overlap in antigens between mouse and humans and other animals that some tests can be conducted, but this is a fairly rare occurrence. While these are not limitations that preclude the use of non-mouse animal models, it does limit the information that can be acquired from using them [46]. There is therefore a huge need to expand our animal model base beyond just the mouse. Genetic evaluation of and the ability to produce inbred strains of other animal models would be an unbelievable advantage to all clinical research beyond just tuberculosis vaccine development.

We can garner important information from all of these animal models and it is clear that their use is absolutely essential for progress in medical researcher to be made. However, it must be remembered that these models are imperfect and there are scientific limitations to the results from studies using them. For instance, in a laboratory setting, animals tend to be exposed only once and to only one strain of pathogen. We know this will not be the case for humans since, as discussed above, *M. tuberculosis* is constantly mutating and in endemic regions a person will likely be exposed to several different strains at multiple times throughout their life [47]. Ultimately, the only way to test out if a vaccine will be effective in a human population is to actually test it in a human population. While it is certainly possible to move on to human trials, there are many steps that must be undertaken before a vaccine can be put into widespread use. This process will be discussed in the next section.

Another important question to consider when examining results from animal models is if we are missing vaccines that would be highly efficacious in a human, but discarding them because they do not act well in our animal models. This is a problem for all areas of clinical research and is, unfortunately, unavoidable given our current knowledge. The only way to overcome this limitation is for research to continue to close the gap in our understanding of how animal and human immune systems differ. The continued refinement of our animal models will provide us with the tools necessary to produce an effective vaccine. This is another reason why the use of multiple animal models is often needed in order to improve the translatability of the research. Most animal models recapitulate some, but not all, aspects of the human features of a disease. If multiple animal models are tested, it increases the likelihood of finding a vaccine that will work in humans.

5. The future of *M. tuberculosis* vaccine development

There is a profound lack of understanding about what exactly a good immune response to *M. tuberculosis* infection actually looks like. This is due, in part, to our limited information about how the immune system contains infection in a latent state as well as how it can revert to active disease. Because our knowledge is incomplete, it complicates decisions regarding which vaccine candidates to pursue in animal models. Our best vaccine, BCG, is not 100% effective in killing off *M. tuberculosis* in a mouse despite eliciting a strong Th1 immune response that is thought to be necessary to produce immunity against the pathogen [1]. In general, if a new vaccine candidate can also elicit a strong Th1 response in a mouse model, it will then move on to challenge studies where an animal model is immunized, then infected. While it is clear that protection from infection does require strong T cell immunity, it is also clear that that form of immunity is not sufficient to prevent disease. Sometimes, even when a vaccine candidate is promising in preliminary trials, this will not lead to protection when challenged with infection. This is why many of the vaccines currently in the approval process pipeline have multiple pathways by which they induce an immune response. The hope is that one of these other pathways, or a combination of various pathways, will give us more and better information about what immunological protection would look like [1].

There are at least 12 new vaccines candidate that have entered the pipeline for efficacy and safety testing and are the first to be put through the approval process in over 100 years [2, 48]. It is encouraging to note that there are so many vaccines being tested as it increases the likelihood of finding a formulation that will be effective. The arrival of these new vaccines, even those that fail, is a promising step forward in our understanding of immunity and what protection will look like. In this section we will discuss some of the characteristics of these vaccines as well as the steps that must be gone through before they can be put into widespread use.

5.1. Common tactics taken for vaccine development

There are two main tactics for the development of a new vaccine against *M. tuberculosis* infection. The first is the prime-boost or enhancing the efficacy of the existing vaccine, BCG. In this approach, an individual can be given an adjuvanted vaccine at the same time or at a specified period of time after BCG vaccination. The other tactic is to develop a whole new vaccine that is given instead of BCG. There are advantages and disadvantages to both strategies and a discussion on the ethics of trial design for both of these can be found in the next section.

Many of the vaccines that are being developed contain one or more of a select group of antigens for the initiation of an immune response. Antigen 85A/B (Ag85A/B) and the 6kD early secreted antigenic target (ESAT-6) are proteins that are commonly included in a vaccine make up [2]. Ag85A/B are *M. tuberculosis* surface proteins that are involved in bacterial cell wall biosynthesis and elicit an immune response in animal models [23]. ESAT-6 is a secreted protein critical for virulence that is not found in BCG and can also stimulates a strong immune response [18, 49]. These proteins, along with several others that have been found to be immunogenic, have been put into various formulations and are currently being tested.

In addition to multiple combinations of proteins found to be immunogenic, there has also been testing of which delivery route will provide the best protection. For instance, some vaccines provide better immune protection if they are delivered via aerosol route rather than through intradermal injection. Therefore, many studies are being conducted looking at both multiple delivery routes as well as vaccine make-up.

5.2. Ethical considerations

There are also important ethical considerations that must be addressed when developing a new vaccine. When testing out a vaccine, it is important to consider the health and safety of the control groups as well as those receiving the novel vaccine. For instance, if you have in your possession a vaccine (i.e BCG) that conveys at least some protection against TB, you ethically cannot withhold access to that vaccine simply because you need a placebo control group for your research study. Additionally, a researcher attempting to test out an entirely new vaccine must also consider the possibility that their vaccine will not work and therefore those test subjects are at an increased risk of developing disease. While there are ways to circumvent these issues and still produce an ethically sanctioned and scientifically sound vaccine trial, it does require additional preparation and manpower to execute. Because of these significant ethical complications, however, much of the recent research into TB vaccines has been for the development of adjuvants to boost BCG rather than to develop completely new vaccines.

5.3. MVA85A

The most notable of these new vaccines is MVA85A, which is the first modern day *M. tuberculosis* vaccine to reach an efficacy trial. MVA85A is a Modified Vaccinia virus Ankara that has been engineered to express Ag85A [1, 50]. In animal models, MAV85A was shown to produce a strong Th1 response and provide better protection against *M. tuberculosis* infection than BCG [47, 51-53]. It was designed as a prime boost, to enhance the efficacy of BCG, by giving it to infants a few months after BCG vaccination. In a Phase 2b clinical trial, MVA85A was found to be quite safe and did produce an immunogenic response, but unfortunately, did not provide better protection against infection than BCG alone [53]. This was despite earlier findings that MVA85A induces the immune responses believed to be necessary for protection [54]. In fact, this (previously assumed to be beneficial) CD4+T cell response to Ag85A is still detectable in individuals given MVA85A up to 6 years after vaccination [55]. Even though MVA85A did not provide the protection that was hoped, there are some promising indications that this vaccine may be useful in other settings. For instance, the authors suggest that this vaccine maybe beneficial in preventing the spread of disease in adults rather than in infants [53]. Clearly further testing of the MVA85A vaccine needs to be conducted. Even though initial results with MVA85A were disappointing, it does represent a promising step in vaccine development. Given the state of the field, any knowledge gained about immunity against *M. tuberculosis*, even if negative, can provide useful information and guide future studies

5.4. Vaccine approval process

The WHO offers a set of guidelines for the approval of a vaccine, and many countries adopt these standards or use them as a basis for their own set of regulations. The point of these regulations is to do as much as possible to ensure the safety and efficacy of the vaccine before it is put into widespread use. In the United States, the Federal Drug Administration (FDA) regulates and oversees the approval process for the development of all vaccines. This discussion will give a quick overview of the FDA regulations specific to the US as an example of what must be undertaken before a vaccine is approved for use. The FDA approval process involves an exploratory stage, a pre-clinical stage, an Investigational New Drug (IND) application, and finally a three phase clinical trial in human subjects [56]. The FDA has the authority to stop a vaccine trial at any point if safety becomes a concern.

The exploratory stage is the basic science side of the vaccine development process. It is in this stage where researchers investigate the potential of various antigens to induce an immune response and are frequently done *in vitro* although some *in vivo* studies may be conducted. This is where the formulation of the vaccine is first tested and the identification of immunogenic proteins is determined.

The pre-clinical stage involves animal model testing of the various antigens that were discovered in the exploratory stage. In this stage, animals are immunized using a new antigen or vaccine make up and then challenged with *M. tuberculosis* infection. The various animal models discussed in the previous section are used in this stage of vaccine development. In order for the vaccine to move on to humans, it must first demonstrate efficacy in multiple animal models. The animal models used can vary depending on pathogen, but for *M. tuberculosis* these models generally include (in order), mouse, guinea pig, and non-human primates. Once a vaccine has been found to be effective, it must pass toxicology and distribution studies in the animal models, as well as demonstration of the ability to produce the vaccine in a lab with Good Manufacturing Practice (GMP) certification [57]. After the completion of these studies an IND application is submitted and, upon approval, human clinical trials will commence.

Phase 1 clinical trials are small studies designed to test the safety and immunogenicity of the vaccine. Phase 2 clinical trials are larger and used for further refine dosage and efficacy of the vaccine as well as determining what population it can be most effectively used on. Phase 3 clinical trials involve thousands of individuals and require additional safety documentation to complete [56].

Once all of these stages have been completed, a cross-disciplinary committee from the FDA must then approve a lengthy Biologics License Application (BLA). The BLA will include not only safety and efficacy information but also guidelines for the mass manufacture and distribution of the vaccine as well. As may be obvious from this brief description, the process of vaccine approval can be quite lengthy and will often last 10-15 years. The enormous cost associated with undertaking such an endeavor often requires the collaboration of both private and public funds at multiple institutions in order to be completed.

6. Conclusions

The development of a vaccine against *M. tuberculosis* has been one of the hardest puzzles facing immunologist for the past century. When examining an infection and an appropriate immune response, the traditional approach, at least in relation to tuberculosis research, has been to try to amplify the immune response of a healthy person in order to clear the bacteria. However, is this really the approach we should take when examining *M. tuberculosis*? In the case of *M. tuberculosis* infection, is it the body's very own defense mechanisms that is causing lung tissue damage and forcing the mycobacteria into a latent stage? Is the body's response to infection actually a good thing or is it contributing to disease progression because it creates an environment that harbors the bacteria (a granuloma) rather than eliminating it? Should we instead be attempting to induce activation of a whole new pathway in order to sterilize the lungs?

The urgency to find of an effective vaccine is nowhere as apparent as the emergence of drug resistant tuberculosis that been appearing with increasing frequency in the last decade. The currently available drugs are expensive and require a lengthy course of treatment; increasing the likelihood of non-adherence by sick people and therefore increasing the possibility of even more resistant strains evolving. Because a person does not naturally develop immunity to the pathogen when they are infected, they can become re-infected if they are exposed to the pathogen a second time and have to endure the same drug regimen as before. Only by providing continuous, protective immunity against recurrent infection can we hope to eradicate this devastating disease from the population.

Acknowledgements

This work was supported by the NIH/NIAD program Advanced Small Animal Models for the Testing of Candidate Therapeutic and Preventative Interventions against Mycobacteria (HHSN272201000009I-003, task order 12) at Colorado State University.

Author details

Elizabeth M. MacDonald and Angelo A. Izzo*

*Address all correspondence to: angelo.izzo@colostate.edu

Mycobacteria Research Laboratories, Department of Microbiology, Immunology and Pathology, Colorado State University, Fort Collins, CO, USA

References

[1] Andersen P, Woodworth JS. Tuberculosis vaccines--rethinking the current paradigm. Trends in immunology. 2014;35(8):387-95.

[2] Brennan MJ, Stone MR, Evans T. A rational vaccine pipeline for tuberculosis. The international journal of tuberculosis and lung disease : the official journal of the International Union against Tuberculosis and Lung Disease. 2012;16(12):1566-73.

[3] World Health Organization. Global tuberculosis report 2013 2013 [cited 2014 23 Sept]. Available from: http://www.who.int/tb/publications/global_report/en/.

[4] Dye C, Williams BG. Eliminating human tuberculosis in the twenty-first century. Journal of the Royal Society, Interface / the Royal Society. 2008;5(23):653-62.

[5] Ernst JD. The immunological life cycle of tuberculosis. Nature reviews Immunology. 2012;12(8):581-91.

[6] North RJ, Jung YJ. Immunity to tuberculosis. Annual review of immunology. 2004;22:599-623.

[7] O'Garra A, Redford PS, McNab FW, Bloom CI, Wilkinson RJ, Berry MP. The immune response in tuberculosis. Annual review of immunology. 2013;31:475-527.

[8] Ritz N, Curtis N. Mapping the global use of different BCG vaccine strains. Tuberculosis. 2009;89(4):248-51.

[9] Luca S, Mihaescu T. History of BCG Vaccine. Maedica. 2013;8(1):53-8.

[10] Brosch R, Gordon SV, Garnier T, Eiglmeier K, Frigui W, Valenti P, et al. Genome plasticity of BCG and impact on vaccine efficacy. Proceedings of the National Academy of Sciences of the United States of America. 2007;104(13):5596-601.

[11] Experiments with Tuberculosis Vaccine on African Apes. Science. 1925;62(1609):xiv.

[12] Professor Calmette on a vaccine for tuberculosis. Science. 1921;53(1363):131-2.

[13] Trunz BB, Fine P, Dye C. Effect of BCG vaccination on childhood tuberculous meningitis and miliary tuberculosis worldwide: a meta-analysis and assessment of cost-effectiveness. Lancet. 2006;367(9517):1173-80.

[14] Zwerling A, Behr MA, Verma A, Brewer TF, Menzies D, Pai M. The BCG World Atlas: a database of global BCG vaccination policies and practices. PLoS medicine. 2011;8(3):e1001012.

[15] Rowland R, McShane H. Tuberculosis vaccines in clinical trials. Expert review of vaccines. 2011;10(5):645-58.

[16] Brennan MJ, Thole J. Tuberculosis vaccines: a strategic blueprint for the next decade. Tuberculosis. 2012;92 Suppl 1:S6-13.

[17] Mangtani P, Abubakar I, Ariti C, Beynon R, Pimpin L, Fine PE, et al. Protection by BCG vaccine against tuberculosis: a systematic review of randomized controlled trials. Clinical infectious diseases : an official publication of the Infectious Diseases Society of America. 2014;58(4):470-80.

[18] Pym AS, Brodin P, Brosch R, Huerre M, Cole ST. Loss of RD1 contributed to the attenuation of the live tuberculosis vaccines Mycobacterium bovis BCG and Mycobacterium microti. Molecular microbiology. 2002;46(3):709-17.

[19] Doffinger R, Dupuis S, Picard C, Fieschi C, Feinberg J, Barcenas-Morales G, et al. Inherited disorders of IL-12-and IFNgamma-mediated immunity: a molecular genetics update. Molecular immunology. 2002;38(12-13):903-9.

[20] Young D, Dye C. The development and impact of tuberculosis vaccines. Cell. 2006;124(4):683-7.

[21] Kaufmann SH. Tuberculosis vaccines: time to think about the next generation. Seminars in immunology. 2013;25(2):172-81.

[22] Pai M, Zwerling A, Menzies D. Systematic review: T-cell-based assays for the diagnosis of latent tuberculosis infection: an update. Annals of internal medicine. 2008;149(3):177-84.

[23] Bekmurzayeva A, Sypabekova M, Kanayeva D. Tuberculosis diagnosis using immunodominant, secreted antigens of Mycobacterium tuberculosis. Tuberculosis. 2013;93(4):381-8.

[24] Centers For Disease Control. Recognizing the Biosaftey Levels [cited 2014 25 Feb]. Available from: http://www.cdc.gov/training/quicklearns/biosafety/.

[25] American Biological Safety Association. Risk Classification criteria for World Health Organization, Australiam Canadam European Union (EU), USA CDC/NIH and NIH for RDNA [cited 2014 25 Sept]. Available from: http://www.absa.org/riskgroups/index.html.

[26] Straus E, Wu N. Radioimmunoassay of tuberculoprotein derived from Mycobacterium tuberculosis. Proceedings of the National Academy of Sciences of the United States of America. 1980;77(7):4301-4.

[27] Salgame P. Host innate and Th1 responses and the bacterial factors that control Mycobacterium tuberculosis infection. Current opinion in immunology. 2005;17(4): 374-80.

[28] Diedrich CR, Flynn JL. HIV-1/mycobacterium tuberculosis coinfection immunology: how does HIV-1 exacerbate tuberculosis? Infection and immunity. 2011;79(4): 1407-17.

[29] Corbett EL, MacPherson P. Tuberculosis screening in high human immunodeficiency virus prevalence settings: turning promise into reality. The international journal of tuberculosis and lung disease : the official journal of the International Union against Tuberculosis and Lung Disease. 2013;17(9):1125-38.

[30] Walker NF, Meintjes G, Wilkinson RJ. HIV-1 and the immune response to TB. Future virology. 2013;8(1):57-80.

[31] Dye C. Tuberculosis 2000-2010: control, but not elimination. The international journal of tuberculosis and lung disease : the official journal of the International Union against Tuberculosis and Lung Disease. 2000;4(12 Suppl 2):S146-52.

[32] Lawn SD, Myer L, Edwards D, Bekker LG, Wood R. Short-term and long-term risk of tuberculosis associated with CD4 cell recovery during antiretroviral therapy in South Africa. Aids. 2009;23(13):1717-25.

[33] Thacher EG, Cavassini M, Audran R, Thierry AC, Bollaerts A, Cohen J, et al. Safety and immunogenicity of the M72/AS01 candidate tuberculosis vaccine in HIV-infected adults on combination antiretroviral therapy: a phase I/II, randomized trial. Aids. 2014;28(12):1769-81.

[34] Geldmacher C, Schuetz A, Ngwenyama N, Casazza JP, Sanga E, Saathoff E, et al. Early depletion of Mycobacterium tuberculosis-specific T helper 1 cell responses after HIV-1 infection. The Journal of infectious diseases. 2008;198(11):1590-8.

[35] Dooley KE, Chaisson RE. Tuberculosis and diabetes mellitus: convergence of two epidemics. The Lancet Infectious diseases. 2009;9(12):737-46.

[36] Martineau AR. Old wine in new bottles: vitamin D in the treatment and prevention of tuberculosis. The Proceedings of the Nutrition Society. 2012;71(1):84-9.

[37] Jayachandran R, BoseDasgupta S, Pieters J. Surviving the macrophage: tools and tricks employed by Mycobacterium tuberculosis. Current topics in microbiology and immunology. 2013;374:189-209.

[38] Abebe F. Is interferon-gamma the right marker for bacille Calmette-Guerin-induced immune protection? The missing link in our understanding of tuberculosis immunology. Clinical and experimental immunology. 2012;169(3):213-9.

[39] Chackerian AA, Behar SM. Susceptibility to Mycobacterium tuberculosis: lessons from inbred strains of mice. Tuberculosis. 2003;83(5):279-85.

[40] Seok J, Warren HS, Cuenca AG, Mindrinos MN, Baker HV, Xu W, et al. Genomic responses in mouse models poorly mimic human inflammatory diseases. Proceedings of the National Academy of Sciences of the United States of America. 2013;110(9): 3507-12.

[41] Acosta A, Norazmi MN, Hernandez-Pando R, Alvarez N, Borrero R, Infante JF, et al. The importance of animal models in tuberculosis vaccine development. The Malaysian journal of medical sciences : MJMS. 2011;18(4):5-12.

[42] Oksanen KE, Halfpenny NJ, Sherwood E, Harjula SK, Hammaren MM, Ahava MJ, et al. An adult zebrafish model for preclinical tuberculosis vaccine development. Vaccine. 2013;31(45):5202-9.

[43] Kaushal D, Mehra S, Didier PJ, Lackner AA. The non-human primate model of tuberculosis. Journal of medical primatology. 2012;41(3):191-201.

[44] Villarreal-Ramos B, Berg S, Chamberlain L, McShane H, Hewinson RG, Clifford D, et al. Development of a BCG challenge model for the testing of vaccine candidates against tuberculosis in cattle. Vaccine. 2014;32(43):5645-9.

[45] Flynn JL, Capuano SV, Croix D, Pawar S, Myers A, Zinovik A, et al. Non-human primates: a model for tuberculosis research. Tuberculosis. 2003;83(1-3):116-8.

[46] Padilla-Carlin DJ, McMurray DN, Hickey AJ. The guinea pig as a model of infectious diseases. Comparative medicine. 2008;58(4):324-40.

[47] McShane H, Williams A. A review of preclinical animal models utilised for TB vaccine evaluation in the context of recent human efficacy data. Tuberculosis. 2014;94(2): 105-10.

[48] Tameris M, McShane H, McClain JB, Landry B, Lockhart S, Luabeya AK, et al. Lessons learnt from the first efficacy trial of a new infant tuberculosis vaccine since BCG. Tuberculosis. 2013;93(2):143-9.

[49] Yu X, Xie J. Roles and underlying mechanisms of ESAT-6 in the context of Mycobacterium tuberculosis-host interaction from a systems biology perspective. Cellular signalling. 2012;24(9):1841-6.

[50] Odutola AA, Owolabi OA, Owiafe PK, McShane H, Ota MO. A new TB vaccine, MVA85A, induces durable antigen-specific responses 14 months after vaccination in African infants. Vaccine. 2012;30(38):5591-4.

[51] Goonetilleke NP, McShane H, Hannan CM, Anderson RJ, Brookes RH, Hill AV. Enhanced immunogenicity and protective efficacy against Mycobacterium tuberculosis of bacille Calmette-Guerin vaccine using mucosal administration and boosting with a recombinant modified vaccinia virus Ankara. Journal of immunology. 2003;171(3): 1602-9.

[52] Williams A, Goonetilleke NP, McShane H, Clark SO, Hatch G, Gilbert SC, et al. Boosting with poxviruses enhances Mycobacterium bovis BCG efficacy against tuberculosis in guinea pigs. Infection and immunity. 2005;73(6):3814-6.

[53] Tameris MD, Hatherill M, Landry BS, Scriba TJ, Snowden MA, Lockhart S, et al. Safety and efficacy of MVA85A, a new tuberculosis vaccine, in infants previously vaccinated with BCG: a randomised, placebo-controlled phase 2b trial. Lancet. 2013;381(9871):1021-8.

[54] Scriba TJ, Tameris M, Mansoor N, Smit E, van der Merwe L, Mauff K, et al. Dose-finding study of the novel tuberculosis vaccine, MVA85A, in healthy BCG-vaccinated infants. The Journal of infectious diseases. 2011;203(12):1832-43.

[55] Tameris M, Geldenhuys H, Luabeya AK, Smit E, Hughes JE, Vermaak S, et al. The candidate TB vaccine, MVA85A, induces highly durable Th1 responses. PloS one. 2014;9(2):e87340.

[56] Administration USFaD. Vaccine Product Approval Process [cited 2014 25 Sept]. Available from: http://www.fda.gov/BiologicsBloodVaccines/DevelopmentApprovalProcess/BiologicsLicenseApplicationsBLAProcess/ucm133096.htm.

[57] McShane H, Pathan AA, Sander CR, Goonetilleke NP, Fletcher HA, Hill AV. Boosting BCG with MVA85A: the first candidate subunit vaccine for tuberculosis in clinical trials. Tuberculosis. 2005;85(1-2):47-52.

2

Application of High Performance Liquid Chromatography for Identification of *Mycobacterium* spp.

Carlos Adam Conte Junior,
César Aquiles Lázaro de la Torre,
Eduardo Eustáquio de Souza Figueiredo,
Walter Lilenbaum and Vânia M. Flosi Paschoalin

1. Introduction

Since 1896, when Lehmann and Neumann described the bacterium responsible for causing tuberculosis and leprosy, about 150 species of *Mycobacterium* have been described. Except for *Mycobacterium leprae*, which does not grow *in vitro*, those species were classified in two distinct groups: species that belong to the *Mycobacterium tuberculosis* complex (MTC), and non-tuberculous mycobacteria (NTM) [1, 2]

Mycobacterium tuberculosis infects over one-third of the human population worldwide, causing nine million new cases of tuberculosis and two million deaths annually [3]. While members of the MTC cause more disease worldwide than any other bacteria [4], NTM are widespread in nature and, with some significant exceptions, are free-living saprophytes and opportunistic pathogens. Although considered to be non-pathogenic, NTM can pose a threat to humans, mainly in patients with underlying conditions such as AIDS or cancer, and there is an increasing awareness of their public-health importance, especially as nosocomial pathogens [5].

Some strategies employed to identify *Mycobacterium* spp. included observations of staining properties of bacilli, cultural morphology, biochemical tests, and, rarely, the inoculation of susceptible animals with live bacilli for observation of animal pathogenicity [6]. At the beginning of mycobacterial research identification the differentiation of species level was performed by traditional culture methods based on phenotypic and biochemical characteristics. The principal disadvantage of this method is the time-consuming evaluation. Currently a genotypic evaluation is more preferred by the mycobacterial species [7]. Different species can display distinct antibiotic resistances and require different prescriptions for treatment. For this reason it is important to identify *Mycobacterium* species in a rapidly and accurately way [8, 9]

Complex high-molecular-weight β-hydroxyl fatty acids with a 22-or 24-carbon alkyl chain at the α-position are structural characteristics of mycolic acids (MAs), a type of fatty acid found in the *Mycobacterium* spp. cell wall. Several methods of fatty-acid analysis have indicated that MAs are species-or group-specific [10]. High-performance liquid chromatography (HPLC) analysis of MAs is a reliable method for the detection of mycobacteria, because of the rapid and reproducible nature of the method and because the MAs elution spectrum observed for each mycobacterial species has generally been found to be unique, except for two species (*M. bovis* and *M. tuberculosis*) that share the same spectrum pattern [11, 12]. The HPLC method has been considered a standard test for chemotaxonomic classification and rapid identification of *Mycobacterium* species by the Centers for Disease Control and Prevention (CDC) since 1990, and has been reported to be more than 96% accurate compared with DNA probe tests [6]. Even HPLC is considered one of the most reliable and cost-effective tools for the rapid identification of *Mycobacterium* spp. isolated in culture based on the presence of different MAs [13] and it was well described and standardized [14], the methodology could be affected by several factors and must be optimized in accordance with local laboratory capabilities in order to assure accurate diagnosis.

In this review are presented the procedures to saponification, extraction (chloroform), derivatization (p-bromophenacyl), separation (C18 column and a gradient of methanol and methylene chloride) and detection (ultraviolet spectrophotometer) of MAs. Also is explored the importance of built a pattern chromatogram library for successful identification of clinical samples based on comparison of the relative retention times (RRT) of the chromatogram patterns with those obtained from reference strains and with those available in external databases. HPLC is necessary for separation of MAs due to their large size and complexity that requires the use of different columns and solvents. Initial methods required manual interpretation of chromatograms with eventual development of automated systems.

2. Mycobacterium species and mycolic acids

The analysis of lipid fractions has contributed significantly to the knowledge of *Mycobacterium* species. The abundance of lipid constituents in mycobacterial cell walls made them classic candidates for early chemical investigations [6, 15]. MAs, 2-alkyl, 3-hydroxy long-chain fatty acids, are the hallmark of the cell envelope of *Mycobacterium tuberculosis* (Figure 1). They are found either unbound, extractable with organic solvents (esters of trehalose or glycerol) or esterifying the terminal pentaarabinofuranosyl units of arabinogalactan, the polysaccharide that, together with peptidoglycan, forms the insoluble cell wall skeleton [16]. Both forms presumably play a crucial role in the remarkable architecture and impermeability of the cell envelope, also called the mycomembrane [17-19].

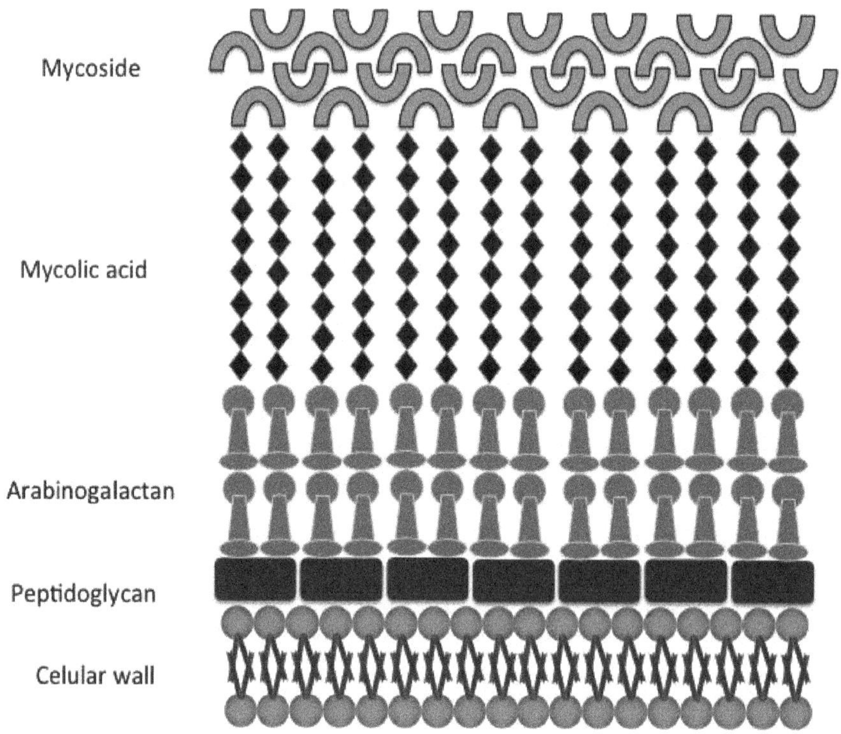

Figure 1. Diagrammatic presentation of mycobacterial cell wall and location of mycolic acids.

Structurally similar substances to MAs have been found in all mycobacterial species, with very few exceptions (e.g., *Corynebacterium amycolatum* and *Corynebacterium kroppenstedtii*). The identification of MAs structure has been addressed through the application of analytical techniques such as thin-layer chromatography (TLC), gas chromatography (GC), HPLC, mass spectrometry, and nuclear magnetic resonance spectroscopy. Based on their structural variability and complexity, MAs were largely used as taxonomic markers [17]. These large fatty acids contain a variety of functional groups and can vary in both qualitative and quantitative characteristics between species. This variety provides the basis for separation and identification of a large number of mycobacterial species using the HPLC.

3. High performance liquid chromatography methodology

Reverse-phase high-performance liquid chromatography of MAs esters has been demonstrated to be a rapid, reproducible, species-specific method for the identification of mycobacterial species. Also this method is relatively inexpensive and has been found to be more rapid alternative laboratory technique than the use of commercial nucleic acid probes [20]. Different methods have been developed for the detection of mycobacteria in clinical samples (e.g., blood, sputum) but they can also be applied to detection in other sources such as water [21] and milk [22]. Standard procedures to HPLC identification of mycobacterial species and most common steps used for different researchers are showed in the Figure 2 and Table 1, respectively.

Saponification	Fatty acid extraction	Stationary phase	Mobile phase/flow rate	Derivatization/ detector	Ref.
25% KOH in 50% ethanol	Chloroform	C18	Chloroform (C) + methanol (M): 10 % C:90%M: 13 min 25% C:75%M: 14 min 70% C:30%M: 20 min Gradient elution: 0.6 mL/min	p-bromophenacyl/UV (254nm)	[13]
25% KOH in 50% methanol	Chloroform	C18	Methanol (M) + methylene chloride (MC): 98% M:2% MC: Initial 80% M:20% MC:1 min 35% M:65% MC: 10 min 98% M:2% MC: 10.5 98% M:2% MC: 12 min Gradient elution: 2.5 mL/min	p-bromophenacyl/UV (260nm)	[20]
50% aqueous potassium hydroxide Autoclaved: 1 h /121 ºC	Chloroform	C18	Methanol (M) + methylene chloride (MC): 98% M:2% MC: Initial 85% M:15% MC:1 min 55% M:45% MC: 1.75 min 55% M:45% MC: 8.75 min 30% M:70% MC: 11.75 98% M:2% MC: 12 min Gradient elution: 2.5 mL/min.	4-bromomethyl- 6,7-dimethoxycoumarin/ FL (Emission: 418nm; Excitation: 240-420nm)	[26]
Methanolic potassium hydroxide	Chloroform	C18	Methanol-methylene chloride Gradient elution	p-bromophenacyl/UV (254nm)	[34]
25% of KOH in 50% ethanol	Chloroform	C18	Methanol (M) + methylene chloride (MC): 98% M:2% MC: Initial 80% M:20% MC:1 min	p-bromophenacyl /UV (254-260nm)	[35]

Saponification	Fatty acid extraction	Stationary phase	Mobile phase/flow rate	Derivatization/ detector	Ref.
Autoclaved: 1 h /121 °C			35% M:65% MC: 10 min 98% M:2% MC: 10.5 98% M:2% MC: 12 min Gradient elution: 2.5 mL/min		
25% KOH in a water methanol (1:1) mixture. Autoclaved: 1 h /121 °C.	Chloroform	C18	Not referenced	p-bromophenacyl /UV	[36]
2 ml KOH 25% in 50% ethanol Autoclaved: 1 h /121 °C.	Chloroform	C18	Methanol (M) + methylene chloride (MC): 80% M:20% MC: Initial 60% M:40% MC:1 min 40% M:60% MC: 5.5 min 40% M:60% MC: 6 min 80% M:20% MC: 8 min Gradient elution: 3 mL/min	p-bromophenacyl /UV (254nm)	[37]
2 ml KOH 25% in methanol:H_2O (v:v) Autoclaved: 1 h /121 °C, 15 psi	Chloroform	C18	Methanol (M) + methylene chloride (MC): 98% M:2% MC: Initial 80% M:20% MC:1 min 35% M:65% MC: 2 min 98% M:2% MC: 17.5 min 98% M:2% MC: 20 min Gradient elution: 2 mL/min	p-bromophenacyl /UV (260nm)	[22]
25% KOH in 50% ethanol	Chloroform	C18	Chloroform (C) + methanol (M): 9 % C:91%M: Initial 70% C:30%M: 65 min Gradient elution: 2 mL/min	p-bromophenacyl /UV (254nm)	[38]
50% KOH in methanol solution	Chloroform	C18	Methanol (M) + 2-propanol (P): 60 % M: 40% P: Initial 60 % M: 40% P: 3 min 6 % M: 94% P: 21 min 30 % M: 70% P: 25 min Gradient elution: 1.5 mL/min	p-bromophenacyl /UV (260nm)	[25]

Table 1. Different chromatographic methods to *Mycobacterium* species identification from bacterial grown medium.

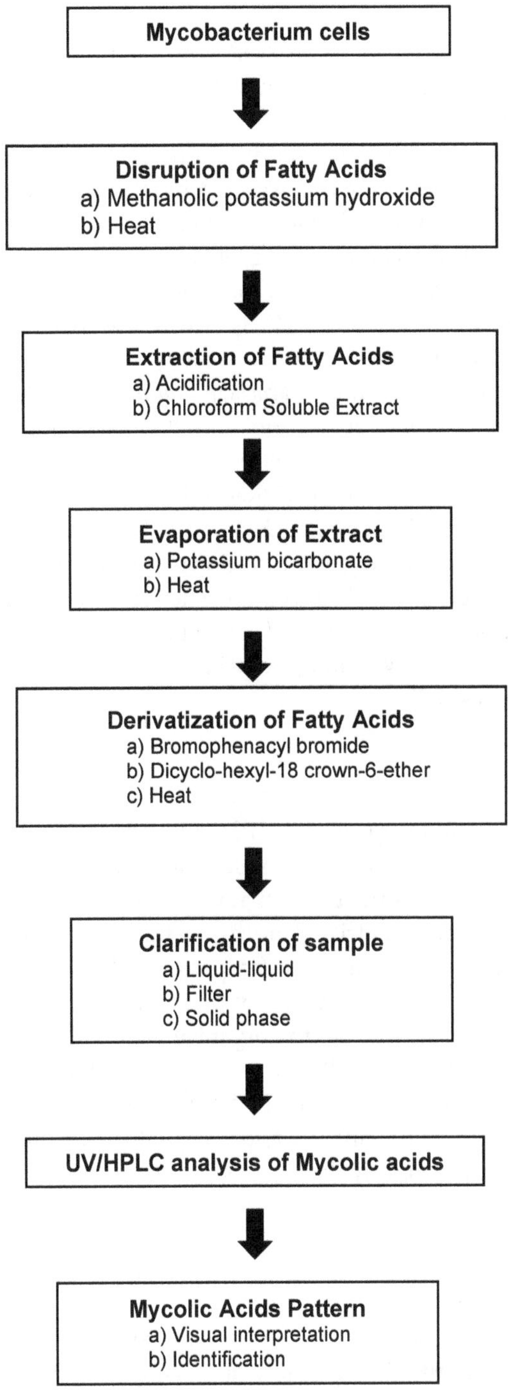

Figure 2. Flowchart for isolation and detection of mycolic acids. Adapted from [6].

3.1. Bacterial culture

HPLC still requires initial culture of isolates on solid medium before analysis. This can be problematic because the slow growth rate of mycobacteria delays full identification and leaves treating physicians with little useful information after the initial report of an acid-fast bacilli (AFB)–positive broth culture [23]. The identification is achieved when Mycobacteriae are grown under standardized culture medium conditions such as Lowenstein-Jensen (L-J) slant, which may be supplemented with additional growth factors for those strains of Mycobacteriae that are unable to grow on L-J. A carbol fuchsin/phenol or fluorochrome stain is performed to verify the presence of AFB. Another common solid medium used for mycobacterial species is the Middlebrook 7 H10 or 7 H11 at 35–37 °C. Currently available databases have been developed which incorporate mycobacterial species which require different growth conditions such as *Mycobacterium haemophilum* and *Mycobacterium marinum* (30 °C) [24]. According the Brazilian National Manual for the Laboratory Surveillance of Tuberculosis and other Myco-bacteria [1], mycobacteria strains are cultured in L-J culture, except for *Mycobacterium bovis* that is grown in Stonebrink media, at 35 °C. Recently Buchan *et al.* [23] explored the use of broth culture for mycobacterial species such as an alternative for the solid medium and demonstrated a rapidly and accurately identification of mycobacteria to the species level from solid medium (7H11) or directly from broth culture such as Myco broth. It is important remark that culturing of *Mycobacterium tuberculosis* must be performed in special laboratorial conditions (Biosafety level 3) and follow and appropriate guidelines for the use and handling of pathogenic microorganisms [25].

3.2. Saponification

The autoclaving-saponification steps in the HPLC procedure is performed for two reasons: frees MAs and kills the mycobacteria, assuring laboratory safety. Also this step is important because it will determine the amount of MAs that will be extracted. MAs are covalently linked to the cell wall arabinogalactan matrix. Removal of the MAs requires saponification with potassium hydroxide (50 % w/v), which is often performed in an autoclave to accelerate the process and provide for the safety of laboratory personnel working with Biosafety Level III mycobacterial species. Once autoclaved, the organisms are killed by the procedure and the mycolic acids released from the cell wall [24]. A standard protocol for HPLC identification of mycobacteria of CDC suggest transfer 1–2 loops of bacterium culture to a glass tube (13 by 100 mm) and add 2 mL of methanolic saponification reagent (25% potassium hydroxide in 50% methanol). The tube is capped tightly, homogenised and autoclaved for 1 h at 121°C and 15 psi [14].

3.3. Extraction

MAs exist in the cell in two basic forms: covalently bound to the cell wall, and loosely associated with an insoluble matrix esterified to a variety of carbohydrate containing molecules. Treatment of intact cells with mixtures of chloroform and methanol is suitable for extracting the smaller quantity of non-covalently attached mycolate [16]. Once autoclaving has been completed, samples are cooled to room temperature, acidified, and extracted into chloroform.

Free MAs are extracted by acidifying with 1.5 ml of a 50% solution of concentrated HCl and H_20 (v/v) and 2 mL chloroform. The chloroform layer is dried under air at 80-100 °C, and 2 mg of potassium bicarbonate is added [14].

3.4. Derivatization

The preparation from extraction step is resuspended in 1.0 mL chloroform, and a derivatize reagent (*p*-bromophenacyl) is added. Derivatization is completed in a water bath at 80-100 °C for 20 min. Tubes are cooled, the mixture is acidified with 1 mL of the acidification solution (concentrated HCl and H_2O; 1:1, v/v), and 1 mL methanol is added. After that the solution is thoroughly mixed, the bottom chloroform layer is transferred to a glass tube and evaporated to dryness. Samples are resuspended in 50 μL methylene chloride before analysis.

Some experiences make done using fluorescence-labeling compounds. According to Butler and Guthertz [6] these compounds evolved as a follow: 4-bromomethyl-7-methoxycoumarin (Br-Mmc), performed in TLC analysis for detection of picomolar amounts; 4-bromomethyl-7-acetoxycoumarin (Br-Mac), suggested for femtomolar detection and finally 4-bromomethyl-6,7-dimethoxycoumarin and 3-bromomethyl-7-methoxy-1,4-benzoxazin-2-1 and 4-bromomethyl-7-acetoxycoumarin. All fluorophores produced mycolic acid patterns similar to the patterns for *p*-bromophenacyl derivatives and were suggested for optimization of the method for clinical mycobacterial species identification. Jost *et al.* [26] reported the excellent analytical sensitivity of fluorescence (4-bromomethyl-6,7-dimethoxycoumarin) for the detection of MAs ester patterns and resulted in a substantial decrease in the time required to identify mycobacteria from cultures.

3.5. HPLC conditions

MAs are analyzed using a HPLC apparatus, in a gradient elution, and a UV detector set at 260 nm. Samples are separated in a C-18 reverse-phase column. The mobile phase is a mixture of methanol and methylene chloride in a flow rate of 2 mL min^{-1}. Authors performed some modifications in a CDC protocol for HPLC identification of MAs. Du et al. [9] tested a column with different dimensions (15.0 cm × 4.6 mm, 5 μm) and also a different elution program (run time 30 min and 1.5 mL min^{-1} flow rate) from the CDC specifications [14]. However, they obtained chromatograms quite similar to those from the CDC protocol. On the other hand, Figueiredo et al. [22] use a C-18 column 33% taller than those used in the CDC protocol (7.5 cm), increased the run time to 20 min. With these changes they observed a superior resolution in an adapted protocol and could be an alternative to discriminate between species with homologous HPLC chromatogram patterns. Special careful must be taken when manual injection is performed. Its is recommended cleaned the syringe at least five times with HPLC-grade methylene chloride and the injection loop be cleaned one time with 1 mL of the mobile phase solvent; it is also recommended that a blank injection be used between samples when the prior MAs signal is high [27].

4. Identification of mycobacteria species

There is a wide range of structures and also concentrations of types or classes of MAs (α, methoxy, keto, epoxy mycolates, etc.) among mycobacterial species. The HPLC methodology is unable to separate all the homologous series of MAs, and for this reason the chemical composition of the chromatogram components could not be precisely identified. Although the individual mycolate cannot be identified, this is not necessary for identification of mycobacteria, since a species-specific chromatographic pattern is generated [10, 28].

In order to identify unknown mycobacteria specimens using HPLC, the laboratory maintains chromatograms of mycobacteria commonly seen in the laboratory. HPLC profiles of unknown mycobacteria are compared to the patterns contained in this spectral library. The chromatographic pattern for each strain is examined for differences in the heights for pairs of peaks. HPLC patterns are grouped according to species, and the values calculated for each ratio are combined, sorted in numerical order, and examined for their ability to discriminate species, using the range of the relative standard deviation (RSD) of the absolute retention times (ART) and the relative retention times (RRT). RRTs are adjusted by comparison with external mycobacterial MA peaks [29]. The *Mycobacterium intracellulare* mycolic acid fingerprint is usually used as a reference standard to help differentiate *Mycobacterium* spp.

The visual pattern recognition method employs only chromatographic criteria, although when available, other identification test results should be included in the decision-making processes. The initial step for identifying a species is determining the overall complexity and number of MA peak clusters. These clusters may consist of a few peaks or many peaks and are further defined as single-, double-, and triple-or multiple-peak clusters [6]. The amount of MA present is related to the amount of light emitted and the structure of the MA is related to the time of elution off the column. Pattern recognition is performed by visual comparison of sample results with MA patterns from reference species of known Mycobacteriae; however, a correct pattern of interpretation requires training. For that reason computer-assisted pattern recognition software, which utilizes retention time, peak width, and peak amount to provide a peak name which can then be compared to a library database, was developed [24].

5. Chromatogram profile database from *Mycobacterium* spp.

Due to the interpretation of chromatographic data can become tedious and time consuming for laboratories that process large numbers of samples, some studies recommend the construction of computer-based file (library) of *Mycobacterium* species. This library is to be used in conjunction with commercially available pattern recognition software packages like a Pirouette [20] or more recently, the Sherlock Mycobacterial Identification System (SMIS; MIDI, Inc.) has been developed for the rapid, computer-assisted identification of mycobacterial species based on the separation and quantification of MAs using HPLC technology [30].

Figueiredo *et al.* [22] grouped 35 strains of *Mycobacterium* species according a fingerprint library into three general patterns (single-, double-and triple-peak clusters) and divided in subgroups according to the chromatogram characteristics of MAs derivatives (Figure 3).

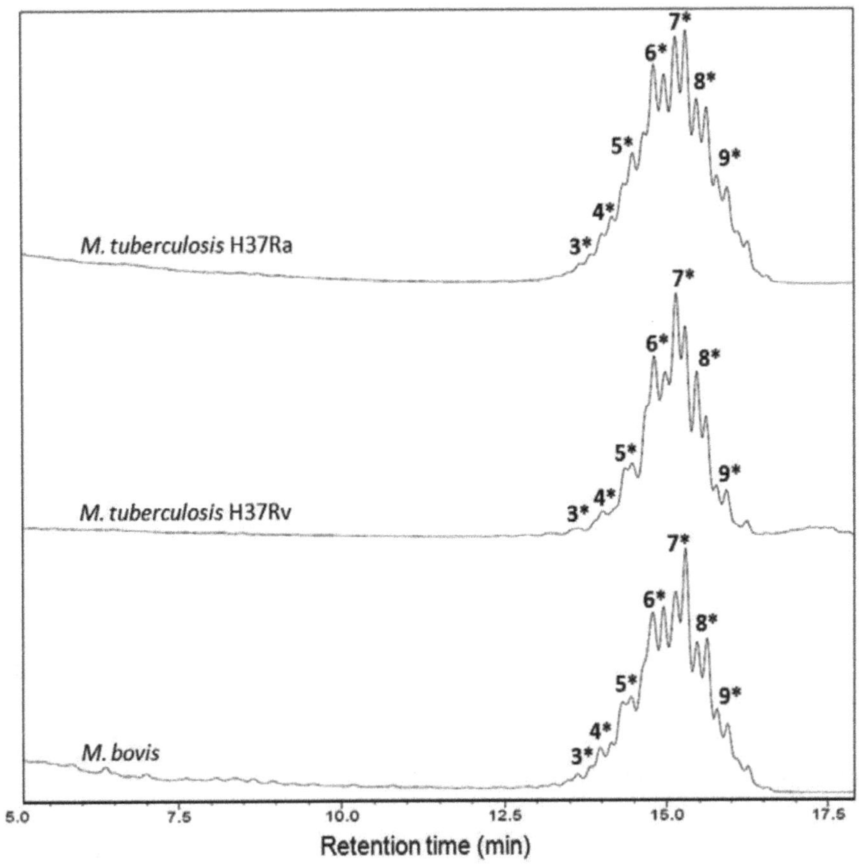

Figure 3. HPLC mycolic acid chromatograms from *Mycobacterium* reference strains, with single-cluster peak. *M. tuberculosis* H37Ra (ATCC 25177) and H37Rv (ATCC 27294) and *M. bovis* (ATCC 19210). *peaks showing a high degree of separation (appearing as a "double peak"), named according to [10]

5.1. Single-peak cluster patterns

Members of the MTC such as *Mycobacterium bovis* (Figure 4) and *Mycobacterium tuberculosis,* and others species such as *Mycobacterium asiaticum, Mycobacterium gordonae* chromotype I and *Mycobacterium. kansasii* showed chromatogram patterns with a single, late-emerging peak cluster. Mycobacteria species within the same taxonomic groups, such as the *M. tuberculosis* complex species, show very similar chromatographic patterns, since they share the same MA structural types. A means to discriminate between the closely related species with similar HPLC chromatogram profiles could further distinguish the MAs that might be present in the same peak. Considerable heterogeneity exists within a particular class of MAs, considering the chain length of individual acids (which can show a mixture of up to 100 structural isomers of α mycolates) and the potential range of heterogeneity in each species or subspecies [16].

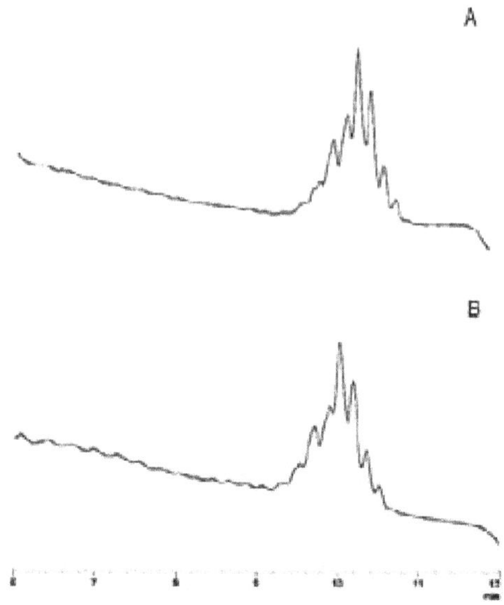

Figure 4. Representative reverse-phase HPLC chromatograms of bromophenacyl esters of mycolic acids from isolates of tissue fragments of Comparative Intradermal Tuberculin Test reactive cows: *M. bovis* ATCC 19210 (A) and *M. bovis* clinical isolates from bovines (B).

5.2. Double-peak cluster patterns

Mycobacterium chitae, Mycobacterium porcinum and *Mycobacterium agri* are representatives of this group that displays late-emerging and close-together clusters of peaks. *Mycobacterium fortuitum, Mycobacterium peregrinum* and *Mycobacterium smegmatis* are members of the *Mycobacterium fortuitum* complex and displayed very similar chromatogram patterns. Therefore, the HPLC results obtained for these species provided insufficient information to distinguish between them. The *Mycobacterium chelonae-Mycobacterium abscessus* taxonomic group has undergone several revisions following the identification of newly recognized species such as *Mycobacterium massiliense,* which was proposed based mainly on genotypic analysis. As expected for closely related species all the members of this group showed a single chromatogram pattern [31, 32].

5.3. Triple-peak cluster patterns

Mycobacterium simiae could be included in this group. The last group included *Mycobacterium chubuense, Mycobacterium obuense, Mycobacterium parafortuitum* and *Mycobacterium vaccae,* which showed early-peak clusters emerging before 10.0 min.

6. Application of high performance liquid chromatography

According to Figueiredo *et al.* [22] the identification of mycobacteria by HPLC is performed by comparing fingerprint patterns obtained from each clinical sample with those from the reference strains. The first criterion for identifying *Mycobacterium* spp. is to match the overall complexity and number of MA peak clusters: single, double and triple peaks. The second criterion is the range of time of elution between multiple peak groups, where the positions of peaks are determined as RRTs, adjusted by comparison to an external mycobacteria MA peak. To increase reliability, the relationships of peak heights of major diagnostic peaks are determined and compared to those from reference strains. Mondragón-Barreto et al. [33] describe the advantages of HPLC method to *Mycobacterium* identification but if results are unclear (problems are principally for inadequate HPLC reference patterns, the isolate should be analyzed using PCR-RFLP. Another interesting application to MAs identification by HPLC is the estimation of bacterial growth [27]. It was described a linear relationship between the total area under the MA chromatographic peaks of a culture of *Mycobacterium tuberculosis* and log CFU per milliliter, suggesting the possibility of using this results as a good estimator of mycobacterial growth.

7. Conclusion

HPLC procedure for MAs separation is a rapid, reproducible and easily way to *Mycobacteria* identification and can be executed by many laboratories, making this approach one of the most appropriate methods to distinguish among the species. A customized database, using locally adapted protocols, must be developed in order to obtain chromatogram spectra from reference strains in the new analytical conditions, accrediting the local methodology and allowing accurate analysis of clinical samples. Although HPLC equipment is too expensive for many laboratories, it is realize that this system is useful to MAs identification. It is recommended that the HPLC can be combined with other techniques like PCR as a confirmatory diagnosis for the identification of clinical isolates where the matching chromatogram fingerprints failed or were inconclusive in differentiating species within the same taxonomic group, such as the *M. tuberculosis* complex species.

Acronyms

AFB=Acid-fast bacilli

ART=Absolute retention time

CDC=Centers for Disease Control and Prevention

CFU=Colony forming unit

DNA=Deoxyribonucleic acid

GC=Gas chromatography

HPLC=High-performance liquid chromatography

L-J=Lowenstein-Jensen

MAs=Mycolic acids

MTC=*Mycobacterium tuberculosis* complex

NTM=Non-tuberculous mycobacteria

RRT=relative retention times

RSD=Relative standard deviation

SMIS=Sherlock Mycobacterial Identification System

TLC=Thin-layer chromatography

Acknowledgements

The authors thank the Fundação de Amparo à Pesquisa do Estado do Rio de Janeiro (process no. E-26/103.003/2012, FAPERJ, Brazil) and the Conselho Nacional de Desenvolvimento Científico e Tecnológico (processes no. 311361/2013-7, 313917/2013-2 and 401922/2013-8, CNPq, Brazil) for the financial support.

Author details

Carlos Adam Conte Junior[1*], César Aquiles Lázaro de la Torre[1,2],
Eduardo Eustáquio de Souza Figueiredo[3], Walter Lilenbaum[4] and
Vânia M. Flosi Paschoalin[2]

*Address all correspondence to: carlosconte@hotmail.com

1 Department of Food Technology, Faculty of Veterinary, Fluminense Federal University, Niterói, Rio de Janeiro, Brazil

2 Faculty of Veterinary Medicine, Universidad Nacional Mayor de San Marcos, San Borja, Lima, Peru

3 Department of Food and Nutrition, Federal University of Mato Grosso, Cuiabá/MT, Brazil

4 Department of Microbiology, Fluminense Federal University, Niterói, Rio de Janeiro, Brazil

References

[1] Brasil. Ministério da Saúde. Secretaria de Vigilância em Saúde. Manual Nacional de Vigilância Laboratorial da Tuberculose e Outras Micobactérias. In: Epidemiológica. V, editor. Brasilia2008. p. 436.

[2] List of Prokaryotic names with Standing in Nomenclature-Genus Mycobacterium. [Internet]. 2011. Available from: http://www.bacterio.cict.fr/m/mycobacterium.htm.

[3] WHO. Response to the global TB epidemic. Global Health Observatory (GHO). 2014.

[4] Dye C. Global epidemiology of tuberculosis. The Lancet. 2006;367(9514):938-40.

[5] Griffith DE, Aksamit T, Brown-Elliott BA, Catanzaro A, Daley C, Gordin F, et al. An Official ATS/IDSA Statement: Diagnosis, Treatment, and Prevention of Nontuberculous Mycobacterial Diseases. American Journal of Respiratory and Critical Care Medicine. 2007;175(4):367-416.

[6] Butler WR, Guthertz LS. Mycolic Acid Analysis by High-Performance Liquid Chromatography for Identification of *Mycobacterium* Species. Clinical Microbiology Reviews. 2001;14(4):704-26.

[7] Furlanetto LV, Figueiredo EES, Conte Júnior CA, Carvalho RCT, Silva FGS, Silva JT, et al. Use of complementary methods in post mortem inspection of carcasses with suspected bovine tuberculosis. Pesquisa Veterinária Brasileira. 2012;32:1138-44.

[8] Furlanetto LV, Figueiredo EES, Conte Júnior CA, Silva FGS, Duarte RS, Silva JT, et al. Prevalence of bovine tuberculosis in herds and animals slaughtered in 2009 in the State of Mato Grosso, Brazil. Arquivo Brasileiro de Medicina Veterinária e Zootecnia. 2012;64:274-80.

[9] Du R, Chen B, Guo L, Li Y, Xie J, G. W, et al. Identification of *Mycobacterium* species using reversed-phase high performance liquid chromatogram analysis of mycolic acid. Chinese Journal of Chromatography. 2008(26):234-9.

[10] Butler WR, Jost KC, Kilburn JO. Identification of mycobacteria by high-performance liquid chromatography. Journal of Clinical Microbiology. 1991;29(11):2468-72.

[11] Hagen SR, Thompson JD. Analysis of mycolic acids by high-performance liquid chromatography and fluorimetric detection implications for the identification of *mycobacteria* in clinical samples. Journal of Chromatography A. 1995;692(1–2):167-72.

[12] Tiwari RP, Hattikudur NS, Bharmal RN, Kartikeyan S, Deshmukh NM, Bisen PS. Modern approaches to a rapid diagnosis of tuberculosis: Promises and challenges ahead. Tuberculosis. 2007;87(3):193-201.

[13] Butler WR, Kilburn JO. Identification of major slowly growing pathogenic mycobacteria and *Mycobacterium gordonae* by high-performance liquid chromatography of their mycolic acids. Journal of Clinical Microbiology. 1988;26(1):50-3.

[14] CDC. Standardized Method for HPLC Identification of *Mycobacteria*. Atlanta: U.S. Department of Health and Human Services. Public Health Service; 1996. p. 99.

[15] Garza-González E, Guerrero-Olazarán M, Tijerina-Menchaca R, Viader-Salvadó JM. Determination of drug susceptibility of *Mycobacterium tuberculosis* through mycolic acid analysis. Journal of Clinical Microbiology. 1997;35(5):1287-9.

[16] Barry Iii CE, Lee RE, Mdluli K, Sampson AE, Schroeder BG, Slayden RA, et al. Mycolic acids: structure, biosynthesis and physiological functions. Progress in Lipid Research. 1998;37(2–3):143-79.

[17] Marrakchi H, Lanéelle M-A, Daffé M. Mycolic Acids: Structures, Biosynthesis, and Beyond. Chemistry & Biology. 2014;21(1):67-85.

[18] Minnikin DE. Mycolic acids. In: Mukherjee KD, Weber N, editors. CRC Handbook of Chromatograpy: Analysis of Lipids. Boca Raton: WILEY-VCH Verlag; 1994. p. 339-48.

[19] Rafidinarivo E, Lanéelle M-A, Montrozier H, Valero-Guillén P, Astola J, Luquin M, et al. Trafficking pathways of mycolic acids: structures, origin, mechanism of formation, and storage form of mycobacteric acids. Journal of Lipid Research. 2009;50(3): 477-90.

[20] Glickman SE, Kilburn JO, Butler WR, Ramos LS. Rapid identification of mycolic acid patterns of mycobacteria by high-performance liquid chromatography using pattern recognition software and a *Mycobacterium* library. Journal of Clinical Microbiology. 1994;32(3):740-5.

[21] Galassi L, Donato R, Tortoli E, Burrini D, Santianni D, Dei R. Nontuberculous mycobacteria in hospital water systems: application of HPLC for identification of environmental *mycobacteria*. Journal of water health. 2003;1(3):133-9.

[22] Figueiredo EES, Conte-Junior CA, Furlaneto LV, Silvestre FG, Duarte R, Lilenbaum W, et al. Molecular Techniques for Identification of Species of the *Mycobacterium tuberculosis* complex: The use of multiplex PCR and an adapted HPLC method for identification of *Mycobacterium bovis* and diagnosis of bovine tuberculosis. In: Pere-Joan C, editor. Understanding Tuberculosis-Global Experiences and Innovative Approaches to the Diagnosis. Rijeta: InTech-Open Access Publisher; 2012. p. 411-32.

[23] Buchan BW, Riebe KM, Timke M, Kostrzewa M, Ledeboer NA. Comparison of MALDI-TOF MS With HPLC and Nucleic Acid Sequencing for the Identification of *Mycobacterium* Species in Cultures Using Solid Medium and Broth. American Journal of Clinical Pathology. 2014;141(1):25-34.

[24] Parrish N, Riedel S. Cellular Fatty Acid-Based Microbial Identification and Antimicrobial Susceptibility Testing. In: Tang Y-W, Stratton CW, editors. Advanced Techniques in Diagnostic Microbiology: Springer US; 2013. p. 177-85.

[25] Vilchèze C, Jacobs WR. Isolation and Analysis of *Mycobacterium tuberculosis* Mycolic Acids. Current Protocols in Microbiology: John Wiley & Sons, Inc.; 2005.

[26] Jost KC, Dunbar DF, Barth SS, Headley VL, Elliott LB. Identification of *Mycobacterium tuberculosis* and *M. avium* complex directly from smear-positive sputum specimens and BACTEC 12B cultures by high-performance liquid chromatography with fluorescence detection and computer-driven pattern recognition models. Journal of Clinical Microbiology. 1995;33(5):1270-7.

[27] Viader-Salvadó JM, Garza-González E, Valdez-Leal R, de los Angeles del Bosque-Moncayo M, Tijerina-Menchaca R, Guerrero-Olazarán M. Mycolic Acid Index Susceptibility Method for *Mycobacterium tuberculosis*. Journal of Clinical Microbiology. 2001;39(7):2642-5.

[28] Butler WR, Thibert L, Kilburn JO. Identification of *Mycobacterium avium* complex strains and some similar species by high-performance liquid chromatography. Journal of Clinical Microbiology. 1992;30(10):2698-704.

[29] CDC. Mycolic Acid Pattern Standards for HPLC Identification of *Mycobacteria*. Atlanta: U.S. Department of Health and Human Services. Public Health Service; 1999. p. 99.

[30] Kellogg JA, Bankert DA, Withers GS, Sweimler W, Kiehn TE, Pfyffer GE. Application of the Sherlock *Mycobacteria* Identification System Using High-Performance Liquid Chromatography in a Clinical Laboratory. Journal of Clinical Microbiology. 2001;39(3):964-70.

[31] Duarte RS, Lourenço MCS, Fonseca LdS, Leão SC, Amorim EdLT, Rocha ILL, et al. Epidemic of Postsurgical Infections Caused by *Mycobacterium massiliense*. Journal of Clinical Microbiology. 2009;47(7):2149-55.

[32] Leao SC, Tortoli E, Viana-Niero C, Ueki SYM, Lima KVB, Lopes ML, et al. Characterization of *Mycobacteria* from a Major Brazilian Outbreak Suggests that Revision of the Taxonomic Status of Members of the *Mycobacterium chelonae-M. abscessus* Group Is Needed. Journal of Clinical Microbiology. 2009;47(9):2691-8.

[33] Mondragón-Barreto M, Vázquez-Chacón CA, Barrón-Rivero C, Acosta-Blanco P, Jost Jr KC, Balandrano S, et al. Comparison among three methods for *mycobacteria* identification. Salud Pública de México. 2000;42:484-9.

[34] Thibert L, Lapierre S. Routine application of high-performance liquid chromatography for identification of *mycobacteria*. Journal of Clinical Microbiology. 1993;31(7): 1759-63.

[35] Tortoli E, Bartoloni A. High-performance liquid chromatography and identification of *mycobacteria*. Reviews in Medical Microbiology. 1996;7:207-19.

[36] Jeong J, Kim S-R, Lee SH, Lim J-H, Choi JI, Park JS, et al. The Use of High Performance Liquid Chromatography to Speciate and Characterize the Epidemiology of *Mycobacteria*. Lab Medicine. 2011;42(10):612-7.

[37] Floyd MM, Silcox VA, Jones WD, Butler WR, Kilburn JO. Separation of Mycobacterium bovis BCG from *Mycobacterium tuberculosis* and *Mycobacterium bovis* by using high-performance liquid chromatography of mycolic acids. Journal of Clinical Microbiology. 1992;30(5):1327-30.

[38] Aravindhan V, Sulochana S, Narayanan S, Paramasivan CN, Narayanan PR. dentification & differentiation of *Mycobacterium avium* & *M. intracellulare* by PCR-RFLP assay using the groES gene. Indian Journal of Medical Research. 2007;126:575-9.

3

Tuberculosis (TB) and Human Rights in Chiapas, Mexico

H.J. Sánchez-Pérez, Anaximandro Gómez-Velasco,
G. Leal, A. Bencomo-Alerm,
N. Romero-Sandoval and M. Martín-Mateo

1. Introduction

Tuberculosis (TB) is a devastating disease from many points of view: from individuals suffering the disease through public health systems, and health cost services [1]. Although TB is a disease that can be prevented and cured, TB is worldwide spread [2]. Despite the universal adopted Directly Observed Therapy Short Course (DOTS) strategy, TB is now more prevalent than in any previous period of human history. According to the most recent report by World Health Organization (WHO) [2], there were an estimated 8.6 million (8.3-9 million) new cases and 1.3 deaths related to TB in 2013 [2]. Nevertheless, a recent study estimated that in 2013, including in HIV-positive individuals, all-form TB incidence was 7.5 million, prevalence was 11.9 million, and number of deaths was 1.4 million [3]. In the same year and in only individuals who were HIV-negative, all-form TB estimated incidence was 7.1 million, prevalence 11.2 million, and number of deaths was 1.3 million [3]. According with Stop Partnership TB Human Rights Task Force, in 2009 1.7 million people died from TB, including nearly 600,000 women, and 150,000 by multidrug-resistant TB (MDR-TB). The vast majority of deaths occur in developing countries. In the same year, there were 440,000 MDR-TB cases (3.3% of all new cases) [4].

In Latin America, 70% of the new cases are concentrated in five countries (Brazil, Peru, Mexico, Haiti and Colombia) [5]. WHO estimated in 2012 that there were 219,349 new and relapsed cases, 56% of them were smear-positives, 57% HIV positives and 1.35% MDR-TB cases [5].

Worldwide, co-infection with HIV-AIDS, co-morbidity with diabetes mellitus (DM), and the emergence of drug-resistant *Mycobacterium tuberculosis* strains –the causal agent of the disease- (DR-TB), MDR-TB, as well as the extensively drug-resistant TB (XDR-TB), and the most recent TB strains, totally drug-resistant TB (TDR-TB) are the most accepted factors that have contributed enormously to the rise of TB [2]. A recent study has highlighted that even in places with substantial decreases in TB incidence, prevalence and deaths, DR-TB could reverse important gains in combatting TB [3]. In this regard, the emergence of DR-TB is iatrogenic and suggests that the current biomedical and public health approaches for TB are failing [6].

However, renaissance of TB in the present days is caused not only by the above-mentioned factors. It is a disease strongly associated with poverty and social inequality [7]. It affects first of all people who have little or no access to basic services such as education, health and food, among others. Furthermore, factors such as reduction to access to diagnostic, prevention and treatment services increase people's vulnerability to get TB.

Although the right to health is universally recognized and guaranteed through a range of international, regional and national laws and treaties that the majority of countries have ratified, the numerous evidences from all over the world indicate that it is ill implemented in the case of TB prevention and treatment [1]. Experts point out that control over TB will require both real compromise of governments to face the disease and the inclusion of people's ability to realize their human rights. However, there is little or poor discussion regarding to human rights and its association to the control and management of TB, perhaps given the complexity of this topic. Therefore, any health system and social security should prevent and control diseases, either chronic or infectious, in a holistic approach (opportune and adequate diagnosis, right treatment, and suitable rehabilitation), benefiting the person and his community.

The state of Chiapas lies in the southeast of Mexico and extends over an area of 74,415 square kilometers [8]. Its estimated population, for 2014, is 5,149,319 inhabitants distributed in 122 municipalities [8]. Chiapas is one of the poorest Mexican states whose majority of population lives in poverty. The state has important ethnographic, social, cultural, historical and socioeconomic characteristics. All these factors are combined and reflect poor health indicators such as: high maternal and child mortality, malnutrition, high prevalence of TB, lack or null access to health services [9,10].

Chiapas has significant indigenous population (27.2% of the total population) from Mayan groups such as Tseltal, Tsotsil, Ch'ol, Zoque and Tojolabal, among others, who are the most marginalized population. A significant percentage (32%) lives in extreme poverty and 54% in overcrowding conditions. Chiapas ranks in the last place among all Mexican states in terms of both infant and child mortality and has the country's highest maternal mortality ratio and the highest proportion of mortality due to infectious diseases [9]. Chiapas historically has been in the firsts places in the country, in mortality associated with diarrheal diseases, acute respiratory infections, maternal mortality and pulmonary tuberculosis (PTB) [9]. Although the state's largest cities have greatly increased in size, 51.3% of Chiapas's population still lives in rural areas (less than 2,500 inhabitants), compared to the national average (23.2%) [11]. In these rural areas, farming small parcels of collectively owned land or working as day laborers on larger plots offers a poor and precarious existence for most residents [9].

In this chapter, we aim to examine situation of human rights compliance in the case of TB patients residing in Chiapas, Mexico, taking into account the Mexican government's obligations to respect, protect and fulfill the right to health of all population. We will address the following topics: human rights, the right to health, principles of health rights, patient rights, TB in several vulnerable populations (children, elderly, women, indigenous groups and migrants); and legal health reforms in Mexico and its impact in DOTS strategy.

2. Chiapas: A brief description of epidemiological TB situation

In Mexico, in 2013 there were registered 21,381 cases of TB (in all its forms) with a incidence rate of 16.7 *per* 100,000 inhabitants [12], from which 92.3% were new cases; 81.7% were PTB; 21% were associated with DM and 5.6% with HIV/AIDS; 1.05% were drug-resistant (any forms) and 8.4% were pediatric [12]. Among the pediatric group, 68.2% were PTB and 31.8% extra-pulmonary-TB [12]. Chiapas, Guerrero, Veracruz, Puebla, and Tabasco, are Mexican states which contribute every year about 5,400 new cases of PTB, and this constitutes 36% of the total national average [12]. Factors that contribute to the high prevalence of PTB in these states are: (a) internal and external migration; (b) problems with accessibility to health services and social security; (c) significant presence of indigenous populations; (d) more than 90% of their municipalities are considered with low human development index [13,14]; (e) inadequate implementation of the DOTS strategy [10]; (f) little or null access to early TB diagnosis [10]. The above-mentioned factors, related to life styles and living conditions also contribute to health inequities increasing the high prevalence of TB in Chiapas and worldwide.

According to official data provided by the Mexican Ministry of Health, in 2012, Baja California, Guerrero and Tamaulipas, were states with the highest incidence rates of TB, all its forms, (54.8, 38.1 and 32.0, respectively, *per* 100,000 inhabitants), while Chiapas ranked eleventh place with an incidence rate of 24.4 *per* 100,000 in the same denominator [15]. On the other hand, Tlaxcala and the State of Mexico were ranked with the lowest incidence rates, 3.9 and 4.4 *per* 100,000, respectively [15]. Regarding to PTB, for the same year, the registered incidence rate for the whole country was 13.6 *per* 100,000 inhabitants, whereas Chiapas ranked eighth with 21.8 incidence rate for the same denominator [15].

For administrative purposes, Chiapas is divided into ten health districts or sanitary jurisdictions. For 2012, the three regions with highest registered incidence rates were Tapachula, Tonala and Pichucalco, having 59.3, 33.1 and 22.3 *per* 100,000 inhabitants, respectively, while San Cristobal and Comitan regions reported the lowest incidence rate with 11.7 and 12.7 *per* 100,000 people, respectively [16]. However, epidemiological studies carried out in the San Cristobal region[1], also known as the Highlands region, have reported high morbidity and mortality rates which doubles the state and national figures [9,10,17–25]. Furthermore, the official epidemiological data is based on notified cases by the health sector systems, and this could lead to under-quantification of cases in great part due to under-diagnosis. In Chiapas, the main and only method to diagnose PTB is bacilloscopy which is well known to have low sensitivity in rural and marginalized areas [26,17,19,9,23]. From the 122 municipalities located in Chiapas, 28 indigenous municipalities reported in 2012, 203 new TB cases, from which 178

1 San Cristobal region is an area with strong presence of Tsotsil and Tseltal population, characterized by high levels of poverty and social exclusion.

were PTB, and 29 deaths associated with the disease [16]. It is important to highlight that San Cristobal region is the place in Chiapas with highest number of smear positive cases with two and three crosses (over 80%), which means both delay in diagnosis and the potential transmissibility of TB in the region [16].

Regarding to TB mortality, official data for 2012, there were 2,253 deaths (in all its forms), representing a mortality rate of 1.9 *per* 100,000 inhabitants [15]. From these deaths, 1,761 were PTB with a rate of 1.5 *per* 100,000 people [15]. In the same year, Baja California, Sonora, Nayarit, and Chiapas were the states with the highest mortality rate associated with TB (all its forms) with 5.68, 4.38, 3.98 and 3.31 *per* 100,000 inhabitants[2] [15]. The states with lower mortality rate were Tlaxcala, State of Mexico, and Guanajuato with rates of 0.0, 0.57, and 0.69 *per* 100,000 inhabitants, respectively [15].

In 2011, the Prevention and Control TB Program reported 838 PTB cases, from which 90.1% were considered as an anti-TB treatment success, while treatment defaulting and failure rates were 4.1 and 1.31, respectively. However, health sector in Chiapas recognizes that between 2010 and 2013, 47 cases were multidrug-resistant (MDR-TB), one of which was extremely resistant [16]. It is alarming to note, that between 2008-2014, the Tapachula Jurisdiction[3] reported 73 cases of drug-resistant TB (DR-TB) (Dr. Julio Cesar de la Cruz, Coordinator of DR-TB and Leprosy, personal communication), from which 17 had died, 5 had defaulted, 4 had been reluctant to receive treatment, 22 were cured, 11 were still in treatment, 8 were awaiting treatment and 6 were served by another health institution (Social Security Mexican Institute) with no information regarding to their situation.

According to Dr. Julio Cesar de la Cruz, the main problems which account for follow-up DR-TB cases are: (a) the lack of mycobacteriological cultures; (b) the lack of adequate medical records by the physician treating the patients, which sometimes are incomplete and erroneous; (c) adverse reactions from the drugs used in anti-TB treatment along with the lack of request in time and form to treat such adverse reactions. Also, the main problems identified to defaulting treatment are: (a) the adverse reactions; (b) the lack of adequate follow-up to patients under treatment; (c) perception by patients who think they are cured; and (d) the lack of financial resources from the patients, who need to continue working.

Statistics by The Population and Housing Census conducted in 2010 in Mexico [11], 38.9% of households in Chiapas have moderate to severe food insecurity (FI)[4]. In 42% of households where the head of family or spouse mentioned speaking an indigenous language, were

---

2 Noteworthy to mention is that in official statistics, there is a discrepancy on the data regarding to TB mortality rate of Chiapas (all its forms); for 2011, when the mortality rate of Chiapas is compared with other states, the notified rate was 2.98 per 100,000 inhabitants (it is not indicated whether or not adjusted rate), but when a trend analysis is carried out for the last years, only for the state of Chiapas, the mortality rate is 3.5 per 100,000 inhabitants, with 163 deaths reported.

3 This Jurisdiction is located in the border with Guatemala and is one of the main migrant passages mainly from Centro American countries such as Guatemala, El Salvador, Honduras to United States of America. Lately is been reported migrants from Asian and African countries. Due to its geographical location, and the number of migrants who cross this region, a high number of TB cases is reported annually by this jurisdiction, which makes it one of the most important area in terms of public health because the migrants poverty and bad health conditions.

4 The Food and Agriculture Organization of the United Nations (FAO) states that food security exists when "all people, at all times, have physical and economic access to sufficient, safe and nutritious food to meet their needs and preferences, to lead an active and healthy life". In contrast, no or uncertain access to food is defined as food insecurity (FI).

classified in the categories of moderate and severe FI. Moreover, 41.7% of population in Chiapas lacks any social security scheme, although this percentage decreased with respect to 2000 (when it was 77.8%) [27], which may be explained by the introduction of the System of Social Protection in Health (65.7%), called "Seguro Popular", a "basic package of health services". However, according to a recent study, this basic package has increased the inequality gap in health services use between indigenous and non-indigenous populations [28].

In Mexico there are 150 municipalities in extreme poverty, and 28 are located in Chiapas. The Highlands region has 11 of these municipalities, whose main characteristic is the important presence of indigenous groups [8,13]. In Chiapas, there are at least 925,000 children (32.86% of its population) aged between 0-14 years old [8] and the majority (60-74%) has not social security scheme [29]. According to a study by Network for the Rights of Children in Mexico [29], the number of children, mainly indigenous, with no social security scheme has increased which make them more vulnerable to acquire any infectious disease. Alarmingly, in Mazapa de Madero (a Chiapas municipality), 97.7% of its children have no access to health services [30].

In Chiapas, in 2013, there was 27,704 deaths from which 350 were children, with an infant mortality rate of 18.16 *per* 1,000 live births [29], the second highest in the country. The Ministry of Health has recognized that the infant mortality in indigenous population is 58% higher than the national average. This figure indicates twice the probability of death of an indigenous child before their first year of life compared to one non-indigenous. This situation is worse in rural and indigenous areas with high socio-economic marginalization in which the infant mortality rate has reached 75 *per* 1000 children, a number equivalent to those reported in Sub-Saharan Africa [31].

Regarding to education, it is estimated that the rate of illiteracy among indigenous peoples is four times higher (over 26% of the population aging 15 years and over) than the national average (6.88%) [32]. Moreover, two out of three indigenous schools are multi-grade, that is, their teachers attend more than one degree [32]. Noteworthy to mention is that in 2005 only 13% of indigenous students of sixth grade of primary school can read compared to that of the national average (33%). On the contrary, 51% of indigenous students of sixth degree are in the lowest level, while the national average is 25%. More alarmingly, indigenous children stop going to school because they are engaged in working at their early age due to socioeconomic issues [11].

3. Patients rights

3.1. What are human rights?

Human rights are universal and considered the birthright of every human being. Human rights are aimed to safeguarding the dignity and equal value of everyone. They are inalienable, they cannot be waived or taken away, and each one is closely related to and often dependent upon the realization of others, and they are indivisible. Human rights are articulated as entitlements of individuals and groups, thereby creating obligations of action and non-action, particularly for states [32]. Universal human rights are often expressed and guaranteed by law, in the forms of treaties, customary international law, general principles and other sources of international law. International human rights law lays down obligations of Governments to act in certain ways or to refrain from certain acts, in order to promote and protect human rights and fundamental freedoms of individuals or groups. Human rights are inherent entitlements to all human beings without discrimination, whatever nationality, citizenship, place of residence, sex, ethnic origin, color, religion, language, or any other status [32].

Human rights involve economic, social, political, health and cultural issues and are guaranteed by law in national and international instruments, from local legislation to constitutions in countries. States assume obligations under international law to respect, protect and fulfill human rights as well as to refrain from interfering with the enjoyment of the right, prevent others from interfering and adopt appropriate measures towards the full realization of the rights [1,4].

The main international human rights treaties that involve the right to health, to which Mexico is a party, are:

- The International Covenant on Economic, Social and Cultural Rights (ICESCR).
- The Convention on the Rights of the Child (the Children's Convention, CRC);
- The Convention on the Elimination of All Forms of Discrimination against Women (the Women's Convention, CEDAW);
- The International Convention on the Elimination of All Forms of Racial Discrimination (Race Convention, ICERD);
- The Additional Protocol to the American Convention on Human Rights in the Area of Economic, Social and Cultural Rights (the Protocol of San Salvador), adopted in 1988, entered into force in 1999), provides for the right to health and the right to a healthy environment, and other health-related rights, such as social security.
- Convention 169 of the International Labor Organization Concerning Indigenous and Tribal Peoples in Independent Countries (ILO Convention 169)
- The Convention against Torture and Other Cruel, Inhuman or Degrading Treatment or Punishment (CAT);
- The International Covenant on Civil and Political Rights (ICCPR);
- The Convention on the Rights of Persons with Disabilities (CRPD);
- The American Declaration of the Rights and Duties of Man (1948), that in it's Article XI, refers to the "right to preservation of health".
- The International Convention on the Protection of the Rights of All Migrant Workers and Members of Their Families (ICRMW);

On the other hand, in Latin American, the Inter-American Commission on Human Rights and the Inter-American Court of Human Rights, make up the Inter-American System of Human Rights.

4. The right to health

According with the ICESCR (Art. 12) the right to health is defined as "the right of everyone to the enjoyment of the highest attainable standard of physical and mental health" [34]. This right involves the right to be free from non-consensual and uninformed medical treatment, medical experimentation, forced HIV testing, and other forms of cruel, inhumane and degrading treatments [38]. In this sense, states have the obligation to provide adequate health services necessary for the realization of the highest attainable standard of health. This include the right to a system of protection (i.e. a system of prevention, treatment and control of diseases) for all population in equal conditions, access to information and education about health, regular provision of essential medicines, and sexual and reproductive health-care services. In fact, two of the main steps that states should take in fulfilling the highest attainable standard of health are the prevention, treatment and control of epidemic, endemic, occupational and other diseases, and the creation of conditions which would assure to all medical service and medical attention in the event of sickness [34]. In Mexico, Article 4 of its Political Constitution establishes that "every person has the right to health protection" [35].

The right to health is dependent on and contributes to enjoy of other human rights. In consequence also comprises the access to healthy occupational and environmental conditions, drinking water, food, housing, education, and protection against epidemic diseases and rights relevant to sexual and reproductive health [36]. The right to health is not an abstract aspiration; on the contrary, international human rights norms provide a concrete set of principles by which to evaluate the design and implementation of health policy-making and programming [1,33,34]. The basic components of the right to health, commit to the states to guarantee that health facilities, goods and services are: available, accessible, acceptable, of good quality and applicable to all sectors of the population, including migrants [1,4,34,37,38]:

Availability means functioning public health and health facilities, goods (general supplies, essential medicines and vaccinations, laboratory equipment, among others), services and programs in sufficient quantity and in a timely manner, as well as to avoid stock shortage. It includes drinking water, sanitation, and other determinants of health.

Accessibility includes several issues related to:

- Non-discrimination: all services and goods must be accessible to all population, especially the most vulnerable and marginalized groups, in law and in practice. This includes migrants, independently if they are regular or irregular, and not only emergence interventions.
- Physical accessibility: provision of safe access to health services and underlying determinants of health for all groups and subgroups of population. It must be considered the location and opening hours of health facilities.

- Economic accessibility: affordable health services (including basic medicines) and health insurance for all population, especially for individuals in poverty or in need of special assistance.
- Equity: that poorer households should not be disproportionately burdened with health expenses as compared to richer households [34].
- The right to seek, receive and impart information and ideas concerning health issues, which includes health information in indigenous languages [38].

Acceptability: respectful of medical ethics and culturally appropriate, sensitive to age and gender in order to reduce socioeconomic, cultural, gender and age barriers. It may include interpretation, translated written materials and cultural mediation in health facilities (both hospitals and health centers). Cultural acceptability requires respect for traditional medicines and practices which have not been shown to be harmful to human health [9]. Barriers can have negative effects on prevention, diagnostic (delays or mistakes) and medical care attention, and affect anti-TB treatment and adequate follow-ups. It is not uncommon that people feel distrust of government services and instances of outright denials of care or mistreatment due to such factors as: bureaucratic arguments, ethnic, social and gender discrimination.

Quality: Health facilities, goods and services must be scientifically and medically appropriate and good quality. It implies: sensitive and trained health professionals at all levels, scientifically approved drugs, trustworthy laboratories, appropriate hospital equipment, adequate sanitation and safe drinking water. In Chiapas, many of the programs administered by the public health system are of inadequate quality [9-10, 17,19]. This situation is reflected in the high levels of subdiagnosis of TB cases, as well as constant lack of appropriate treatment for PTB [9-10, 17,19]

The perspective of human rights in the health services place people as the principal element of any activity, program, policy and legislation. Thus, human rights regarding to health is defined as: everyone should enjoy the highest possible standard of physical and mental health, which include access to timely, acceptable, satisfactory quality and affordable health care, and create conditions that allow people to live as healthy as possible. This is related and in function of access to housing, jobs, clean and drinkable water, food security and education services, among other basic services.

4.1. Principles of the right to health

The main principles of the right to health, are: principle of non-discrimination, principle of Non-retrogression and adequate progress, principle of meaningful participation, accountability and multi-sectorial strategies [9].

4.1.1. Principle of non-discrimination

This principle is the core for the full realization of the right to health, as for all human rights. In consequence all forms of discrimination create obstacles for the realization of the right to health. The ESC Rights Committee stated that: "By virtue of article 2.2 and article 3, the

Covenant proscribes any discrimination in access to health care and underlying determinants of health [34]. Discrimination can adopt a lot of forms: sex, age, ethnic/race, color, language, national or social origin, economic, political, religion, migrant status, sexual orientation, property, physical or mental disability, health status (including HIV-AIDS, among other status, which has the intention or effect of nullifying or impairing the equal enjoyment or exercise of the right to health. Health personnel must not make distinction among persons in any form because international human rights specify that all individuals, without discrimination, must have access to health-care facilities, goods and services, especially the most vulnerable groups [39]. Governments are obligated to ensure it. In Mexico, the Political Constitution states the right to health in its Article 4 [35].

In addition, State responsibilities include: (a) ensuring equal protection and opportunity under the law, as well as in policies, programs, etcetera, for the enjoyment of rights, including to health and social security [36]; (b) to monitor the effects of their public health and social policies and actions; and, c) to ensure that these are anchored in a system which does not allow inequalities in the enjoyment of human rights. In order to achieve this, states are compelled to gather disaggregated data on the realization of the rights to health, social security and education, among others. The indicators under study must include special measures that recognize the diversity of population groups and assist states in meeting their human rights obligations by eliminating all forms of discrimination [38].

A study carried out in the conflict zones of Chiapas [9][5], found some of the effects of discrimination and structural inequalities faced by the largely indigenous populations. The fragmentation of communities and politicization of care and other governmental services has had serious implications for the accessibility and utilization of health services in the region, such as discrimination and denial of health services against patients on the basis of political and religious affiliation, as well as on the basis of indigenous ethnicity. In Chiapas, it is common that indigenous people feel discrimination in health services, and they claim that non-indigenous patients are treated better than indigenous patients with better quality care, more medicines, and a shorter wait time to be treated [10].

Other forms of discrimination are: (a) the availability of resources and programs –including of the health sector- depending on political filiation. The effects of these discriminatory policies have been the creation of a cycle of fragmentation and polarization among and within communities that affect the utilization and access to health services in opposing groups to the government; (b) the amazing differences among states in Mexico as well as between for the insured and uninsured population with respect to distribution of health resources and health care *per* capita spending: the allocation of health resources is inversely related to poverty, and levels of unsatisfied health needs [40]; (c) indigenous people are disproportionately represented among poor and uninsured, studies have shown that the availability of health care resources increases when the proportion of indigenous people in a county is very low [41]; and (d) the discrimination faced by women in Chiapas. The women's health is affected by structural

5 In January 1, 1994, the Zapatista Army for National Liberation (EZLN) staged an armed uprising in Chiapas, Mexico on behalf of the indigenous populations of the state, whose rights they claimed to be defending.

problems in the health system, for example, they not participate at all in planning of health services and the high levels of poverty in the majority of them in rural and indigenous areas, constitutes a serious obstacle to enjoyment their rights [9] Mexico's Constitution prohibits discrimination in the enjoyment of all rights, including the right to health protection, and recognizes that every person in the country shall enjoy the guarantees granted by this Constitution, and that "men and women are equal before the law", but in practice, in Chiapas it is not occurring. People with TB often are discriminated with exclusion and rejection, by both society and health personnel [10,15,17,19,20,31], mainly because they are considered as source of infection [10,23]. Health personnel avoid contact with patient with consequences in adequate timely diagnosis, treatment and follow up, and even refusal to provide health care [43].

4.1.2. Principle of non-retrogression and adequate progress

Realizing the right to health requires not only avoiding retrogression but also deliberate steps to make adequate progress. The ICESCR obligates States parties such as Mexico to take steps "toward the progressive realization" of all rights contained in the Covenant to the "maximum available extent of its resources" [34]. One of the principal governmental programs intended to address the health conditions of marginalized people in Chiapas and elsewhere is the "Prospera" program (firstly named Solidaridad, afterwards called Oportunidades and nowadays Prospera). The program serves individuals who are not covered by formal health insurance. It has an assistance perspective, which can have contradictory results since incentives do not lend recipients to have self-sufficiency or improve communal conditions. In order to receive funding from this program, recipients must continually demonstrate that they live in conditions of extreme poverty. As a result, women and families receiving benefits from the program often reject other programs aimed at the improvement of their standard of living, which may be community-oriented, so that they can continue benefiting from Oportunidades Program (recently named Prospera) [9].

4.1.3. Principle of meaningful participation

Realization of the right to health entails providing individuals and communities with an authentic voice in decisions defining, determining or affecting their well-being. According to the United Nations Development Program [44] "participating in the rules and institutions that shape one's community is a basic human right and part of human development. More inclusive governance can be more effective. When local people are consulted about the location of a health clinic, for example, there is a better chance it will be built in the right place". In Chiapas, the socioeconomic and health situation require meaningful participation by all its citizens, and should recognize indigenous autonomy and self-determination.

International instruments to which Mexico has voluntarily bound itself require inclusiveness and democratic participation. People have the right to participate in the design and management of their health care services, as set forth under relevant international law. The Mexican government has adopted international instruments related to genuine participation of indigenous people's in their own affairs, including health. The San Andrés Accords, an agreement between the government and EZLN issued in 1996, but never implemented, would have provided some self-determination for indigenous communities in Chiapas and Mexico [45]. However, in contrast to other states in the region, the government of Mexico has never adopted national legislation to incorporate its international obligations into domestic law [9]. Nor has it recognized some meaningful degree of autonomy for indigenous communities, in relation to the organization and delivery of social services [9].

Under international human rights law, participation requires more than using local health promoters, on the contrary, states should provide resources and support for that communities be able to define their own health priorities, design, deliver and control their health services [9]. True rights-based participation requires programs that enable people to be active, informed and critical agents and citizens, rather than objects of charity [46].This include formulation, implementation and monitoring of health policies and programs. In Chiapas, genuine participation of population (indigenous, civil society, women, etcetera) in matters relating to health decisions, except Zapatistas communities, is poor or absent.

4.1.4. Principle of access to information

Three main aspects are important to have access to information. Firstly, every person must have accessibility to health information, that include the right to seek, receive impartial information and professional opinions in an accessible social and cultural format, easy to understand, and according to different groups of society. In the case of TB, breach of this right may result in misinformation about the disease, causing much greater probability of infection to closer, stigma, and social discrimination. As a consequence, chain of transmission of the disease is not interrupted, and increase the probabilities to defaulting because of lack of both family and social understanding and support, and with the possibility that patients are not cured, continue to infect other people, and even worse, die [10,24].

Secondly, social participation and monitoring health issues are impossible without access to information. In Chiapas, the compliance of this principle is inadequate. On the one hand, there is not transparency in information: government data is not easily accessible by the public, academics or interested non-governmental organizations. Public servants tend to not proportion health information because they feel that, if indicators for example, are "not good", they can be affected and be the cause that they have to leave their job. On the other hand, health data collected is usually no disaggregated by variables of great useful and interest. For example, in an study to analyze TB mortality, we reviewed the registers of the TB Prevention and Control Program, and data about ethnicity, occupation and schooling of patients, were absent [10].

Finally, in Chiapas there is a consistent pattern of under-diagnosis and under-reporting health data, including TB and others health problems as maternal deaths. In several studies carried out by our work team, we have detected cases of PTB at least three times than the official state level [9]. In addition, we have observed that many health workers do not keep any medical records of their patients –especially in those cases when patients come from other villages- and that patients complain of not being made aware of their most basic rights, such as their right to their medical records or to informed consent in medical procedures.

4.1.5. Principle of accountability

It is important that all states ratify international instruments which provide protection for the right to health, and of enacting and implementing legislation in domestic legal orders, as well as incorporate enables courts to adjudicate violations of the right to health to provide sanctions for violations to human rights and, in this case, the right to health. Additionally, accountability needs the adoption of a framework law to operationalize and monitoring the right to health. For example, a human rights ombudsman with authority to investigate and sanction perpetrators in cases of violations to the right to health. In Mexico, in spite of Mexico's General Health Law ensures health protection, and contains programmatic provisions, which commit the State to action on health matters, in practice there is no effective monitoring and oversight, as well as remedies for victims of violations [33]. Medical negligence cases are generally brought to the National Commission on Human Rights (CNDH), state human rights commissions, and the National Medical Arbitration Commission (CONAMED). Although they can review negligence claims brought against individual providers, these institutions only deliver mechanisms to enforce the patient rights against malpractice set out under Mexican law. Mechanisms such as the *amparo* (protection writ), which is commonly used in civil and political rights violations cases, would need to be reformed in order to: (1) provide people and groups with a collective remedy; and (2) establish precedent for other related cases. Even in individual cases, Mexican judges have been inappropriately reluctant to use the *amparo* to enforce the right to health under the apparent misconception that "programmatic rights" are not actionable [9].

4.1.6. Principle of multi-sectorial strategies

The right to health goes beyond the provision of medical care as well as the health sector. States must have institute coherent with development and food security policies, which incorporate health affairs. It includes the promotion of adequate living conditions, access to sufficient safe drinking water, to basic sanitation for disposal of excreta, access to educational opportunities (especially for women) and access to arable land, among other issues. In spite of Mexico's General Health Law sets out an integrated, multi-sectorial approach to health, calling on ministries of health, education, and labor to work jointly to, *inter alia*, to fulfill goals of the National Health System. This coordination efforts seeks to integrate biological and socioeconomic factors essential to good health, however, in practice this is not materialized. Evidence of this, are the high rates of diseases associated with poverty –including TB- in Mexico as a whole, but particularly in Chiapas, as a result of a failure of the Mexican government to establish a coherent rural development policy, which should incorporate health issues [9]. Therefore, coordination efforts among health, agricultural, educational, socioeconomic sectors should combat the unfavorable health conditions of vulnerable populations. Likewise, governments at different levels (Federal, State, and local) should coordinate efforts to strength social security programs that met communities' health needs and adopt approaches that encourage cooperation and capacity-building. In Chiapas there is not adequate coordination between health sector and government and non-government sectors. There are fragmentation, dispersion and, sometimes, objectives in one direction in some programs, and in other direction in others [9]. For example, the "Vida Mejor (Better life)" program focused for women and child in Chiapas, does have multi-sectorial components, and is directed towards the community. Its impact has been limited because it competes with the federal program Oportunidades (now named Prospera), which provides incentives for individuals and individual families to opt out of Vida Mejor in order to retain their benefits from the Oportunidades. The lack of coordination between these programs undermines potential progress in advancing the affected populations' right to health.

In summary, as we stated before, the perspective of human rights in the health services should place people as the principal element of any activity, program, policy and legislation. However, most human rights are far from being met for the majority of the population. The right to health is among rights which have tendency not to be considered as universal human right, but as a merchandise [47]. This view of right to health emphasize on lifestyles promoting health consumption, where individuals are victims and murders of their health-disease process.

5. The right to social security

According to the ICESCR, the States parties "recognize the right of everyone to social security, including social insurance (Art. 9)". This right encompasses the right to access and maintain benefits, whether in cash or in kind and without discrimination, in order to secure protection, *inter alia,* from (a) lack of work related income caused by sickness, disability, maternity, employment injury, unemployment, old age, or death of a family member; (b) unaffordable access to health care; and (c) insufficient family support, particularly for children and adult dependents [48].

Social protection strategies such as cash transfers, microcredit, and training might be harnessed to improve social and health conditions of vulnerable groups and therefore preventing and mitigating causes and effects of TB. However, in some regions of Chiapas health programs - including TB diagnosis and treatment- have been politicized threatening patients life and hindering prevention and control of disease transmission [9,10].

6. Patient rights and TB

The five elements of DOTS and the six components of the TB Stop strategy should ensure TB prevention, diagnosis and treatment to achieve early case detection and successful treatment [49,50]. Nevertheless, those elements are not satisfied due to inadequate implementation of DOTS in highly marginalized settings, where TB is often endemic or with high prevalence, such as in Chiapas, Mexico.

It might be considered that TB is a disease that can be "easily" diagnosed (mainly the pulmonary form), prevented, treatable and curable, but it may lead to death if neglected. How TB might be neglected? The failure of BCG to prevent *M. tuberculosis* infection, the appearance of

DR-TB *M. tuberculosis* strains, the lack of an effective and affordable diagnostic methods, and the growing HIV-AIDS as well as DM, threaten to overwhelm current TB control strategies in many endemic areas where resources, human and material, are scarce.

6.1. Right to prevent TB: The failure of the BCG vaccine

Active immunization is one of the essential components of TB control. The bacilli Calmette-Guérin (BCG) live vaccine was developed in 1909 by Albert Calmette and Camille Guérin and is still the only worldwide vaccine used to protect against TB [51]. Despite its global use, with over 100 million doses given annually, its efficacy remains controversial since in randomized controlled trials and case control-studies range from detrimental effect to 80% protective benefit [52], and 50% in a meta-analysis of the literature [53]. However, other studies have shown its efficacy against severe forms of childhood TB, principally milliary and meningitis [54], but limited benefit in preventing adult PTB, the form that is the most contagious and hence fuels the continuing epidemic [52]. This variation has been attributed to genetic and antigenic differences between BCG strains, geographic localization, and previous exposure to environmental mycobacteria and genetic variation of the human population [51].

The WHO recommends that BCG is given at birth, or shortly after birth [55]. However, some countries do not follow this guideline. BCG vaccination is not used at all in Netherlands and USA [52]. In Norway, BCG is given only to school age or older children, while in the United Kingdom, Sweden, and Switzerland is administered to risk groups only (health care workers, people with positive tuberculin skin test, etc.) [52]. The WHO also recommends applying BCG vaccination in countries with high burden of TB, including in HIV endemic areas, but vaccination of adults is not normally recommended [37, 38].

In Mexico, the BCG vaccine started to be used in 1951, but its massive application to the Mexican population was on 1973 [57]. Although BCG vaccination is part of the national childhood immunization program [57–59] and provided free by the state, its coverage remains uncertain and impact of BCG vaccination on transmission of *M. tuberculosis* is therefore limited, especially in regions such as Chiapas, with poor or null access to health services.

The Mexican National Council for Vaccination (Consejo Nacional de Vacunación, CONAVA) and the state vaccine programs organize the vaccination campaigns all over Mexico [58]. Application of vaccines is considered a universal human right, regardless whether children are engaged in an official health service. Thus, in Mexico and Chiapas children under five years old must have vaccination booklet, a certificate that documents all vaccines, including BCG, offered by official health services. According to official data, Chiapas' BCG vaccination coverage for children was 97.6% in 2012, while coverage at the national level in this year was 96.7% [27]. However, the percentage of vaccinated children might be lower due to several regions of the state have null or lack of access to health services as well as political or religious conflicts that act as barriers to the health services. To exemplify this situation, a study carried out in three regions of Chiapas (North, Highlands, and Jungle), between 2001 and 2002, only 76.4% children under five years old had received their complete scheme vaccination [9]. This study also documented that official health services did not vaccinate children because parents either were not registered in an official program or belonged to a distinct political affiliation

[19]. Furthermore, there was no BCG vaccine available because vaccine campaigns have ended at the time parents took their children to the clinic [19]. Unfortunately there is no a current study assessing the actual vaccination coverage in Chiapas.

Since there is uncertainty regarding to the protection time, some countries undertake BCG revaccination programs. However, such programs have been considered highly costly [60–62], because the price of preventing a single case of TB appears to be nine times greater than treating a single patient with PTB [61]. Furthermore, revaccination has been associated with the decrease childhood and adolescent TB in Hungary and Poland [52], but not in Chile [63] and Brazil [62].

Independently of benefit-cost ratio effectiveness, meningeal TB (MTB) sometimes yields a variety of complications, including permanent disability [64]. If BCG vaccine is a cost-effective intervention against severe childhood TB, as based *per* disability-adjusted life year (DALY), its prevention could be an important reason to continue revaccination [46].

One of the highest priorities of TB research is to develop vaccines that are more efficacious for preventing TB than BCG. Novel vaccine development has accelerated in the past years, with at least 16 candidates entering human trials, and a few vaccines have entered into Phase 2b efficacy studies. However, different vaccines may be needed due to the varying disease states (latently infected, or active), the ages affected (infants, adolescents, young and the elderly), and patient health status (HIV and immunocompromised patients especially) [65,66]. It has been argued that the development of a new vaccine is highly costly due to the relatively regional incidence of TB, despite the high worldwide prevalence. It has been estimated that proof-of-concept trials that use clinical endpoints are necessarily very large (1000-35,000 subjects) and highly expensive, a cost that countries with high incidence cannot afford in the development of a new vaccine [67].

On the other hand, the satisfaction of the following rights prevent vulnerability to TB: Non-discrimination, right to health, to work, to adequate housing, food and safe drinking water and sanitation, right to education and right to information [4].

6.2. Active case contact finding and prophylaxis

Clinical manifestations of TB are simply divided into a binary classification: active disease and latent infection. *M. tuberculosis* is transmitted to person to person through aerosols, but not all develop the active disease [68,69]. Healthy individuals might suppress *M. tuberculosis* following infection, with only a 10% lifetime risk of latent TB infection (LTBI) reactivating into active TB disease, most commonly within a few years after exposure [68,69]. Persons closely exposed to individuals with active infection (i.e. index case) are at higher risk for infection and to ultimately develop active TB [70]. Risk is largely determined by the frequency and duration of exposure to the index case, and increases in persons with HIV-AIDS, DM, and tumor necrosis factor (TNF) neutralization therapy for other diseases [68,69]. Identifying and prophylactically treating close contacts at higher risk, such as children and people with DM and HIV-AIDS, has therefore become priority to disrupt transmission chain.

Contact investigation involves the systematic evaluation of the contacts of known TB patients to identify active disease or LTBI [71]. The WHO has launched guidelines, which should be applied according to specific settings and among risk groups [53]. However, screening depends on many conditions: (a) capacity of health systems (availability of human and material resources as well as infrastructure); (b) focus risk group; (c) objective of screening; and (d) epidemiological situation.

WHO has recommended that screening should be carried out in settings where the TB prevalence in the general population is 100 *per* 100,000 population or higher and in subpopulations that have very poor access to health care, such as people living in urban slums, homeless people, people living in remote areas with poor access to health care, and other vulnerable or marginalized groups including some indigenous populations, migrants and refugees [53].

Chiapas met all the above conditions to perform screening to search for active and latent TB infection. It is well known that marginal groups are the ones presenting the highest TB morbidity and mortality rates; however, their characterization is not usually considered in the design of programs for their prevention and control. Thus, TB continues to cause high rates of transmission, death and rising health costs in these marginalized groups, which represents a violation of their human rights as a consequence of the governmental incapability of preventing this situation. Our research team has performed active case finding in diverse regions of Chiapas and has found worrisome high morbidity and mortality rates due to PTB [13-15, 17-23] (Table 1). It is alarming to note that in some regions of Chiapas, high PTB incidence have reached 276.9 *per* 100,000 in inhabitants aged 15 and over [21], one of the highest in the world for 1998. It is also probable that PTB incidence in Chiapas is underestimated, in part due to under-diagnosis. TB cases, and therefore incidence rates notified by health sector systems, basically corresponds to cases detected in health services by smear microscopy examination, that it is well known, to have low sensitivity in rural and marginalized areas [9,10,17,19].

TB control programs are emphasized in adults. However, children contribute to the caseload related to the disease and experience morbidity and mortality. In 2013, Chiapas, reported 1,238 new TB cases, from which 129 (10.4%) were pediatric (defined as those aged ≤19 years old) (Dr. Alied Bencomo-Alerm, records of Prevention and Control TB Program at the Highlands region). Yet, these estimations might not reflect the real magnitude of TB in children because of the technical challenges in diagnosing pediatric TB. In an attempt to identify TB in children, the local TB prevention and control program performed a pilot study in the Highlands region using a point-based scoring system to aid in detecting TB in this vulnerable population. This pilot study detected two TB cases in children < 5 years old. However, the study was limited to only health services settings. This point-based scoring system has become an invaluable tool for detecting pediatric TB at the community level. Nevertheless, health staff and mothers should be trained and supervised through the application of this point-score system to ensure its reliability and validity (Dr. Alied Bencomo-Alerm, unpublished data)

Region studied[a]	Study population	Number of population studied	Prevalence of pulmonary tuberculosis (PTB)	Year	Reference
Border (Second level Hospital)	Considerable percentage were indigenous people (Mayan Tojolabal)	221	21% of chronic coughers studied, hospital users, aged 15 years and over,	1994	[18]
[b]Border	Considerable percentage were indigenous people (Mayan Tojolabal)	2,203	11.1% of chronic coughers studied users of primary care services	1997	[19]
[c]Border	19% indigenous (Tojolabal)	11,274	276.9 *per* 100,000 people aged 15 and over	1998	[22,26]
[d] Los Altos	Mainly indigenous (Tsotsil and Tseltal Mayan)	529	78 people deceased for whom the cause of death was associated with TB.	1998-2009	[10,24]
[e] Los Altos, Selva and Norte regions	Mainly indigenous (Tsotsil, Tseltal Mayan Lacandon, Chol)	2,997 households	161.2 *per* 100,000 persons aged 15 years and over.	2000-2001	[9]
[f] Soconusco		710,716[f]	59.3 *per* 100,000 inhabitants	2013	[16]
[g] Central		705, 201[g]	19.7 *per* 100,000 inhabitants	2013	[12]

[a] Local Ministry of Health divides Chiapas into ten administrative regions. In 1994, an armed uprising begun led by the Zapatista Army for National Liberation (EZLN or Zapatistas) on behalf of the indigenous population of the state, which claimed the compliance of their human rights, including health services. After twenty years, the socioeconomic situation of majority of indigenous people has not undergone significant changes.

[b] Active case finding of patients with chronic cough (15 days or more) was carried out among all patients aged over 14 years seeking consultation in a random sample of seven primary care centers; 573 coughers were found.

[c] The PTB incidence rate was extremely high in relation to official statistics reported during 1998 for Chiapas and Mexico (as a whole), 34.2 and 19.1 *per* 100,000 inhabitants. Authors also estimated that TB incidence rate might have reached 400 *per* 100,000 inhabitants aged 15 and over, if extrapulmonary cases were considered. The study included 32 communities.

[d] This study aimed to analyze the PTB mortality of a cohort of patients in Los Altos Region of Chiapas, who had been diagnosed with PTB from January 1998 to December 2002. The records of the TB Program were reviewed, and patients were located through a search attempting to locate them in their homes. Of the 40 deceased due to PTB found, 33 died without having received any medical care. Advanced age was associated with higher PTB mortality, and this indicates that among older patients, the accumulation of unfavorable living conditions (malnutrition and poverty) together with the probably deficient medical care by health services, make them an especially vulnerable group. Furthermore, only five of them had been treated via DOTS. The difference in the death proportion between those not treated via DOTS and those treated via DOTS was considerable (93.6% versus 6.4%, respectively).

[e] This study undertook the first comprehensive population-based health research in the conflict zone. The study carried out household survey in the municipalities most affected by the armed conflict among three types of communities: opposition, pro-government and divided communities, i.e. which contained both opposition and pro-government groups. The PTB rate found, at the time of the study, was at least three times greater that registered for Chiapas State as a whole.

[f] Data taken from Ministry of Health (Secretaría de Salud, SSA). In 2013, according to official statistics, the Soconusco and Central regions have the highest incidence rates of PTB in Chiapas, with 59.3 and 19.7 *per* 100,000 inhabitants, respectively. The Soconusco region is another border area and limits Mexico and Chiapas from Guatemala; it is characterized for its high migration of Centro American people crossing Chiapas to United States of America.

[g] In the Central region is located the capital of Chiapas; the high incidence might be explained due to centralized health services.

Table 1. Research projects carried out, from 1994 to 2010, at different regions of Chiapas, Mexico, to assess the epidemiological situation of TB.

On the other hand, the tuberculin skin test (TST) and interferon gamma release assays (IGRAS) have been proposed as a means to identify people with LTBI. Yet, in many countries including Mexico, efforts are focused in detecting active cases, despite the effect of isoniazid treatment for LTBI to reduce the risk of progression to active TB. In resource-poor settings TST is rarely available, and IGRAS are not even considered due to their high cost and complexity to interpret [68]. Downsides that are common to both TST and IGRAS are that they do not differentiate active from latent infection, nor do they provide any direct evidence of the presence of viable bacilli, and are not specific to *M. tuberculosis* (for example, *M. avium* may cause false positive test); all those factor hinders IGRAS useful in detecting LTBI in poor resource settings [72]. They simply determine that infection has at some point led to an acquired immune response that is detectable following re-challenge with antigen.

Mexico does not have an efficient program to follow-up close TB contacts; consequently, no reliable records exist to determine the prevalence of LTBI at national level. This situation is especially true in Chiapas, which is one of the poorest states of the country, as well as one of the most highly indigenous, marginalized, with high number of rural and dispersed communities, as well as presence of socioeconomic, political, and religious conflicts, and lack of health care resources. All these factors combine and reflect poor health indicators, including TB, for the state [9,10].

The Mexican official norm (NOM-006-SSA2-1993) continues to state that healthy adults with positive TST should not receive prophylactic treatment unless people are HIV positive and/or with DM [73]. TST is the only screening test used in Mexico to determine LTBI [74,75]. When resources are available, and when cost-effectiveness is assessed against a range of other expensive health interventions, TB screening in selected risk groups may be affordable and have relatively low opportunity costs. Whether a country is struggling to eliminate TB, and needs to invest additional resources to effectively provide those who are hardest to reach (see section: vulnerable populations), screening selected high-risk groups may be a key part of the response to tackle TB. In this regard, some studies have used IGRAS in Mexican population, but those studies have been focused in some risk groups such as injection drug users [76], migrant agricultural workers [77], PTB contacts [78,79], dairy farm and abattoir workers [80], and HIV-infected people [81,82]. Controversial results have emerged when comparing TST and IGRAS [83]. In Chiapas there is no a single study assessing the levels of LTBI, but it might be expected to be high due to endemic prevalence of the disease as we described previously.

Some studies suggest that use of IGRAS is indicative of an approximately eight-fold higher risk of progression to TB disease within two years on a cohort of adolescents in a high-TB burden setting [84] and in low income countries [85,86]. Although neither TST nor IGRAs has real value to diagnose TB among adults from low- and middle-income countries, TST appears to perform well to identify LTBI among close contacts of individuals with TB in Mexico. If the detection of people with active and LTBI is improved, as well as the adequate anti-TB treatment, situation of TB in Chiapas could be much better than today.

6.3. Right to receive free, timely and appropriate diagnosis and treatment

Due to the increase of TB worldwide during the 1990's, WHO launched the DOTS strategy which comprises free TB diagnosis and treatment specified in five components: (a) political commitment with increased and sustained financing by governments; (b) case detection through quality-assured bacteriology, (c) standardized treatment, with supervision and patient support, (d) an effective drug supply and management system, and (e) monitoring and evaluating system, and impact measurement [49]. National governments that have adopted this strategy, including Mexico, must ensure all the above elements in order to provide adequate TB diagnosis and treatment. However, there are hidden costs assumed by patients. In a study conducted in Malawi [87], the cost of obtaining diagnosis for TB could represent up to 244% of the total monthly family income. These expenses were related to transport and the loss of working hours.

Although DOTS has been the landmark of TB control, many people with TB remain undiagnosed or are diagnosed only after long delays. This strategy was developed only from a biomedical orientation without including other dimensions such as social, economic, cultural, linguistic and physical access to TB services as well as migration and stigmatization [10,17,19,21,23,26].

The high burden of undiagnosed TB causes much suffering and economic hardship, not only for the individuals who have TB but also their families [88]. This burden is determined by a range of factors, such as socioeconomic status, clinical needs, health system structure, TB service delivery model, distance to health services, insurance coverage, capacity to work, existence of any social protection scheme, and effectiveness of informal social networks supporting patients and families [88].

Most countries aim to provide TB diagnosis and treatment free of charge within public health services. Access to free TB care has expanded substantially over the past two decades through national efforts and global financial support [88]. However, many TB patients and their families are still facing very high direct and indirect costs due to TB illness and care-seeking, hampering access and putting people at risk of financial ruin or further impoverishment. Total costs for TB diagnosis and treatment might range from 55 to 8,198 United States Dollars (USD), which include the following components: direct medical costs (consultations, tests, medicines and hospitalization, etcetera), direct non-medical cost (transport, food, and accommodation during healthcare visits) and indirect costs (lost income) [88].

The following rights increase access to quality TB diagnosis, treatment, care and support: Non-discrimination, access to health services and anti-TB treatment, right to participation, information, education, right to social security and financial protection, right to privacy, freedom of movement, right to body integrity and freedom from torture and inhuman or degrading treatment, right to due process protection, Siracusa principles, and right to enjoy the benefits of scientific progress and its applications [4].

Chiapas was one of the first Mexican states which adopted DOTS strategy [89] and therefore Mexican and state governments assumed the responsibility to provide free diagnosis and treatment. Although it is stipulated that the anti-TB treatment is free for all population, it is quite often that anti-TB drugs supply is not available for local TB programs during large periods of time, even weeks. Chiapas is considered a high priority for prevention and control of TB due to the presence of many DR-TB cases [16]. Moreover, a study carried out in three different regions of Chiapas identified serious deficiencies in both the detection and treatment of PTB, as well as alarming conditions that expose people to risk to PTB [9]. This study found 29 cases of PTB, from which four had not received any medical care. Of the 25 that had received medical care, 22 had done in government health services and three in private services. Of these 25 cases, ten had not received any diagnosis, thirteen had been diagnosed with PTB, and two received diagnosis other than PTB. From the 13 who were diagnosed by health services, one had not received any treatment, six were receiving anti-TB drugs, and six had failed to comply due to several irregularities and deficiencies in their treatment [9]. Furthermore, the study also highlighted that patients with PTB did not seek health care due to lack of money, great walking distance to nearest clinic, denial of health service, and mistreat by health personnel [9]. Whether TB patients receive free and adequate treatment by health services, their socioeconomic conditions (poverty, malnutrition, overcrowding, marginalization, etcetera) makes them at high risk for defaulting treatment, either by the need to work and support their family, or by the adverse effects of anti-TB drugs [10,19,23,90].

Economically productive people affected by TB are unable to work, and this has immediately consequences for the family. Patients with TB and their family are condemned to a higher level of poverty that often has a negative impact on their living conditions. Incapacity to work reduces access to food, and forces other members of the family into the labor market. In many occasions, children become the work force for the family and drop out their education. WHO [1] has stated that if the social determinants of disease such as poverty, social exclusion, poor working conditions and food insecurity, are not tackled, TB will remain a major public health. Poverty has strongly been associated with prevalence of TB. In Mexico, in 2012, almost half (45.5%) of its population lives in poverty [91], whereas Chiapas has 74.7% of its population in poverty conditions [92]. The fact that Chiapas is one of poorest Mexican states and the considerable shortage of health resources in the country, suggests that TB is, and will continue to be a serious public health issue in terms of morbidity and mortality with impact in health costs care. Our studies reflect this epidemiological situation in which we have reported high incidence and mortality rates (See Table 1).

6.4. Public or individual health rights?

TB is transmitted to person to person and this implies and requires both individual and public rights [93,94]. A fundamental function of government is public health protection that requires formulation and implementation of policies in order to prevent transmission of diseases such as TB [93,94]. Public health is sometimes used by States as a ground for limiting the exercise of human rights. In the case of TB, governments have traditionally focused on preventing transmission of disease by controlling the movement of infected persons [93,94]. However, this causes a tension between individual rights and public health security, because governments must protect public health as well as safeguard legal rights of individuals [93,94]. PTB poses a serious demonstrable threat to the public health, especially when any DR-TB strains are being transmitted from endemic to global settings [95].

International law provides rights-limiting principles, which might justify enforcing compulsory measures against TB patients who refuse to have diagnostic procedures or who refuse to be monitored and treated once disease is confirmed [93,94]. Restrictions of human rights are permitted, on limited duration and subject to review, if there is a need to protect public health, but these limitations must fulfill the five criteria of the Siracusa Principles [96]:

a. The restriction is provided for and carried out in accordance with the law;

b. The restriction is in the interest of a legitimate objective of general interest;

c. The restriction is strictly necessary in a democratic society to achieve the objective;

d. There are no less intrusive and restrictive means available to reach the same objective;

e. The restriction is based on scientific evidence and not drafted or imposed arbitrarily i.e. in an unreasonable or otherwise discriminatory manner.

Since interaction between infectious people and those susceptible to infection is a strategy to interrupt TB transmission, some countries have adopted two approaches: (a) isolation, the segregation of presently infectious people; and (b) quarantine, the segregation of people exposed to TB but who are not yet infectious [97]. Isolation might be acceptable under appropriate and effective means of preventing transmission if patients are released as soon as transmission becomes unlikely [97]. However, quarantine is unethical for TB [97]. Either way there are implications in both individual and collective human rights. The high incidence rates of MDT-TB and XDR-TB in South Africa has challenged both points of view [98].

7. TB in several vulnerable populations: Children, elderly, indigenous groups, migrants, and women

All societies are vulnerable in several ways and factors that contribute to this are: physical, economic, social, cultural, ethnicity, religious, language, and political, among others. All these conditions might determine people's level of vulnerability. Poverty is one of the major contributors to vulnerability, because poor people are more likely to live and work in areas exposed to potential hazards, while they are less likely to have resources to affront such hazards. Since the vast majority of people living with TB are from the poorer and vulnerable segments of the society, the global TB control goals cannot be met unless these populations segments have sufficient social and economic empowerment [1]. Key social determinants of TB that include food insecurity, malnutrition, hunger, poor housing and environmental conditions, as well as financial, geographical, cultural and linguistic barriers to health care access, should also be addressed in order to achieve TB control and management [99]. Thus, TB is deeply associated with vulnerability conditions such as: (a) poverty because of the low socioeconomic status which implies legal, structural and social barriers that impede access to health services and, in consequence, difficult TB prevention, diagnosis and treatment care; (b) demographic factors like age, sex and ethnic group; and, (c) socioeconomic issues as migration, among others.

7.1. TB in children

In Chiapas, as in worldwide, TB in children is a crucial issue that has not received enough attention despite that this state has a very high TB mortality rate among adult population –as was stated before- and adult persons with TB can transmit the bacteria to their family members, including children.

In 2012, WHO estimated that TB incidence among children (aged <15 years old) was 530,000, from which the total number of deaths from TB among HIV-negative children was estimated to be 74,000 [2]. However, these figures do not show the real burden of TB in children because TB prevention and control programs are emphasized in adults, who mainly having the PTB form. In this regard, TB in children is not considered a source of infection and therefore they are a vulnerable population whose rights are violated for not receiving appropriate diagnosis and treatment. TB diagnosis and treatment for children is difficult due to the following reasons: (a) non-specific symptoms and problems in confirming diagnosis, requiring more expensive diagnostic methods and experienced physicians; and (b) treatment is challenging due to the lack of child-friendly formulations and difficulties in monitoring toxicity [100].

Globally, TB in children represents 5% to 30% of all cases, but regions with incidence greater than 15% indicates poor TB control [2]. In Mexico, 8.4% new cases registered in 2013 were pediatric [15]. The most common forms of TB in children in Mexico are pulmonary, lymphatic, renal and meningeal, while miliary TB continues to be present. From these, miliary and meningeal forms of TB are the most dangerous to the child. The risk of developing the disease varies according to age, increasing overall for those 10 years and over, while severe forms predominate among children under five. The Mexican states that reported highest incidence rates of TB among children in 2013, were: Baja California (18.5%), Chiapas (12%) Guerrero (8.5%), Tamaulipas (8.5%), and Nuevo Leon (7.7%) [15]. However, the Highlands region, which is characterized by large presence of indigenous groups, the incidence rate of TB in children has reached up to 22% [101]. The latter figure contrasts to that reported by official statistics, in which this region had the lowest incidence rate (11.7 *per* 100,000 inhabitants), even below the national rate [16]. Despite these numbers, the burden of TB in children for Chiapas and Mexico is unknown and is expected to be much greater due to the high prevalence of disease, lack or null access to health services, and problems in diagnosis, preventing and treating patients [9,10].

Finally, it is important to remember that in the "International Childhood Tuberculosis Meeting" [102] carried out in 2011, were set out, among others, the next key aspects:

- Children with TB infection today represent the reservoir of TB disease tomorrow.
- Children are more likely to develop more serious forms of TB such as meningeal and miliar, resulting in high morbidity and mortality.

- Despite policy guidelines, the implementation of contact tracing and delivery of isoniazid preventive therapy (IPT) to young and HIV-infected children is often neglected by public health programs.
- Most public health programs have limited capacity to meet the demand for care and high-quality services for childhood TB.
- BCG, the only licensed TB vaccine, has limited efficacy against the most common forms of childhood TB and its effect is of limited duration.
- Due to inadequate case detection it is estimated that a large number of children suffering from TB are not appropriately treated. This is further compounded by drug stock outs and the lack of child-friendly formulations of drugs for TB treatment and prevention.
- Children are rarely included in clinical trials to evaluate new TB drugs, diagnostics or preventive strategies.

7.2. TB in elderly population

The demographic transition worldwide has resulted also in an ageing population. A weakening in immunity and age related physiological changes leads to an increased burden of communicable and non-communicable diseases in the elderly. Hence, elderly population is the group that most suffer TB, independently of development degree and the efficacy of the fight against TB in the past. At present, as the elderly population's growth in numbers, there has been an increase in number of TB cases among this vulnerable group. In elderly patients, many clinical features of TB are subtle or absent, making diagnosis difficult. Autopsy among the elderly suggests that TB often remains unrecognized [103,104]. This population group is also at greater risk for re-activation of LTBI and for acquisition of new TB infection. Furthermore, the elderly also present challenging to receive treatment due to adverse effects (i.e. hepatoxicity), and the poor outcome of treated TB in this age group warrants more aggressive treatment [103,104]. Therefore, it is not surprising that compared with younger individuals, the mortality rate of TB in elders is six times higher [103,104].

In Mexico, there are 10 million older adults (≥ 60 years old) representing 9% of the total population [11]. Its annual growth rate is 3.8%, which means that there will be 14 million in 2018. A recent report has highlighted that there is an increase of up to 5% of chronic diseases, primarily DM in this age group [105]. In 2012, there were 2,253 deaths associated to TB from which 34.7% were people aged ≥ 65 years old, both women and men. However, epidemiological studies carried out in different regions of Chiapas have found that people aged ≥45 years old are in high risk to die due to PTB [10,24]. Factors that might explain why TB affects the elderly are: (a) the cumulative prevalence of TB through their lifetime; (b) their immune system become weak as they grow up older; (c) the presence of other diseases, mainly chronic such as DM, which form comorbidities with TB.

DM is one of the leading causes of deaths in Mexico, and has significantly increased the number of TB cases in the elderly. The association between DM and TB is 20.9% in TB cases, versus 5.6% people infected with HIV [15]. Patients with DM respond late to the anti-TB treatment, and they have higher risk to become DR-TB [106]. It has been stated that DM increases three times the risk of PTB, either by reactivation or new infections. However, a study carried out in southeast of Mexico, people having DM had ten times risk to be infected by TB, than patients having HIV. This study also found that the incidence rate was significantly higher in patients with DM compared to the rest of the population (209.5 versus 30.7 *per* 100,000 inhabitants/year) [107]. In Chiapas, the elderly group is the most affected by TB. Thus, in 2013, 15.44% of the reported cases were people aged over 65 years old, and the association of TB and DM among elder people was 18% [16]. However, the real burden determined by both diseases is unknown because not all people have access to health services to measure its glucose levels.

7.3. TB in women

Worldwide, women have more probabilities to be poor than men because they suffer the more generalized discrimination, more assistance work non remunerated, violence, violation of their rights and less levels of income, among others gender inequalities [108].

Globally, in 2012, there were an estimated 2.9 million new cases of TB among women, from which more than half (1.5 million) neither were diagnosed nor treated. Of the 2.9 million, it was estimated that 410,00 died, of which 54% occurred in Africa [2]. In this sense, a study carried out in Bangladesh, India and Malawi, identified gender and illness related factors of diagnostic delay of TB [109] Furthermore, TB is one of the main causes of women's death in reproductive years, and kill more women that all causes of maternal mortality [110]. In fact, in the age group 15-44 years, TB figures in the top three causes of death, and represents 9% of deaths in this age group, versus 3% for HIV and heart diseases [4].

However, the burden of TB morbidity and mortality among women is larger than often realized. Gender discrimination, even when not directly related to health care (for example denying girls and women access to education, information, and various forms of economic, social and political participation) can create increased health risk. Even if the best public health services are available, a woman has to be able to decide when and how she is going to access them, and that implies that she must have the ability to control and make decisions about her life [111]. Unfortunately, in practice, TB-related stigma and discrimination affect women's access to health care, delaying seeking care [4].

Stigma associated with TB may be greater for women than men, and its consequence include ostracism, abandonment by the husband and/or her family, divorce or the husband's taking of a second wife, and loss of social and economic support, housing, access to one's children, etc. [1]. Marriage chances may be affected if women are known to have TB, or even if they have a family member with TB, since stigma associated with the disease may affect all household members. In situations of poverty, women have the least access to food, health, education, training and opportunities for employment and other basic needs [1]. This highlights the social structural inequalities resulting from the arbitrary assignment of biological, cultural, political, and economic roles to women, which make them vulnerable in different situations, and particularly the gain to access to health [111].

The natural history of TB is different in both sexes. Women in reproductive age (15-40 years old) are more susceptible to developing TB with twice the probability to progress to an active phase after the infection, than men. Maternal and neonatal complications increase in pregnant women with TB, who require up to 12 times more hospitalizations compared to women who do not have the disease [110]. Risks of perinatal and neonatal deaths increase ten times in women with TB, and risk of transmission of VIH from mother to child increases 2.5 times [110].

In Mexico, in 2013, of 19,738 new cases registered of TB (in all its forms), 38% were women, with a ratio men/women of 1.6:1 [15] and a similar trend also observed in Chiapas [16]. Regarding to mortality, from the total number of deaths (2,253) related to TB reported in 2012, 652 were women [15]. However, the exact numbers of morbidity and mortality is unknown among women because of the stigma associated with the disease with consequences in delays in diagnosis and treatment, as well as null or lack of family support.

In a study of gender differences regarding to social support networks among people with PTB in the State of Veracruz, Mexico, concluded that women struggle to receive either diagnosis or treatment due to their family role (housekeeping, care of child, they have to attend sick persons, go out to work, they are very busy and have no time to go to the doctor), fear to be stigmatized, and lack of family support [112].

Another study [113] documented that men can influence women –negative or favorably- for receiving diagnosis and adequate treatment, because their lack of empowerment to make decisions about their health. Furthermore, the same study also documented more deficiencies in care quality in women than men, such as: (a) they were not examined properly; (b) they were not informed of the causes of and the required treatment for TB; and (c) their diagnosis took a considerable amount of time [113]. A study carried out in the Highlands of Chiapas, documented the case of an indigenous woman whose husband did not let her to take anti-TB treatment [23].

In summary, It may be considered that female deaths due to TB is a form of gender and structural violence given the high number of women TB-deaths avoidable, because a lot of them occur as consequence of differences constructed by gender roles created by society. It is necessary to examine disaggregated data of TB morbidity and mortality by age and sex in order to emphasize the nature and extent of inequality between men and women [114]. The differences in the prevalence of TB among women and men might be explained in terms of socio-economic and cultural factor such as: (a) Level and time exposure and risk of infection; (b) delay in seeking care; (c) difference in quality services; (d) compliance with treatment; (e) impact of disease on individuals and their families [114].

7.4. TB in indigenous people

Disparities in health, including differences in TB risk and burden, between indigenous and non-indigenous people, are the result of the complex interplay between the individual, the community, and the social determinants of health. In Mexico, as in many Latin American countries, the majority of indigenous people live in extreme poverty. Official statistics estimates that in the country there are 13.7 million indigenous people, from which 76.1% live in conditions of poverty [13]. This socio-economic situation has favored migration from rural areas to urban centers, where the population tends to settle on unfavorable living conditions.

Mexico has 2,443 municipalities of which 871 (35.7%) are considered indigenous or with presence of indigenous population. Among these 871, 75.2% (655) have 40% and over of indigenous population, and almost are classified as high or very high poverty level [115].

Studies have estimated that municipalities with over 70% indigenous populations contain approximately 80% of the population living below the poverty line. Additionally, some of the indigenous groups in Chiapas face even greater degrees of poverty than others in the country. For example, 58% of the Mixtec population (in Central Mexico) live in municipalities classified as having "very high" marginalization, compared with 93% of the Tseltal population in Chiapas [9].

Chiapas, Oaxaca, Veracruz, Yucatan and Puebla, are Mexican states having large indigenous population [11]. Indigenous populations represent 27% of the Chiapas population [11]. Most of indigenous settlements are in remote communities, which have a negative impact on the realization of human rights of these populations [9,10]. Indigenous condition in Mexico is not only a demographic indicator, but also a socioeconomic one, because reflects socioeconomic condition and level of accessibility to health services with quality, as well to social security, among other basic human rights.

The life expectancy in indigenous population is 65 years, while in the general population is 74.70 [11]. In Chiapas, infant mortality is greater compared to other states and national average. For example, the likelihood of one infant from Chiapas die before his first year of life is 80% greater than one child from Mexico City and Nuevo Leon. Furthermore, 79% of indigenous infant deaths could be prevented [116]. These statistics show that indigenous people are highly vulnerable in terms of right to access to any social security, including health services [117]. In this sense, there is strong evidence that poverty influence in the utilization of health services and delay in seeking care [118,119].

Health coverage apparently increased among Mexican indigenous people due to the implementation of the so-called "Seguro Popular", however, this did not reflect in health services utilization, neither better living conditions for indigenous populations [28]

Although northern Mexican states, such as Baja California, Tamaulipas, Sinaloa, reported high number of new TB cases [15], a great number of cases are from indigenous people who have migrated from southern states, such as Chiapas. Therefore, the burden of TB in northern Mexican states is influenced due to migratory movements from the south of the country, a region with high proportion of indigenous population.

In terms of TB morbidity and mortality, there are three important sanitary jurisdictions in Chiapas: the Soconusco region (main region of migratory movements from Central America to USA), the Centre (where is located the capital of the state) and the Highlands (with strong presence of indigenous people). It is interesting to highlight that the incidence rate of TB for these regions, in 2013, were: 59.3, 19.7, and 11.7 *per* 100, 000 inhabitants, respectively; the latter figure was the lowest incidence rate reported for the whole state [16]. The TB epidemiological situation in these regions is controversial. Apparently the Soconusco and the Centre regions hold the TB burden for the state, which might be explained as follows: (a) the Soconusco region, which is a border with Guatemala, favors the continuous transmission of TB between countries; (b) the Centre region is becoming rapidly urbanized without planning, with many poverty surroundings. The marked difference of incidence rates of TB between the Soconusco and the Centre regions with respect to the Highlands is unlikely because the latter one possesses socioeconomic conditions that favors high TB burden. Our epidemiological studies show this affirmation (See Table 1). The main factors that can contribute to explain such asymmetry, is precisely the ethnic composition of each region: the Highlands is mainly indigenous, with low human index, and the other ones are "mestizos". This situation is the result of significant differences in levels of under-diagnosis due to inequalities of health resources allocation, both material and human, which violate people's right to health. Noteworthy to mention is that in a study carried out by our work team in the Highlands, we found that the only variable "protective" in people with PTB to avoid MDR-TB form, it was being indigenous due to less contact with health services compared to non-indigenous population [25].

The International Labour Organization (ILO) Convention 169, of which Mexico is party, specifies in its Art. 25 the rights of indigenous persons to health: "Government shall ensure that adequate health services are made available to the peoples concerned, or shall provide them with resources to allow them to design and deliver such services under their own responsibility and control, so that they may enjoy the highest attainable standard of physical and mental health". In Chiapas, these obligations are not being honored in practice [9].

7.5. TB and migrants

Migration, just after poverty, is one of the principle aspects that contribute to the continue spread of TB [120]. Many migrants are likely to move into social and economic conditions characterized by overcrowded, substandard housing, poor sanitation, and lack of access to medical services [1]. Migrants often fall to the lower end of the social structure where they may be at high risk to get TB, together with HIV-AIDS, DM, and the abandonment of programs of TB prevention and control [1,6,37].

Chiapas is an important route of migration. The state shares more than 660 kilometers border with Guatemala [8]. A large number of Central Americans and South Americans people pass through this state on their way to the United States of America (USA). Many peasants and indigenous people from Chiapas have migrated to the USA. Migration from the southern Mexican states of Chiapas, Oaxaca, Guerrero and Veracruz is an important factor for the high morbidity and mortality rates found in the northern states of Mexico, such as Baja California [15,101].

In Chiapas, international migration is an evident phenomenon in the last years [121]. Migration is commonly linked to an image of prosperity and well-being, however, not always international migration increases the ability of migrants and their families to overcome poverty [122]. Migrants from Chiapas, who recently begun migratory movements, are considered a vulnerable subgroup due to their inexperience in migration. They neither have networks nor the resources to guarantee successful border crossings into the USA, they are unfamiliar with the strategies and operations of the border guards, and they are ignorant of the climate, orography and geography of the border region [123].

Additionally, a considerable number of migrants do not recuperate the expenses paid out for their trip, resulting in increased debt. In these circumstances, migration represents a net loss in various senses: monetary, labor, and health. Therefore, the family continues to worsen further into poverty and into conditions of great vulnerability, which only are remedied when the remittances begin to arrive with regularity. The vulnerability of the family can worse when the unsatisfied needs have to be attended for all household members –including children and the elderly- into the work force, or with the sale of the few belongings the family possesses. For a great number of migrants, the conditions of the trip itself, and of the housing available upon arrival, as well as work conditions, reinforce the vulnerability at each step in the process [124].

As we can see, in general terms, migrants suffer conditions of vulnerability. So, states must take into account this condition, and guarantee their human rights, in this case, in the access to TB prevention, diagnosis and treatment without discrimination of any kind, either countries of origin, transit or destination [1,4,44].

The main human rights issues associated with TB with regard to migrants, refugees and internally displaced persons, are [4]:

- Migrants in irregular situations often fall to the lower end of the social structure. Migrants, refugees and internally displaced persons may be at risk of TB due to poor housing (crowed living conditions), inadequate nutrition, lack of access to health facilities, information and services and/or exploitative working conditions;
- Migrants may be denied access to diagnosis and treatment for TB because of their legal status. They may avoid accessing health services for fear of deportation and delay seeking treatment because of lack of education and information;
- Continuity of care is often unavailable to forcibly returned migrants.
- Prevention, diagnosis and continuity of TB care, can be affected in the context of protracted humanitarian emergencies.

Unfortunately, despite the existence of national and international laws that protect their human rights, many states constrain the effective and full realization of the right to health of migrants, particularly those in an irregular situation. These practices include [4]:

- Legal barriers to accessing health services, based on the view that: it would be expensive for taxpayers to shoulder the costs of irregular migrants health, and that excluding this particular group from receiving social benefits would deter future irregular migration.
- Excluding migrants and their families from national health systems, limiting migrants' access to emergency care, with which increases their susceptibility to ill health, but on the other hand, may pose a public health risk to host communities. A person with active TB can infect 20 people each year. Migratory movements facilitate the dissemination of the

infection, especially when the migrant works and lives in overcrowded and in unsanitary places, which greatly complicates its control. In addition, a person undergoing anti-TB treatment who migrates will most likely abandon the treatment and not conclude it. At the same time, migrants can contaminate each other with TB, either during transit to their destination (many migrants travel in subhuman conditions of overcrowding) [125].

- Deny admission and residence to migrants with bad health conditions.
- Lack of health workers sensitized and trained in intercultural issues as well as on migrants' rights. From a human rights perspective, accurate communication and, if necessary, the use of professional interpretation services, are essential when obtaining consent for health interventions and treatment and guaranteeing confidentiality and privacy about health information [126].
- Involve health professionals in migration control. Due to the lack of financial and legal protection in accessing health services, many migrants postpone seeking medical care until they are seriously ill.

8. Legal health reforms in Mexico: Any impact in DOTS strategy?

In Mexico, the socioeconomic situation has led to setbacks in people's to have right to health due to the implementation of neoliberal economy policies followed by structural adjustments. Such policies are driven by structural reforms, economic regulations, trade opening and law markets, instead of health needs [40]. From 2009 to 2012, there was a reduction of 6.5% to 6.1% of gross domestic product (GDP) in the total health expenditure [127]. The immediate consequence is the deterioration of public institutions, which provide services to the Mexican people, and this includes the delivery of health services. These policies are impacting all structural bases, from legal reforms to the substantial reduction of budget [128]. The structural reforms in health sector only seek to reduce financial cost, but not to improve people living conditions [40]. Our epidemiological studies investigating diverse epidemiologic and public health issues in many regions of Chiapas show that the proposal changes by the Mexican government will worsen the so-called social determinants for TB. Therefore, such reforms will impact in the enjoyment of Human Rights to the majority of population, including the right to health. It is highly probably that reduction of financial expenditure on health (worse if expenditures are solely based on political and administrative criteria) will affect local prevention and control TB programs, due to lack of resources such as: physicians, shortage of anti-TB drugs, low resources to follow up TB patients, scarcity of equipment to prevent and diagnosis of TB, among others.

9. Conclusions

Health is a human right, and the right to health is indispensable to the exercise of other human rights, that is, it is also closely related to and dependent upon the realization of, among others rights. The right to health is equally tied to the key principle of non-discrimination, which recognizes the "inherent dignity" of every human being. Through Mexico's General Health Law, and the National Health System theoretically guarantees both the availability and quality of health services, particularly to vulnerable groups, such as indigenous persons. However, in practice health care is not sufficiently available or accessible to many persons in Chiapas. In consequence, the high levels of incidence, mortality and MDR-TB cases, are the reflection that health services is not functioning adequately, and that the right to health in Chiapas is far away to achieve. Therefore, it is necessary:

a. To guarantee that all federal, state, and municipal government programs and activities related to health, be carried out without discrimination.

b. In keeping with the fulfillment of its obligations under the International Covenant on Economic, Social and Cultural Rights, the Mexican federal and Chiapas state governments should improve the availability, accessibility, acceptability and quality of health facilities, goods and services in Chiapas. To achieve this, it is necessary to train and sensitize health personnel about human rights considering local differences such as ethnic, culture, language, social and political structures, among others social determinants of the disease. Including these factors in DOTS strategy, it would be possible to improve diagnosis and treatment and view people with respect and dignity.

c. To improve surveillance and detection systems related to prevention and control of TB on disaggregated basis, so that disparities based on gender, socioeconomic indicators, and ethnicity may be detected and addressed in order to review either progress or failure of the local and regional TB programs.

d. The program of TB Prevention and Control in Chiapas should be strongly reinforced, with more resources, sensitizing, training, supervising, evaluating a comprehensive DOTS program, and incorporating mechanisms to ensure adequate follow-up of patients in accordance with international standards.

Nomenclature

DR-TB (drug resistant-TB): TB strains that are resistant to the one or more drugs used to treat it.

MDR-TB (multidrug-resistant TB): defined as TB that is resistant to at least rifampicin and isoniazid, the most powerful first-line anti-TB drugs [129].

PTB (pulmonary TB): it is the common and most infectious form of TB affecting primarily the lungs [130].

TDR-TB (totally drug-resistant TB): is defined as TB strains that showed *in-vitro* resistance to all first and second line drugs tested (isoniazid, rifampicin, streptomycin, ethambutol, pyrazinamide, ethionamide, para-aminosalicylic acid, cycloserine, ofloxacin, amikacin, ciprofloxacin, capreomycin, kanamycin) [131]. TDR-TB has been identified in the following countries: India, Iran, and Italy. However, it is not yet recognized by WHO.

XDR-TB (extensively drug-resistant TB): is defined as TB that has developed resistance to at least rifampicin and isoniazid (resistance to these first line anti-TB drugs defines MDR-TB) as well as to any member of the quinolone family and at least one of the following second-line anti-TB injectable drugs: amikacin, capreomycin or kanamycin [132].

TB: this term usually does not define the kind of TB. Since *Mycobacterium tuberculosis* primarily infects the lungs, this form is called pulmonary TB, while extrapulmonary TB involves the infection of other organs or tissues [130].

Acknowledgements

Part of this work was sponsored by the Prometeo Project (Ministry of Higher Education, Science, Technology and Innovation, Republic of Equator) and GRAAL. Anaximandro Gómez-Velasco is recipient of a Postdoctoral Fellowship Program from the Mexican National Council for Science and Technology (CONACyT).

Author details

H.J. Sánchez-Pérez[1,2,3*], Anaximandro Gómez-Velasco[1,3,4], G. Leal[5], A. Bencomo-Alerm[6], N. Romero-Sandoval[3,7] and M. Martín-Mateo[3,7,8]

*Address all correspondence to: hsanchez@ecosur.mx

1 Health Department, The College of the Southern Border (El Colegio de la Frontera Sur, Ecosur), San Cristobal de Las Casas, Chiapas, Mexico

2 Prometeo researcher, Loja National University, Loja, Ecuador

3 Research Groups for Africa and Latin Americas (GRAAL), Barcelona, Spain

4 Postdoctoral Research Fellow, Mexican National Council for Science and Technology (CONACyT), Mexico

5 Health Care Department, Health and Society Area, Autonomous Metropolitan University, Xochimilco Campus, Mexico, Distrito Federal., Mexico

6 Mycobacteriology Laboratory, Health Jurisdiction II, Chiapas Institute of Health, San Cristobal de Las Casas, Chiapas, Mexico

7 School of Medicine, Faculty of Medicine, Health and Life Sciences, International University of Ecuador, Quito, Ecuador

8 Faculty of Medicine, Autonomous University of Barcelona, Bellaterra, Barcelona, Spain

References

[1] WHO Regional Office for Europe. Tuberculosis, ethics and human rights. Report of a regional workshop. Copenhagen, Denmark; 2013 p. 31.

[2] WHO. Global Tuberculosis Report. Geneva, Switzerland: WHO; 2013 p. 306.

[3] Murray CJL, Ortblad KF, Guinovart C, Lim SS, Wolock TM, Roberts DA, et al. Global, regional, and national incidence and mortality for HIV, tuberculosis, and malaria during 1990–2013: a systematic analysis for the Global Burden of Disease Study 2013. The Lancet. 2014 Sep;384(9947):1005–70.

[4] Stop TB Partnership, TB Human Rights Task Force. Tuberculosis and human rights. Working Document on TB and Human Rights. 2009 p. 5.

[5] PAHO. Tuberculosis in the Americas: Regional Report 2012. Epidemiology, Control, and Financing. Washington, D.C., USA; 2013.

[6] Isaakidis P, Smith S, Majumdar S, Furin J, Reid T. Calling tuberculosis a social disease—an excuse for complacency? The Lancet. 2014 Sep;384(9948):1095.

[7] Ugarte-Gil C. Tuberculosis: Un enfoque de Derechos Humanos. Acta Médica Peru. 2009;26(1):55–57.

[8] CEIEG. Compendio de Información Geográfica y Estadística de Chiapas. http://www.ceieg.chiapas.gob.mx/home/sintesis-estadistica-y-geografica-de-chiapas/?maccion=9571 (accessed 3 October 2014).

[9] Sanchez-Perez H, Arana-Cedeño M, Ely-Yamin A, Ford D. Excluded people, eroded communities. Realizing the right to health in Chiapas, Mexico. United States of America; 2006 p. 73.

[10] Nájera-Ortiz JC, Sánchez-Pérez HJ, Ochoa-Díaz H, Arana-Cedeño M, Lezama MS, Mateo MM. Demographic, health services and socio-economic factors associated with pulmonary tuberculosis mortality in Los Altos Region of Chiapas, Mexico. Int J Epidemiol. 2008 Aug;37(4):786–95.

[11] INEGI. Censo de Población y Vivienda 2010. http://www.censo2010.org.mx/ (accessed 4 October 2014).

[12] DGIS. Cubos Dinamicos de Morbilidad y Mortalidad. http://www.sinais.salud.gob.mx/basesdedatos (accessed 3 October 2014).

[13] CONAPO. Índice de marginación por Entidad Federativa y Municipio 2010. http://www.conapo.gob.mx/es/CONAPO/Indices_de_Marginacion_2010_por_entidad_federativa_y_municipio (accessed 3 October 2014).

[14] PNUD. Índice de Desarrollo Humano Municipal en México: nueva metodología. Mexico, D.F.; 2014 p. 104.

[15] Castellanos-Joya M, García-Avilés M, Romero-Pérez R, Martínez-Olivares M. El Control de la Tuberculosis en México: en donde estamos?. Querétaro, México: SSA; p. 37. http://www.cenaprece.salud.gob.mx/programas/interior/micobacteriosis/descargas/pdf/controlTbMexico_DrMartinCastellanos.pdf (Accessed on 3 October 2014).

[16] Enríquez-Ríos N. Panorama Epidemiológico: Chiapas. Motozintla, Chiapas, Mexico: Secretaría de Salud, Gobierno del Estado de Chiapas; 2014.

[17] Sánchez-Pérez HJ, Halperin Frisch David D. Problems of diagnosis of pulmonary tuberculosis. The case of the border region of Chiapas (Mexico). Atencion Primaria Soc Esp Med Fam Comunitaria. 1997 Mar 31;19(5):237–42.

[18] Sánchez-Pérez HJ, del Mar Garcia Gil M, Halperin D. Pulmonary tuberculosis in the border region of Chiapas, Mexico. Int J Tuberc Lung Dis Off J Int Union Tuberc Lung Dis. 1998 Jan;2(1):37–43.

[19] Sánchez-Pérez HJ, Prat-Monterde D, Jansà JM, Martín-Mateo M. Pulmonary tuberculosis and use of health services in zones of high socioeconomic marginalization in Chiapas, Mexico. Gac Sanit SESPAS. 2000 Aug;14(4):268–76.

[20] Sánchez-Pérez HJ, Prat-Monterde D, Jansà JM, Martín-Mateo M. Tuberculosis pulmonar y uso de servicios del primer nivel de atención en zonas de alta marginación socioeconómica de Chiapas, México. Gac Sanit. 2000;14(4):268–76.

[21] Sánchez-Pérez H, Flores-Hernández J, Jansá J, Caylá J, Martín-Mateo M. Pulmonary tuberculosis and associated factors in areas of high levels of poverty in Chiapas, Mexico. Int J Epidemiol. 2001 Apr;30(2):386–93.

[22] Sánchez-Pérez HJ, Hernán MA, Hernández-Díaz S, Jansá JM, Halperin D, Ascherio A. Detection of pulmonary tuberculosis in Chiapas, Mexico. Ann Epidemiol. 2002 Apr;12(3):166–72.

[23] Reyes-Guillén I, Sánchez-Pérez HJ, Cruz-Burguete J, Izaurieta-de Juan M. Anti-tuberculosis treatment defaulting: an analysis of perceptions and interactions in Chiapas, Mexico. Salud Pública México. 2008 Jun;50(3):251–7.

[24] Nájera-Ortiz JC, Sánchez-Pérez HJ, Ochoa-Díaz-López H, Leal-Fernández G, Navarro-Giné A. The Poor Survival among Pulmonary Tuberculosis Patients in Chiapas, Mexico: The Case of Los Altos Region. Tuberc Res Treat. 2012;2012:708423.

[25] Sánchez-Pérez HJ, Díaz-Vázquez A, Nájera-Ortiz JC, Balandrano S, Martín-Mateo M. Multidrug-resistant pulmonary tuberculosis in Los Altos, Selva and Norte regions, Chiapas, Mexico. Int J Tuberc Lung Dis Off J Int Union Tuberc Lung Dis. 2010 Jan; 14(1):34–9.

[26] Sánchez Pérez HJ, Halperin Frisch D. Obstacles to overcome in the control of pulmonary tuberculosis in the border region of Chiapas, Mexico. Gac Sanit SESPAS. 1997 Dec;11(6):281–6.

[27] Gutiérrez J, Rivera-Dommarco J, Shamah-Levy T, Villalpando-Hernández S, Franco A, Cuevas-Nasu L, et al. Encuesta Nacional de Salud y Nutrición 2012. Resultados por entidad federativa: Chiapas. Cuernavaca, Morelos, Mexico: Instituto Nacional de Salud Pública (INSP); 2012.

[28] Meneses-Navarro S. ¿Acceso universal a la atención obstétrica?. El Seguro Popular de Salud frente al reto de la muerte maternal en Los Altos de Chiapas. In: Díaz D, editor. Muerte Materna y Seguro Popular. México, D.F.: Fundar, Centro de Análisis e Investigación A.C.; 2014. p. 13–64.

[29] Red por los Derechos de la Infancia en Mexico (REDIM). La Infancia cuenta en México 2013. Hacia la construcción de un sistema de información sobre derechos de infancia y adolescencia en México. México; 2013. p. 206.

[30] CEIEG. Concentrado de Datos Municipales. http://www.ceieg.chiapas.gob.mx/home/consulta-de-indicadores-municipales/ (accessed 4 October 2014).

[31] Tasa de mortalidad infantil por país - Mapa Comparativo de Países - Mundo http://www.indexmundi.com/map/?v=29&l=es (accessed 8 October 2014).

[32] INEGI. México en Cifras. Información nacional, por entidad federativa y municipios: Chiapas INEGI. http://www3.inegi.org.mx/sistemas/mexicocifras/default.aspx?e=7 (accessed 3 October 2014).

[33] United Nations Human Rights. Human Rights. http://www.ohchr.org/en/issues/pages/whatarehumanrights.aspx (accessed 4 October 2014).

[34] United Nations Human Rights (UNHR), Office of the High Commissioner for Human Rights (OHCHR). International Covenant on Economic, Social and Cultural Rights. 1966. http://www.ohchr.org/en/professionalinterest/pages/cescr.aspx (accessed 4 October 2014).

[35] Cámara de Diputados, H. Congreso de la Unión,LXII Legislatura. Constitución Política de los Estados Unidos Mexicanos. Constitución publicada en el Diario Oficial de la Federación el 5 de Febrero de 1917. http://www.diputados.gob.mx/LeyesBiblio/htm/1.htm (accessed 4 October 2014).

[36] WHO. World Conference Against Racism, Racial Discrimination, Xenophobia and Related Intolerance: Health and Freedom from Discrimination. WHO/SDE/HDE/HHR/01.2, p. 6. Geneva, Switzerland; 2001.

[37] UNAIDS Reference Group on HIV and Human Rights. HIV and Tuberculosis: ensuring universal acces and protection of human rights.

[38] Office of the High Commissioner for Human Rights (OHCHR). Report on Indicators for Promoting and Monitoring the implementation of Human Rights. 2008, HRI/ MC/ 2008/3. United Nations Human Rights; 2008.

[39] Committee on Economic, Social, and Cultural Rights (CESCR). General Comment

No. 20 on Non-Discrimination in Economic, Social and Cultural Rights (Art. 2, para. 2), E/C.12/GC/20. CESCR, United Nations; 2009.

[40] Leal G, Sánchez-Pérez H. Seguridad social "Universal" 2013: Plan Nacional de Desarrollo y Sector Asegurador. Universidad Autónoma Metropolitana, El Colegio de la Frontera Sur; 2014.

[41] Hernández Peña P, Zapata O, Leyva R, Lozano R. Equity and health: research needs for the development of a social policy. Salud Pública México. 1991 Feb;33(1):9–17.

[42] Menegoni L. Conceptions of tuberculosis and therapeutic choices in Highland Chiapas, Mexico. Med Anthropol Q. 1996 Sep;10(3):381–401.

[43] Grosse U. Health professionals: fighting TB stigma. 37th World Conference on Lung Health of the International Union Against Tuberculosis and Lung Disease (The Union). Paris, France: Int J Tuberc Lung Dis; 2006. p. 313.

[44] United Nations Development Programme (UNDP). Chapter 2. Democratic governance for human development. In: Human Development Report. Deepening Democracy in a Fragmented World [Internet]. New York, USA; 2002; p. 51–61.

[45] The San Andrés Accords. Joint Proposals that the Federal Government and the EZLN agree to remit to the National Debating and Decision - Making Bodies in Accordance with Paragraph 1.4 of the Rules of Procedure. San Andrés Larrainzar, Chiapas, Mexico; 1996 p. 11. Available from: http://peacemaker.un.org/mexico-jointproposals96

[46] VeneKlasen L, Miller V, Clark C, Reilly M. Rights-based approaches and beyond: challenges of linking rights and participation. Brighton, Sussex, England: Institute of Development Studies; 2004 p. 62.

[47] Laurell A, Zepeda E, Mussot L. Eliminating Economic Barriers in Health Care. In: Mackintosh M, Koivusalo M, editors. Commercialization of Health Care. New York, USA: Palgrave-MacMillan; 2005. p. 216–33.

[48] Committee on Economic, Social and Cultural Rights (CESCR). General Comment No. 19 on the Right to social security (Art. 9), E/C.12/GC/19, para. 2. 2008. http://www.ohchr.org/EN/HRBodies/CESCR/Pages/CESCRIndex.aspx (accessed 5 October 2014).

[49] WHO. Pursue high-quality DOTS expansion and enhancement. http://www.who.int/tb/dots/en/ (accessed 5 October 2014).

[50] WHO. The Stop TB Strategy [Internet]. WHO. http://www.who.int/tb/strategy/en/ (accessed 5 October 2014).

[51] Andersen P, Doherty TM. The success and failure of BCG - implications for a novel tuberculosis vaccine. Nat Rev Microbiol. 2005 Aug;3(8):656–62.

[52] Abubakar I, Pimpin L, Ariti C, Beynon R, Mangtani P, Sterne J a. C, et al. Systematic review and meta-analysis of the current evidence on the duration of protection by

bacillus Calmette-Guérin vaccination against tuberculosis. Health Technol Assess Winch Engl. 2013 Sep;17(37):1–372, v – vi.

[53] Colditz GA, Berkey CS, Mosteller F, Brewer TF, Wilson ME, Burdick E, et al. The efficacy of bacillus Calmette-Guérin vaccination of newborns and infants in the prevention of tuberculosis: meta-analyses of the published literature. Pediatrics. 1995 Jul; 96(1 Pt 1):29–35.

[54] Trunz BB, Fine P, Dye C. Effect of BCG vaccination on childhood tuberculous meningitis and miliary tuberculosis worldwide: a meta-analysis and assessment of cost-effectiveness. Lancet. 2006 Apr 8;367(9517):1173–80.

[55] WHO. BCG vaccine: WHO position report. Geneva, Switzerland; 2004 p. 27–38. Report No.: 4.

[56] WHO. Revised BCG vaccination guidelines for infants at risk for HIV infection. Geneva, Switzerland; 2007 p. 193–6. Report No.: 21.

[57] SSA. Manual de Vacunación 2008-2009. Mexico, D.F.; 2008.

[58] CENSIA. Esquema de Vacunación Actual. http://www.censia.salud.gob.mx/contenidos/vacunas/esquemavacunas.html (accessed 5 September 2014).

[59] SSA. NORMA Oficial Mexicana NOM-036-SSA2-2012, Prevención y control de enfermedades. Aplicación de vacunas, toxoides, faboterápicos (sueros) e inmunoglobulinas en el humano. http://dof.gob.mx/nota_detalle.php?codigo=5270654&fecha=28/09/2012 (accessed 5 September 2014).

[60] Rahman M, Sekimoto M, Takamatsu I, Hira K, Shimbo T, Toyoshima K, et al. Economic evaluation of universal BCG vaccination of Japanese infants. Int J Epidemiol. 2001 Apr;30(2):380–5.

[61] Rahman M, Sekimoto M, Hira K, Koyama H, Imanaka Y, Fukui T. Is Bacillus Calmette-Guerin revaccination necessary for Japanese children? Prev Med. 2002 Jul;35(1): 70–7.

[62] Rodrigues LC, Pereira SM, Cunha SS, Genser B, Ichihara MY, de Brito SC, et al. Effect of BCG revaccination on incidence of tuberculosis in school-aged children in Brazil: the BCG-REVAC cluster-randomised trial. Lancet. 2005 Oct 8;366(9493):1290–5.

[63] Sepulveda RL, Parcha C, Sorensen RU. Case-control study of the efficacy of BCG immunization against pulmonary tuberculosis in young adults in Santiago, Chile. Tuber Lung Dis Off J Int Union Tuberc Lung Dis. 1992 Dec;73(6):372–7.

[64] Kumar R, Dwivedi A, Kumar P, Kohli N. Tuberculous meningitis in BCG vaccinated and unvaccinated children. J Neurol Neurosurg Psychiatry. 2005 Nov;76(11):1550–4.

[65] Andersen P, Kaufmann SHE. Novel Vaccination Strategies against Tuberculosis. Cold Spring Harb Perspect Med. 2014 Jun 1;4(6):a018523.

[66] Montagnani C, Chiappini E, Galli L, de Martino M. Vaccine against tuberculosis: what's new? BMC Infect Dis. 2014;14 Suppl 1:S2.

[67] Ditkowsky JB, Schwartzman K. Potential cost-effectiveness of a new infant tuberculosis vaccine in South Africa--implications for clinical trials: a decision analysis. PloS One. 2014;9(1):e83526.

[68] Barry CE 3rd, Boshoff HI, Dartois V, Dick T, Ehrt S, Flynn J, et al. The spectrum of latent tuberculosis: rethinking the biology and intervention strategies. Nat Rev Microbiol. 2009 Dec;7(12):845–55.

[69] WHO. Guidelines for intensified tuberculosis case-finding and isoniazid preventive therapy for people living with HIV in resource- constrained settings. Geneva, Switzerland; 2011 p. 187.

[70] Fox GJ, Barry SE, Britton WJ, Marks GB. Contact investigation for tuberculosis: a systematic review and meta-analysis. Eur Respir J Off J Eur Soc Clin Respir Physiol. 2013 Jan;41(1):140–56.

[71] WHO. Systematic screening for active tuberculosis: principles and recommendations. Geneva, Switzerland; 2013 p. 146.

[72] Ra SW, Lyu J, Choi C-M, Oh Y-M, Lee S-D, Kim WS, et al. Distinguishing tuberculosis from Mycobacterium avium complex disease using an interferon-gamma release assay. Int J Tuberc Lung Dis Off J Int Union Tuberc Lung Dis. 2011 May;15(5):635–40.

[73] SSA. Norma Oficial Mexicana NOM-006-SSA2-1993 para la prevencion y control de la tuberculosis en la atencion primaria a la salud. http://www.salud.gob.mx/unidades/cdi/nom/006ssa23.html (accessed 5 September 2014).

[74] Serrano-Escobedo CJ, Enciso-Moreno JA, Monárrez-Espino J. Performance of tuberculin skin test compared to QFT-IT to detect latent TB among high-risk contacts in Mexico. Arch Med Res. 2013 Apr;44(3):242–8.

[75] García-Sancho F MC, García-García L, Jiménez-Corona ME, Palacios-Martínez M, Ferreyra-Reyes LD, Canizales-Quintero S, et al. Is tuberculin skin testing useful to diagnose latent tuberculosis in BCG-vaccinated children? Int J Epidemiol. 2006 Dec; 35(6):1447–54.

[76] Garfein RS, Lozada R, Liu L, Laniado-Laborin R, Rodwell TC, Deiss R, et al. High prevalence of latent tuberculosis infection among injection drug users in Tijuana, Mexico. Int J Tuberc Lung Dis Off J Int Union Tuberc Lung Dis. 2009 May;13(5):626–32.

[77] Garfein RS, Burgos JL, Rodriquez-Lainz A, Brodine S, Pietrucha A, Rondinelli A, et al. Latent tuberculosis infection in a migrant agricultural community in Baja California, Mexico. J Immigr Minor Health Cent Minor Public Health. 2011 Oct;13(5):940–7.

[78] Castaneda-Delgado JE, Cervantes-Villagrana A, Serrano-Escobedo CJ, Frausto-Lujan I, Rivas-Santiago C, Enciso-Moreno JA, et al. Tuberculin skin test and interferon-

gamma release assay values are associated with antimicrobial peptides expression in polymorphonuclear cells during latent tuberculous infection. Mem Inst Oswaldo Cruz. 2014 Jun;109(3):330–4.

[79] Chittoor G, Arya R, Farook VS, David R, Puppala S, Resendez RG, et al. Epidemiologic investigation of tuberculosis in a Mexican population from Chihuahua State, Mexico: a pilot study. Tuberc Edinb Scotl. 2013 Dec;93 Suppl:S71–7.

[80] Torres-Gonzalez P, Soberanis-Ramos O, Martinez-Gamboa A, Chavez-Mazari B, Barrios-Herrera MT, Torres-Rojas M, et al. Prevalence of latent and active tuberculosis among dairy farm workers exposed to cattle infected by Mycobacterium bovis. PLoS Negl Trop Dis. 2013;7(4):e2177.

[81] Garfein RS, Laniado-Laborin R, Rodwell TC, Lozada R, Deiss R, Burgos JL, et al. Latent tuberculosis among persons at risk for infection with HIV, Tijuana, Mexico. Emerg Infect Dis. 2010 May;16(5):757–63.

[82] Velasquez MG, Laniado-Laborin R, Rodwell TC, Cerecer P, Lozada R, Cuevas-Mota J, et al. Tuberculosis testing among populations with high HIV risk in Tijuana, Baja California, Mexico. Rev Panam Salud Pública Pan Am J Public Health. 2012 Jul;32(1): 30–5.

[83] González-Salazar F, Vargas-Villarreal J, Garcialuna-Martínez FJ, Rivera G, Moreno-Treviño MG, Montfort-Gardeazabal JM, et al. Snapshot of Quantiferon TB gold testing in Northern Mexico. Tuberc Edinb Scotl. 2011 Dec;91 Suppl 1:S34–7.

[84] Machingaidze S, Verver S, Mulenga H, Abrahams D-A, Hatherill M, Hanekom W, et al. Predictive value of recent QuantiFERON conversion for tuberculosis disease in adolescents. Am J Respir Crit Care Med. 2012 Nov 15;186(10):1051–6.

[85] Diel R, Loddenkemper R, Nienhaus A. Predictive value of interferon-γ release assays and tuberculin skin testing for progression from latent TB infection to disease state: a meta-analysis. Chest. 2012 Jul;142(1):63–75.

[86] Trajman A, Steffen RE, Menzies D. Interferon-Gamma Release Assays versus Tuberculin Skin Testing for the Diagnosis of Latent Tuberculosis Infection: An Overview of the Evidence. Pulm Med. 2013;2013:601737.

[87] Kemp JR, Mann G, Simwaka BN, Salaniponi FM, Squire SB. Can Malawi's poor afford free tuberculosis services? Patient and household costs associated with a tuberculosis diagnosis in Lilongwe. Bull World Health Organ. 2007 Aug;85(8):580–5.

[88] Tanimura T, Jaramillo E, Weil D, Raviglione M, Lönnroth K. Financial burden for tuberculosis patients in low- and middle-income countries: a systematic review. Eur Respir J. 2014 Jun;43(6):1763–75.

[89] SSA. Programa de Accion: tuberculosis. Mexico; 2001 p. 62.

[90] Daniel TM. The impact of tuberculosis on civilization. Infect Dis Clin North Am. 2004 Mar;18(1):157–65.

[91] Consejo Nacional de Evaluación de la Política de Desarrollo Social (CONEVAL). Medición de la pobreza. Estados Unidos Mexicanos. http://www.coneval.gob.mx/Medicion/Paginas/Medici%C3%B3n/Pobreza%202012/Pobreza-2012.aspx (accessed 5 October 2014).

[92] Consejo Nacional de Evaluación de la Política de Desarrollo Social (CONEVAL). Medición de la pobreza: Chiapas http://www.coneval.gob.mx/coordinacion/entidades/Paginas/Chiapas/pobreza.aspx (accessed 5 October 2014).

[93] Harris A, Martin R. The exercise of public health powers in an era of human rights: the particular problems of tuberculosis. Public Health. 2004 Jul;118(5):313–22.

[94] Coker RJ, Mounier-Jack S, Martin R. Public health law and tuberculosis control in Europe. Public Health. 2007 Apr;121(4):266–73.

[95] Boggio A, Zignol M, Jaramillo E, Nunn P, Pinet G, Raviglione M. Limitations on human rights: are they justifiable to reduce the burden of TB in the era of MDR- and XDR-TB? Health Hum Rights. 2008;10(2):121–6.

[96] WHO. Guidance on human rights and involuntary detention for xdr-tb control. http://www.who.int/tb/features_archive/involuntary_treatment/en/ (accessed 5 October 2014).

[97] Kraemer JD, Cabrera OA, Singh JA, Depp TB, Gostin LO. Public health measures to control tuberculosis in low-income countries: ethics and human rights considerations. Int J Tuberc Lung Dis Off J Int Union Tuberc Lung Dis. 2011 Jun;15 Suppl 2:S19–24.

[98] Singh JA, Upshur R, Padayatchi N. XDR-TB in South Africa: No Time for Denial or Complacency. PLoS Med. 2007 Jan 23;4(1):e50.

[99] Hargreaves JR, Boccia D, Evans CA, Adato M, Petticrew M, Porter JDH. The social determinants of tuberculosis: from evidence to action. Am J Public Health. 2011 Apr; 101(4):654–62.

[100] Cuevas LE, Petrucci R, Swaminathan S. Tuberculosis diagnostics for children in high-burden countries: what is available and what is needed. Paediatr Int Child Health. 2012 Nov;32 Suppl 2:S30–7.

[101] Sánchez-Pérez H, Bencomo-Alerm A, Gómez-Velasco A. Migration, tuberculosis and the survival rate of children in the Highlands region of Chiapas, Mexico. (Unpublished document). El Colegio de la Frontera Sur; 2014.

[102] Stop TB Partnership. Call to Action for Chilhood TB. http://www.stoptb.org/getinvolved/ctb_cta.asp (accessed 6 October 2014).

[103] Zevallos M, Justman JE. Tuberculosis in the elderly. Clin Geriatr Med. 2003 Feb;19(1): 121–38.

[104] Chand N, Bhushan B, Singh D, Pandhi N, Thakur S, Bhullar SS, et al. Tuberculosis in the elderly (aged 50 years and above) and their treatment outcome under dots. Chest. 2007 Oct 1;132(4_MeetingAbstracts):640b – 640.

[105] Gutiérrez J, Rivera-Dommarco J, Shamah-Levy T, Villalpando-Hernández S, Franco A, Cuevas-Nasu L, et al. Encuesta Nacional de Salud y Nutrición 2012. Resultados nacionales. Cuernavaca, Morelos, Mexico: Instituto Nacional de Salud Pública (INSP); 2013 p. 200.

[106] Pan American Health Organization (PAHO). Diabetes and Tuberculosis. http://www.paho.org/hq/index.php?option=com_content&view=article&id=8979:diabetes-tuberculosis&Itemid=40045&lang=en (accessed 8 October 2014).

[107] Ponce-De-Leon A, Garcia-Garcia Md M de L, Garcia-Sancho MC, Gomez-Perez FJ, Valdespino-Gomez JL, Olaiz-Fernandez G, et al. Tuberculosis and diabetes in southern Mexico. Diabetes Care. 2004 Jul;27(7):1584–90.

[108] United Nations Development Programme (UNDP). Human Development Report 2014. Sustaining Human Progress: Reducing Vulnerabilities and Building Resilience. New York, USA: UNDP; 2014 p. 239.

[109] Gosoniu GD, Ganapathy S, Kemp J, Auer C, Somma D, Karim F, et al. Gender and socio-cultural determinants of delay to diagnosis of TB in Bangladesh, India and Malawi. Int J Tuberc Lung Dis Off J Int Union Tuberc Lung Dis. 2008 Jul;12(7):848–55.

[110] Mathad JS, Gupta A. Tuberculosis in pregnant and postpartum women: epidemiology, management, and research gaps. Clin Infect Dis Off Publ Infect Dis Soc Am. 2012 Dec;55(11):1532–49.

[111] Hartigan P. Communicable Diseases, Gender, and Equity in Health. USA: Harvard School of Public Health; 1999 p. 36.

[112] Romero Hernández C. Diferencias de género en las redes de apoyo social entre los pacientes con tuberculosis pulmonar: estudio cualitativo en dos poblados del estado de Veracruz, México. Rev Inst Nac Enfermedades Respir. 2004 Jun;17(2):80–90.

[113] Mendoza EM, Martelo EZ, García VV, Nazar AB, Pérez HJS. Tuberculosis en la Sierra Santa Marta, Veracruz: un análisis desde la perspectiva de género. Papeles de Población. 2001; 31 (1-2): 105-124.

[114] Hudelson P. Gender differentials in tuberculosis: the role of socio-economic and cultural factors. Tuber Lung Dis Off J Int Union Tuberc Lung Dis. 1996 Oct;77(5):391–400.

[115] Comisión Nacional para el Desarrollo de los Pueblos Indígenas (CDI). Los números: Indicadores Socioeconómicos. http://www.cdi.gob.mx/index.php?option=com_content&task=view&id=217 (accessed 9 October 2014).

[116] SSA. Programa Nacional de Salud 2007-2012. Secretaria de Salud; 2007 p. 188.

[117] Sánchez Pérez H, Vargas-Morales G, Jansà JM. The conditions of life and health for indigenous women in areas of high marginalization, Chiapas, México. In: Eversole R, McNeish J, Cimadamore A, editors. Indigenous peoples and poverty: an international perspective. London, United Kingdom: Comparative Research Programme on Poverty (CROP), International Studies in Poverty Research; 2005. p. 32–52.

[118] Bindman AB, Grumbach K, Osmond D, Komaromy M, Vranizan K, Lurie N, et al. Preventable hospitalizations and access to health care. JAMA. 1995 Jul 26;274(4):305–11.

[119] Ochoa-Díaz López H, Sánchez-Pérez HJ, Martínez-Guzmán LA. Use of an index of social welfare for health planning at a municipal level. Salud Pública México. 1996 Aug;38(4):257–67.

[120] Migration Health Division, International Organization for Migration. Migration and Tuberculosis: A Pressing Issue. Geneva, Switzerland: International Organization for Migration (IOM); 2014 p. 4.

[121] Freyermuth G. El señuelo del norte. Migración indígena contemporánea. CIESAS; 2007.

[122] Lozano A. Tendencias recientes de las remesas de los migrantes mexicanos en Estados Unidos,. The Center for Comparative Innmigration Studies, University of California, San Diego, United States.; 2004.

[123] Jáuregui-Díaz J, Ávila-Sánchez M. Estados Unidos, lugar de destino para los migrantes chiapanecos. Migr Inter. 2007;4(1).

[124] Escobar A. Pobreza y migración internacional en el México rural: un enfoque antropológico. Pobreza y migración internacional. San Cristóbal de las Casas, Chiapas, México: CIESAS, Publicaciones de la Casa Chata; 2008. p. 39–84.

[125] Soto D. Amnistía Internacional, Sección México (personal communication), San Cristóbal de Las Casas, Chiapas: 14 de diciembre de 2010. 2010.

[126] Flores G. The impact of medical interpreter services on the quality of health care: a systematic review. Med Care Res Rev. 2005;62(3):255–99.

[127] Organization for Economic Co-operation and Development (OECD). Health Expenditure Trends: Mexico. http://www.oecd.org/centrodemexico/estadisticas/ (accessed 7 October 2014).

[128] Leal G. Seguro "universal": justificación "social" para generalizar el IVA. La Jornada. Mexico, D.F.; 2013; http://www.jornada.unam.mx/2013/08/03/opinion/018a2pol (accessed 9 October 2014).

[129] WHO. What is multidrug-resistant tuberculosis and how do we control it?. http://www.who.int/features/qa/79/en/ (accessed 7 October 2014).

[130] ATS. Diagnostic Standards and Classification of Tuberculosis in Adults and Children. This official statement of the American Thoracic Society and the Centers for Disease Control and Prevention was adopted by the ATS Board of Directors, July 1999. This statement was endorsed by the Council of the Infectious Disease Society of America, September 1999. Am J Respir Crit Care Med. 2000 Apr;161(4 Pt 1):1376–95.

[131] Velayati AA, Farnia P, Masjedi MR, Ibrahim TA, Tabarsi P, Haroun RZ, et al. Totally drug-resistant tuberculosis strains: evidence of adaptation at the cellular level. Eur Respir J Off J Eur Soc Clin Respir Physiol. 2009 Nov;34(5):1202–3.

[132] WHO. Global Task Force outlines measures to combat XDR-TB worldwide. http://www.who.int/mediacentre/news/notes/2006/np29/en/ (accessed 7 October 2014).

4

Vaccines – Recent Advances and Clinical Trials

Marisol Ocampo C.

1. Introduction

Short description of the chapter: The chapter gives an overall view of attempts at preventing tuberculosis; this disease has a high impact on public health worldwide. Aspects concerning the development of anti-tuberculosis vaccines being tested by different research groups around the world are analysed in this chapter. The current vaccine is described, as is the search for new antigens, the use of adjuvants, the approaches adopted to date for designing new vaccines, and current trials in their different phases of research. An analysis is made of the results obtained to date and comments are made about the future regarding the development of an effective anti-tuberculosis vaccine.

Tuberculosis is considered the second worldwide cause of mortality after AIDS; it is caused by an infectious agent (*Mycobacterium tuberculosis*) and 8.6 million people were reported as having acquired tuberculosis in 2012 and 1.3 million people died from tuberculosis in the same year [1].

Even though tuberculosis is curable and can be prevented, it has been calculated that a third of the world's population has latent tuberculosis (i.e., they are infected by *Mycobacterium tuberculosis* (*Mtb*) but have not yet become ill nor can they transmit the infection). *Mtb* usually affects the lungs (pulmonary tuberculosis) but can affect other sites (extra-pulmonary tuberculosis). People infected with the tubercle bacilli have around a 10% risk of developing the disease throughout their lifetimes, and this risk becomes much greater for smokers or people who have a deficient immune system, as happens with cases of infection caused by the human immunodeficiency virus (HIV), malnutrition or diabetes.

The best way to avoid the disease is to find a totally efficient vaccine which can prevent mycobacteria entering the target cell for infection, vaccines which can protect individuals from initial infection, those which can prevent progression to active tuberculosis in recently infected individuals, or else those which can reduce the ability of those having active disease to transmit it to others.

Tuberculosis is currently controlled by using antibiotics; however, the socioeconomic panorama of endemic areas, the extensive period of time represented by treating it, together with intense secondary effects produced by anti-tuberculosis drugs, as well as the appearance of cases of multi-resistant tuberculosis, make this a limited solution regarding the enormous problem which this disease represents.

The publication of the H37Rv strain genome in 1998 [2], more than 100 years after Robert Koch discovered the existence of *Mtb* (in 1882), provided information with great potential for identifying its gene repertory, some of which is key when ascertaining mycobacterial virulence, pathogenesis, survival and latency. Such an advance has led to thinking about designing new drugs against this disease, overcoming resistance to drugs and, above all, obtaining an effective vaccine. However, despite around 4,000 of the genes forming this microorganism already being known and the pertinent data being already available in enormous databases, functional information regarding the proteins encoding them is still very limited.

The *Mycobacterium bovis* Bacillus Chalmette–Guerin (BCG) vaccine has been used for almost 100 years for preventing tuberculosis. This vaccine may offer protection against serious forms of tuberculosis in children (tuberculous meningitis and miliary tuberculosis) [3], but it continues to be controversial regarding the variability of protection results (0% to 80%), being especially effective in preventing infant tuberculous meningitis but not pulmonary tuberculosis in adults [4]. BCG use is not recommended in HIV patients due to the risk of infection being disseminated by the *Mycobacterium bovis* strain used in this vaccine. Even though around 12 anti-tuberculosis vaccine candidates are currently in clinical trials, the following should be born in mind as obstacles preventing the development of efficient anti-tuberculosis vaccines. There is a poor correlation among protection in animal models which could be applied to studies in humans, there is the impossibility of validating an animal model since an efficient vaccine for preventing pulmonary tuberculosis has still not been found, and there is the cost and sample size regarding clinical trials due to a low regional incidence despite the disease's high prevalence. Many aspects concerning a natural immune response in humans following infection remain unknown and it is not clear which model would be suitable in choosing the best antigens for an anti-tuberculosis vaccine [5]. However, it is becoming clearer that there are substantial differences in humans' immunological responses to tuberculosis (as well as concerning other inflammatory diseases) which cannot be found in or predicted by studies in animals [6].

The complicated natural history of tuberculosis suggests that at least three vaccination strategies are possible. One would prevent primary infection and disease followed by exposure to the mycobacteria, another would prevent reactivation in cases of already infected individuals, while a third would advocate immunotherapeutic treatment complemented by normal procedures against tuberculosis directed at patients who are already ill from this disease [7, 8].

Research into prophylactic methods against tuberculosis has been based on antigens which are recognized by tuberculosis patients and which produce a cellular immune response;

however, more recent results have led to the conclusion that *Mtb* is a very complex pathogen, and it seems that the T-cell response is not strong enough for controlling the disease in humans. As part of the search for antigens with prophylactic or diagnostic potential, *in vitro* culturing of *Mtb* has led to a set of culture filtrate proteins (CFPs) being recognized whose main characteristic is their immunodominance. Some antigens have been implicated in a protective immune response or in T-cell activation in infected humans and animal models, which is why they have been considered good vaccine candidates. Such antigens have been identified by biochemical approaches and have been characterized by being abundant proteins, secreted by a culture medium [9, 10]. Despite efforts having been made in the field of research into antigens with immunoprophylactic potential, only a few have passed experimentation Phase II; it has been reported recently that one of the vaccines being developed, which has been in the most advanced clinical studies (MVA85A), has not provided greater protection than that currently offered by BCG [11]. Some antigens with immunogenic potential have been identified by using synthetic peptides; their versatility has been shown in developing alternatives against tuberculosis [9, 12-14].

Another has involved bioinformatics as a recent discipline integrating the large amount of biological information which has been obtained regarding different microorganisms and which can be found in large-scale databases, along with their biological significance. This approach has been used for rationally selecting sequences from the best immunomodulator candidates from among the thousands of genes which microorganisms have. Bioinformatics can thus contribute towards limiting the amount of candidates to be tested [15, 16].

Tuberculosis (TB), a disease caused by *Mycobacterium tuberculosis* (*Mtb*) infection, remains a major public health problem. The *Mycobacterium bovis* strain-derived Bacillus Chalmette–Guerin (BCG) vaccine is the only one currently available against this disease; it effectively protects against TB disseminated in younger children, but it has not managed to reduce infection prevalence and it has only shown variable protection against pulmonary TB, which constitutes the global disease burden [3]. Several facts highlight the urgent need for an efficient vaccine against this disease:

- A lack of knowledge regarding the mechanisms by which the BCG vaccine has not provided sufficient protection against *Mtb*;
- *Mtb* is responsible for almost two million deaths annually and remains in a latent stage in a third of the world's population;
- TB is one of the diseases with the greatest potential for evolutionary adaptation; and
- The slow decline in TB incidence globally and the emergence of multidrug-resistant forms of TB is devastating for patients (especially HIV-positive individuals) and healthcare providers.

WHO data reports that efforts at developing new diagnostic tests, new vaccines and drugs against TB have increased considerably during the last decade [1]. Twelve anti-TB preventative vaccine candidates were reported as being in trial Phases I, II or IIb, and two more immuno-therapeutic vaccines in Phases II or III by 2013.

The Phase IIb results for vaccine candidate MVA85A published in February 2013, which was tested in children and administered as a BCG backup, were seen to provide no additional protection when comparing the results with those obtained when just applying the BCG vaccine [11]. However, this study showed that the vaccine had an acceptable safety profile in the study population, and that a high quality trial could be carried out in a high TB load setting after solid results were found.

Even though the nature of protective immunity which must be produced against TB has not been completely understood to date, and despite that biomarkers of protection have not been clearly established, it has been suggested that *Mtb* antigens included in a possible vaccine must induce a strong Th1 cell immune response. It has usually been held that antigens which are immunogenic are recognized by TB patients or else are those which are expressed during *Mtb* infection; however, more recent results have led to concluding that *Mtb* is a very complex pathogen, and it seems that the T-cell response is not strong enough for controlling the disease in humans. As part of the search for antigens with prophylactic or diagnostic potential, the *in vitro* culturing of *Mtb* has led to a set of culture filtrate proteins (CFPs) being recognized whose main characteristic is their immunodominance. Some antigens have been implicated in a protective immune response or in T-cell activation in infected humans and animal models, which is why they have been considered good vaccine candidates. Such antigens have been identified by biochemical approaches and have been characterized by being abundant proteins, secreted by a culture medium [9, 10]. Despite efforts having been made in the field of research into antigens with immunoprophylactic potential, only a few have passed experimentation Phase II; it has been reported recently that one of the vaccines being developed, which has been in the most advanced clinical studies (MVA85A), has not provided greater protection than that currently offered by BCG [11]. Some antigens with immunogenic potential have been identified by using synthetic peptides; their versatility has been shown for developing alternatives against TB [9, 12-14].

Another approach has involved bioinformatics as a recent discipline integrating a large amount of biological information which has been obtained regarding different microorganisms and which can be found in large-scale databases, along with their biological significance. This approach has been used for rationally selecting sequences from the best immunomodulator candidates from among the thousands of genes which microorganisms have. Bioinformatics can thus contribute towards limiting the number of candidates to be tested [15-17], and a new approach has been proposed based on a functional approach involving the pathogen–host interaction in the search for antigens to be included in designing an efficient, minimal, subunit-based anti-TB vaccine [16, 18].

It should be born in mind, here, that vaccines must perform well in a series of clinical phases, thereby establishing vaccine candidate efficacy and safety, encompassing the following phases [19]:

- *First-in-human clinical trials*: First-in-human studies are small studies in healthy adults (usually 20-80 subjects) to evaluate a vaccine candidate's safety and immunogenicity;

- *Phase I clinical trials*: Phase I clinical trials are small safety studies in different target populations. These may include a preliminary assessment of dose-range and/or age de-escalation;
- *Phase IIa clinical trials*: Phase IIa clinical trials are larger studies (usually 100-300 subjects) exploring dose-range in target populations aimed at identifying the optimum dose, the dosing schedule and/or administration route based on safety, immunogenicity and/or biological end-points. These are focused studies designed to provide evidence of biological activity in the target population;
- *Phase IIb clinical trials*: Phase IIb clinical trials are larger, well-controlled studies evaluating safety and proof-of-concept/efficacy. These trials usually include more than 1,000 subjects and are designed to demonstrate evidence of disease prevention or treatment in the target population; and
- *Phase III clinical trials*: Phase III clinical trials are pivotal registration studies to support licensure. They are designed to demonstrate statistically significant evidence of disease prevention or treatment and long-term safety in target populations as required by national regulatory authorities. These studies are conducted with the final manufactured product.

2. The existing BCG vaccine

The established vaccine referred to as 'Bacille de Calmette et Guérin' (BCG), a live-attenuated bacterial vaccine developed in 1921, efficiently protects children against disseminated disease, and this is probably the most convincing argument for its use; however, it induces highly variable protection against TB. Even though the mechanisms have not been identified to date which allow this vaccine to protect against severe forms of TB in children (TB meningitis and miliary TB), while its efficacy in preventing pulmonary TB in adults remains highly variable, it continues to be the gold standard regarding prevention against TB caused by *Mtb*, being given to more than 80% of neonates and nursing infants in countries where it forms part of their national infant immunization programme.

Continued emphasis has thus been placed on understanding the mechanisms behind the failure of BCG to provide sufficient protection against *Mtb* in the lungs, and to designing new vaccines to be used in conjunction with BCG as booster strategies for installing protective immunity at the site of infection. It seems that protective immunity with the current vaccine requires mycobacterial replication in the host, meaning that a pre-existing immune response could lead to a cross-reaction with BCG.

Trials have indicated that BCG has 60-80% protective efficacy against severe forms of TB in children, particularly meningitis [20, 21], and controversial attempts have been made to relate its efficacy against pulmonary diseases with the vaccinated population's geographical location and exposure to environmental mycobacteria [22, 23]. It has also been proposed that different BCG strains induce different levels of protection.

Greater BCG vaccine efficiency regarding protection against pulmonary, miliary and meningeal TB has been associated with the absence of prior *Mtb* infection or sensitization to environmental mycobacteria. This fact is relevant when designing new vaccines against TB since prior infection could mask or block their effects [23]. Other authors have shown the BCG vaccine's efficacy against leprosy and against TB itself [24].

Recent systematic studies have concluded that the BCG vaccine protects against *Mtb* infection as well as its progression towards active disease, determined by interferon-gamma release assays (IGRAs) in children [25]. These IGRAs were based on INF-γ release by T-cells from individuals who had been infected by *Mtb*, and led to the clear differentiation of individuals who had been previously vaccinated with BCG or who had been infected by other mycobacteria [26].

It could be concluded that the BCG vaccine has shown great variety regarding its efficiency concerning protection against TB, thereby creating great controversy and encouraging numerous efforts aimed at producing better vaccines against this disease. However, it cannot be ignored that BCG is the most used vaccine around the world – more than three thousand million doses having been administered to date – and that this fact must be taken into account when designing new vaccines which must necessarily be compared to classic BCG efficacy.

3. Different approaches

Bearing in mind the results obtained in animal models regarding protective immunity concerning TB, most vaccine candidates have been based on vectors, adjuvants and antigens, inducing classical cytokines for a Th1 profile, such as INF-γ and TNF-α, produced by CD4+ and CD8+ T-cells. The main immunization strategies used for developing vaccines against TB would include:

- Prime vaccines are those seeking to be more efficient than the current BCG and which might replace it. These would include those which have improved on the *M. bovis* BCG strain or new vaccines based on live attenuated *M. tuberculosis*. Attempts have also been made to improve the safety of the actual BCG so that it can be used with children exposed to HIV, since using the actual vaccine is not recommended. They prevent infection and are considered pre-exposure, are prophylactic and their intention is to obtain a longer-lasting and more effective immune response;
- Vaccines administered after BCG has been applied to the new born are known as boost or prime-boost vaccines for improving efficiency and extending the protection time produced with the first immunization with classical BCG. They form part of a prophylactic booster strategy for classical BCG vaccination for prolonging the immunity induced by it;
- Post-exposure vaccines include those which prevent the disease's primary progression or latent TB reactivation. They are directed towards individuals with latent tuberculosis infection (LTBI), meaning that it should be considered that any *Mtb* infection could become a clinically active disease or a latent infection (as it is believed that mycobacteria could persist in metabolic stages of slow replication until practically remaining inactive), depending upon the host's immune state. The antigens require careful selection; if the antecedents provoked

by immunization with tuberculin in the past are born in mind [27], proteins are selected in this strategy which are expressed during the infection's latent state and which are recognized by individuals with dormant *Mtb* infection. It is thought that vaccination is a more effective means than antibiotics for eliminating mycobacteria in a latent state. A consideration to be born in mind when selecting antigens is the fact that it has been described how antigens recognized by the immune systems of individuals with latent infection differ from those recognized by patients with active disease [28]; and

- Immunotherapeutic vaccines include whole-cell and fragmented mycobacteria and might become synergized with chemotherapy to shorten treatment for active TB or LTBI.

Subunit vaccines offer great advantages in all cases as they allow for the selective design of antigens which could induce an effective protective immune response. Using these vaccines is justified as only a few antigens are needed to achieve the same protection obtained with complete bacteria, and their use leads to obtaining safe, reproducible vaccines, and no problems have been foreseen regarding their application to immunocompromised individuals.

While DNA-based vaccines offer the induction of robust MHC class I-restricted cytotoxic T-lymphocyte (CTL) cells, due to their strong potential for inducing memory responses, DNA vaccines are particularly suited for priming immune responses. The co-administration of BCG with plasmid DNA encoding immunodominant, subdominant and phase-specific antigens – poorly expressed by BCG – may lead to the development of improved TB vaccines [29].

4. Vaccines currently being developed

Regarding vaccine candidates currently in experimental clinical phases (Figure 1), there are a great variety of strategies for inducing the desired protective response; these would include complete microorganisms, cell extracts and non-pathogenic mycobacteria (*M. vaccae*, RUTI, *M. smegmatis*) [30, 31], candidates included with viral vectors (MVA85A, AERAS-402 and AdAg85A) [11, 32], fusion proteins with Th1 response-inducing adjuvants (M72/AS01, Hybrid 1/CAF01, Hybrid 1/IC31 and HyVac 4) [33, 34], and BCG-based live recombinant vaccines (VPM 1002, Aeras 422, rBCG30) [35, 36] and those based on *Mtb* (MTBVAC) [37].

A broad range of vaccine candidates are already being evaluated pre-clinically, which contributes towards broadening clinical portfolio diversity and filling current scientific gaps. Consensus has been achieved among investigators regarding new TB vaccines to rationalize and streamline advancing TB vaccine candidates, with increased emphasis being placed on global coordination among key stakeholders to advance a common research agenda. A re-prioritized focus on early-stage research is also underway to supplement existing efforts. In this way, resources and research efforts must be devoted to the search for new alternatives for vaccine design, the deepening of immunological mechanisms in humans, and the development of reliable biomarkers that would predict vaccine efficacy and disease progression; using these strategies together we can find new vaccine alternatives and progress towards successful future clinical trials [5].

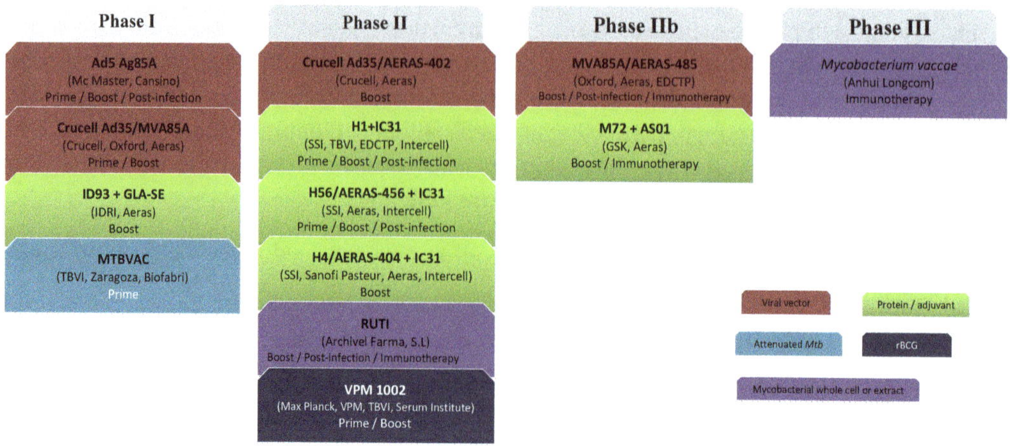

Based on Global tuberculosis Report.WHO. 2013 [1]

Figure 1. The development pipeline for new TB vaccines, 2013

4.1. Phase I clinical trials:

Ad5 Ag85A is a human adenovirus serotype 5 vector expressing Ag85A (*fbpA*, Rv3804c, secreted antigen 85-A, mycolyl transferase 85A), an immunodominant antigen produced by all mycobacterial species. It has been developed by McMaster University with support from Tianjin CanSino Biotechnology Inc. The vaccine was evaluated in a Phase I trial in 12 BCG-naive and 12 previously BCG-immunized, healthy, Canadian adults, which demonstrated no vaccine-related serious adverse events. It showed that Ad5Ag85A was immunogenic in both groups and that it stimulated polyfunctional T-cell responses, but it more potently boosted both CD4+ and CD8+ T-cell immunity in previously BCG-vaccinated volunteers compared to BCG-naive volunteers, supporting its further clinical development as a booster vaccine after BCG priming [38, 39].

ID93/GLA-SE is being developed by the Infectious Disease Research Institute (IDRI) in collaboration with Aeras. It consists of a recombinant fusion protein expressing the antigens Rv2608, Rv3619 and Rv3620 associated with virulence and the Rv1813 Mtb latency antigen; all of them are combined with a stable oil-in-water emulsion incorporating glucopyranosyl lipid adjuvant, a synthetic TLR-4 agonist (GLA-SE), together with the recombinant protein. ID93ID93/GLA-SE induced multifunctional CD4+ Th1 cell responses (IFN-γ, TNF-α, IL-2) in mice and protected both mice and guinea pigs against *Mtb* [40]. It is beginning a Phase Ib trial in adults to assess safety and immunogenicity in such a population. The purpose of this Phase I trial is to determine ID93/GLA-SE safety, tolerability and immunogenicity in BCG-vaccinated healthy adult subjects in South Africa for preventing pulmonary TB; results have yet to be published for this clinical trial.

MTBVAC is being developed by the University of Zaragosa, Institut Pasteur, BIOFABRI and the Tuberculosis Vaccine Initiative (TBVI). It is a live *Mtb* strain which has been attenuated via deletion of the *phoP* gene encoding a transcription factor, which is key to virulence regulation, and *fadD26* which is essential for the synthesis of the lipid complex involving phthiocerol dimycocerosate (DIM), one of the major mycobacterial virulence factors [37]. MTBVAC has been shown to be safe in all preclinical studies and has conferred better protection than BCG in mice. It has been the first live attenuated *Mtb* vaccine to enter a Phase I clinical trial in Lausanne; 36 healthy volunteers participated to ensure the vaccine candidate MTBVAC's safety and immunogenicity.

4.2. Phase II trials:

AERAS-402/Crucell Ad35 is an adenovirus-vectored vaccine formed by replication-deficient adenovirus serotype 35 (Ad35), which functions as a viral vector expressing a fusion protein with three *Mtb* antigens: Ag85A, Ag85B and TB10.4. The antigen 85 complex is highly conserved among different species of mycobacteria and consists of multiple secreted components, Ag85A and Ag85B being highly homologous and the most immunogenic. The TB10.4 antigen (low molecular weight protein antigen 7 ESXH, *cfp7* or Rv0288) has been shown to be an immunodominant antigen. AERAS-402/Crucell Ad35 is designed as a booster vaccine for infants, adolescents and adults. It has been shown to induce polyfunctional CD4T cells and strong CD8T-cell responses when given to adults after priming with BCG, which were fiftyfold higher than those detectable pre-boost [41]. A single AERAS-402 dose has induced CD4T cells predominantly expressing single IFN-γ, whereas two doses induced CD4T cells predominantly expressing IFN-γ, TNF-α and IL-2 together. Although begun as a Phase IIb proof-of-concept trial, preliminary data has led to it now being revised as a smaller Phase II trial, having safety and immunogenicity in healthy infants previously vaccinated with BCG at birth as its primary end-points [42]. AERAS-402/Crucell Ad35 and MVA85A are also being tested in combination to try to drive a balanced CD4+/CD8+ immune response. One or two doses of AERAS-402/Crucell Ad35 followed by a dose of MVA85A are being evaluated for safety and immunogenicity in a combined Phase I/Phase II trial in adults in the United Kingdom. Three vaccines are protein subunit adjuvanted vaccines which were initially developed by the Statens Serum Institute in Copenhagen, Denmark.

Hybrid 1 + IC31 is based on a fusion protein containing Ag85B and ESAT-6 in adjuvant IC31. IC31 (Intercell) is a new adjuvant containing two components (an immunopotentiating cationic peptide (KLKL$_5$KLK) and a single-stranded oligodeoxynucleotide ODN$_1$) and has been shown to induce potent, sustained, antigen-specific cellular immunity via the Toll-like receptor-9/ MyD88 signalling pathway [43], as well as humoral responses to a variety of peptides and antigens. ESAT-6 (in contrast to antigen 85 complex members) is a virulence factor which is restricted to mycobacteria from the *Mtb* complex. The two proteins fused in Hybrid 1 contain epitopes recognized by TB patients' T-cells with a broad range of HLA from different types; this has been determined by the high number of INF-γ-secreting T-cells specific for these antigens. The results from a clinical Phase I study have shown that the vaccine is well-tolerated, highly immunogenic in naïve individuals, and that it has induced strong Th1 responses persisting for more than two-and-a-half years after vaccination [34].

Hybrid 56 + IC31 contains a fusion protein which includes the antigens 85B and ESAT6 (as Hybrid 1) as well as antigen Rv2660c, which has been described as a hypothetical protein, originally identified on the basis of enhanced transcription in a starvation model of *Mtb* growth arrest [44]. The strong induction of Rv2660c has been associated with hypoxia-induced, non-replicating persistence and an enduring hypoxic response. However, it has been proposed, recently, that there could have been a fortuitous crossed reaction between the response of T-cells induced by recombinant protein Rv2660c and a yet-to-be-defined *Mtb* antigen, and it is expected that results will be obtained for Hybrid 56 + IC31 providing relevant information about latent infection physiology [45]. This vaccine combines antigens characteristic of early infection and latency, and seems to have protected mice against TB – as would be ideal – before and after exposure to infection [46].

Hybrid 4 + IC31 uses adjuvant IC31. However, this Sanofi Pasteur candidate includes a fusion protein candidate which expresses Ag85B and TB10.4; the latter antigen is from the same gene family as ESAT-6 and has been included in vaccine candidate AERAS-402.

RUTI is a therapeutic vaccine developed in Badalona (Catalonia, Spain) by Archivel Farma; it is formed by biotransformed *Mtb* cell fragments, delivered in liposomes. The original idea of introducing this vaccine was to boost the dominant immunological response against growing *Mtb* which already exists in a host. RUTI has already demonstrated its efficacy in controlling LTBI in experimental mice and guinea-pig models after a short period of chemotherapy; such experiments in animals have shown the induction of a mixed Th1/Th2/Th3, polyantigenic response involving no local or systemic toxicity [30].

The Phase I clinical trial showed that vaccination was reasonably well-tolerated as judged by local and systemic clinical evaluation, although dose-dependent local adverse reactions were noted; it also trigged a specific immunological response against *Mtb* in healthy subjects compared to a placebo [47]. It has also been shown that it can induce a cellular immune response measurable as IFN-γ secretion.

The results of a double-blind, randomized, placebo-controlled Phase II clinical trial for assessing the safety, tolerability and immunogenicity of three doses of RUTI vaccine administered after completion of one month of isoniazid treatment in HIV-infected and –uninfected subjects with LTBI have been reported recently [48]. The study involving 111 subjects was carried out at three South African sites (Bloemfontein, George and Port Elizabeth); the RUTI safety profile was considered acceptable. As some HIV-positive individuals were found in the group, this suggested that the RUTI vaccine did not cause any variation in the HIV viral load or CD4 count. Vaccination thus did not affect HIV infection evolution.

VPM 1002 is a recombinant Δ*ure*C *hly*+ BCG (rBCG) strain which expresses *Listeria monocytogenes* membrane-perforating listeriolysin (hly) and which is devoid of urease C. This rBCG construct induces superior protection against aerogenic challenges with MTB compared to parental BCG. Phase I clinical trials in adults in Germany and South Africa have proven safe and immunogenic for B-cell and T-cell responses [49], and a current Phase IIa trial is ongoing for assessing immunogenicity and safety in its target population (i.e., the new born in a high TB incidence setting). A second Phase II trial will assess the vaccine's safety and immunogenicity in HIV-exposed and -unexposed new-borns.

4.3. Phase IIb studies:

M72/AS01E is a protein subunit vaccine, formulated in a novel adjuvant system which induces type I to enhance cell-mediated immunogenicity. It contains a fusion protein containing *Mtb* antigens Mtb32A (*pepA*, probable serine protease pepA, Rv0125) and Mtb39A (Rv1196, a PPE family protein) in adjuvant system AS01E, which is a liposome formulation with monophosphoryl lipid A (MPL) and QS21 immunostimulants. The M72 antigen expressed in BCG and *Mtb* mycobacteria contains human CD4+ and CD8+ T-cell epitopes and induces proliferation and INF-γ production by T-cells from PBMC in TB-infected individuals. Although no immune-correlate regarding protection has been identified, T-cells expressing Th1 cytokines (INF-γ and TNFα) are associated with protection. Safety and immunogenicity were tested in different populations: as a booster to BCG in Gambian infants [50], in HIV-infected adults on combination antiretroviral therapy in Switzerland [51] and healthy PPD-positive adults in the Philippines [52]. The Phase IIb study will be the largest trial of a novel TB vaccine in adults, aiming to enrol 4,500 HIV-negative adults in TB-endemic countries in Africa. The primary end-point will be the protective efficacy of two doses of M72/AS01E against pulmonary TB. Secondary end-points will include safety and immunogenicity.

MVA85A is the first virally vectored TB vaccine to be tested in humans. It is a recombinant, attenuated vaccinia-vectored vaccine candidate expressing *Mtb* Ag85A. It was designed as a booster vaccine for BCG-vaccinated infants and this vaccine's first Phase IIb trial was conducted in South Africa from 2009 to 2012, results being published in early 2013 [11]. An additional MVA85A Phase IIb trial was conducted in adults infected with HIV-1, at two clinical sites, in Cape Town, South Africa and Dakar, Senegal; the trial concluded that MVA85A was well-tolerated and immunogenic in adults infected with HIV-1. However, it was detected as offering no efficacy against *Mtb* infection or disease [53].

Although the MVA85A vaccine has produced some protection in murine models of TB, the recent trial in BCG-vaccinated children in South Africa revealed that, although it could generate a high level of multifunctional CD4+ T cell response in the host and produce IFN-γ, failed to prevent either TB infection or disease in vaccinated subjects.

4.4. Phase III studies:

Vaccae consists of a heat-inactivated *Mycobacterium vaccae* preparation, developed by Anhui Zhifei Longcom Biopharmaceutical. It has been approved for TB adjuvant therapy and is the only drug recommended for TB immunotherapy by the WHO [54]. Killed *M. vaccae* is safe and does not present any adverse side-effects, except for local reaction at the injection site. Injectable *M. vaccae* (Vaccae) was approved in 2001 for sale in China as adjunct immunotherapy for TB drugs; nevertheless, *M. vaccae* appeared to produce a measurable improvement in some geographical regions but not in others; such inconsistency has led some researchers to doubt its efficacy [55]. The cell wall seems to be responsible for *M. vaccae* immunostimulating effects, which have been greater than those produced by inactivated complete mycobacteria, and this would partly explain the variability of results obtained in different studies.

The purpose of the Phase III study is to add new indications for Vaccae, mainly to prevent TB for high-risk groups of infection; it has passed this phase, including testing in MDR-TB and HIV co-infected individuals.

5. Conclusion

Even though significant achievements have been made in research into different aspects related to the prevention, diagnosis and treatment of TB, and the group of researchers dedicating their time to the topic has grown worldwide, it has been recognized that a more effective vaccine is needed for reducing the high levels of mortality caused by this disease.

Several development stages and clinical trials are involved in developing new vaccines and, while new vaccine candidates emerge, it is essential that work continues on discovering new approaches. It is considered that immunization is one of the most profitable interventions regarding health, despite this leading to significant investment in terms of time and money. Candidates selected during the design phase must pass the preclinical phase to advance to clinical Phase I, clinical Phases IIa and IIb and clinical Phase III.

Research in this field has involved different approaches regarding the selection of the best antigens, adjuvant use, antigen dose, and immunization strategy. For the development of TB vaccines, two strategies have been mainly suggested: in the first case, the widely-used BCG vaccine is substituting by an improved vaccine, either a recombinant BCG or an attenuated *Mtb* strain. The other strategy implies a boosting vaccine which improves the protection provided by the actual BCG vaccine. It must thus be born in mind that different groups of the population are exposed, so that emphasis is placed on vaccines to be administered to children, the new born and suitable vaccine candidates for adolescents and adults. A search is also being made for therapeutic vaccines which will lead to the potentiating treatment of drug-resistant TB. All vaccines must be safe for people affected by HIV and those suffering latent TB infection.

Trying to find effective vaccines against TB continues to be a significant challenge as a greater understanding of a protective immune response is still required and there remain gaps regarding the mechanisms regulating *Mtb* immunopathology in human hosts [56]. An additional complication concerns the fact that TB may be the only pathogen manipulating the host's immune response in promoting its transmission. Some aspects needing to be clarified are related to protective immunity in humans, making surrogate end-points inadequate for evaluating TB vaccine efficacy. To date, no biomarker has been validated in TB, thereby hampering selection during the early phase and the clinical evaluation of new vaccine candidates.

Even though the systematic study and selection of vaccine antigens has led to the development of promising candidate vaccines [40, 46], these vaccines' efficacy in preventing TB in the human population remains to be determined. Studies carried out so far have suggested that TB vaccine development should not be limited to the most antigenic proteins during natural infection. It is hoped that Phase I and II clinical trials data with different antigens and vaccine delivery systems will be crucial to understanding which immunological parameters are important for vaccine efficacy.

The animal models which have helped during the early phases of research into protective antigens against TB and which have provided valuable information about vaccine candidate safety, immunogenicity and efficacy have not so far led to predictive results being obtained in developing vaccines which can be used with human beings.

Despite consensus having been achieved regarding the fact that only a vaccine is the solution which will lead to eradicating TB from the world, there remain many unanswered questions in this field which must be resolved to ensure obtaining an efficient and safe vaccine against this emergent disease, which causes a large number of deaths annually. Significant advances have been made regarding basic and applied research directed towards finding definitive solutions against this disease, showing that a vaccine against TB can be obtained in the mid-term.

Acknowledgements

I would like to thank Dr Manuel A. Patarroyo and Professor Manuel E. Patarroyo for their invaluable comments and suggestions, and Jason Garry for translating and reviewing this manuscript.

Author details

Marisol Ocampo C.[1,2]

Address all correspondence to: marisol.ocampo@urosario.edu.co

1 Head of the Tuberculosis Department, Fundación Instituto de Inmunología de Colombia, FIDIC, Carrera, Bogotá, Colombia

2 School of Medicine and Health Sciences, Universidad del Rosario, Bogotá, Colombia

References

[1] WHO. Global tuberculosis report. 2013. Geneva: World Health Organization; 2013 http://apps.who.int/iris/bitstream/10665/91355/1/9789241564656_eng.pdf.

[2] Cole ST, Brosch R, Parkhill J, Garnier T, Churcher C, Harris D, et al. Deciphering the biology of Mycobacterium tuberculosis from the complete genome sequence. Nature. 1998;393:537-44 http://www.ncbi.nlm.nih.gov/entrez/query.fcgi?cmd=Retrieve&db=PubMed&dopt=Citation&list_uids=9634230.

[3] Fine PE. Variation in protection by BCG: implications of and for heterologous immunity. Lancet. 1995;346:1339-45 http://www.ncbi.nlm.nih.gov/pubmed/7475776.

[4] Dietrich J, Lundberg CV, Andersen P. TB vaccine strategies--what is needed to solve a complex problem? Tuberculosis (Edinb). 2006;86:163-8 http://www.ncbi.nlm.nih.gov/entrez/query.fcgi?cmd=Retrieve&db=PubMed&dopt=Citation&list_uids=16678489

[5] Evans TG, Brennan MJ, Barker L, Thole J. Preventive vaccines for tuberculosis. Vaccine. 2013;31 Suppl 2:B223-6 http://www.ncbi.nlm.nih.gov/pubmed/23598486.

[6] McShane H, Williams A. A review of preclinical animal models utilised for TB vaccine evaluation in the context of recent human efficacy data. Tuberculosis (Edinb). 2014;94:105-10 http://www.ncbi.nlm.nih.gov/pubmed/24369986.

[7] Aagaard C, Dietrich J, Doherty M, Andersen P. TB vaccines: current status and future perspectives. Immunology and cell biology. 2009;87:279-86 http://www.ncbi.nlm.nih.gov/entrez/query.fcgi?cmd=Retrieve&db=PubMed&dopt=Citation&list_uids=19350048

[8] Skeiky YA, Sadoff JC. Advances in tuberculosis vaccine strategies. Nat Rev Microbiol. 2006;4:469-76 http://www.ncbi.nlm.nih.gov/entrez/query.fcgi?cmd=Retrieve&db=PubMed&dopt=Citation&list_uids=16710326.

[9] Nagai S, Wiker HG, Harboe M, Kinomoto M. Isolation and partial characterization of major protein antigens in the culture fluid of Mycobacterium tuberculosis. Infect Immun. 1991;59:372-82 http://www.ncbi.nlm.nih.gov/entrez/query.fcgi?cmd=Retrieve&db=PubMed&dopt=Citation&list_uids=1898899.

[10] Andersen AB, Hansen EB. Structure and mapping of antigenic domains of protein antigen b, a 38,000-molecular-weight protein of *Mycobacterium tuberculosis*. Infect Immun. 1989;57:2481-8 http://www.ncbi.nlm.nih.gov/entrez/query.fcgi?cmd=Retrieve&db=PubMed&dopt=Citation&list_uids=2545626

[11] Tameris MD, Hatherill M, Landry BS, Scriba TJ, Snowden MA, Lockhart S, et al. Safety and efficacy of MVA85A, a new tuberculosis vaccine, in infants previously vaccinated with BCG: a randomised, placebo-controlled phase 2b trial. Lancet. 2013;381:1021-8 http://www.ncbi.nlm.nih.gov/pubmed/23391465.

[12] Launois P, DeLeys R, Niang MN, Drowart A, Andrien M, Dierckx P, et al. T-cell-epitope mapping of the major secreted mycobacterial antigen Ag85A in tuberculosis and leprosy. Infect Immun. 1994;62:3679-87 http://www.ncbi.nlm.nih.gov/entrez/query.fcgi?cmd=Retrieve&db=PubMed&dopt=Citation&list_uids=7520418

[13] Mustafa AS, Al-Attiyah R, Hanif SN, Shaban FA. Efficient testing of large pools of Mycobacterium tuberculosis RD1 peptides and identification of major antigens and immunodominant peptides recognized by human Th1 cells. Clin Vaccine Immunol. 2008;15:916-24 http://www.ncbi.nlm.nih.gov/entrez/query.fcgi?cmd=Retrieve&db=PubMed&dopt=Citation&list_uids=18400977

[14] Seghrouchni F, Contini S, Markova R, Drenska R, Sadki K, Baassi L, et al. Design of immunogenic peptides from Mycobacterium tuberculosis genes expressed during

macrophage infection. Tuberculosis (Edinb). 2009;89:210-7 http://www.ncbi.nlm.nih.gov/entrez/query.fcgi?cmd=Retrieve&db=PubMed&dopt=Citation&list_uids=19447677

[15] Vivona S, Gardy JL, Ramachandran S, Brinkman FS, Raghava GP, Flower DR, et al. Computer-aided biotechnology: from immuno-informatics to reverse vaccinology. Trends in biotechnology. 2008;26:190-200 http://www.ncbi.nlm.nih.gov/entrez/query.fcgi?cmd=Retrieve&db=PubMed&dopt=Citation&list_uids=18291542

[16] Ocampo M, Patarroyo MA, Vanegas M, Alba MP, Patarroyo ME. Functional, biochemical and 3D studies of Mycobacterium tuberculosis protein peptides for an effective anti-tuberculosis vaccine. Critical reviews in microbiology. 2014;40:117-45 http://www.ncbi.nlm.nih.gov/pubmed/23445450.

[17] Vizcaino C, Restrepo-Montoya D, Rodriguez D, Nino LF, Ocampo M, Vanegas M, et al. Computational prediction and experimental assessment of secreted/surface proteins from Mycobacterium tuberculosis H37Rv. PLoS computational biology. 2010;6:e1000824 http://www.ncbi.nlm.nih.gov/pubmed/20585611.

[18] Patarroyo ME, Bermudez A, Patarroyo MA. Structural and immunological principles leading to chemically synthesized, multiantigenic, multistage, minimal subunit-based vaccine development. Chem Rev. 2011;111:3459-507 http://www.ncbi.nlm.nih.gov/pubmed/21438608.

[19] AERAS. www.aeras.org. 2014

[20] Rodrigues LC, Mangtani P, Abubakar I. How does the level of BCG vaccine protection against tuberculosis fall over time? BMJ. 2011;343:d5974 http://www.ncbi.nlm.nih.gov/pubmed/21964347.

[21] Trunz BB, Fine P, Dye C. Effect of BCG vaccination on childhood tuberculous meningitis and miliary tuberculosis worldwide: a meta-analysis and assessment of cost-effectiveness. Lancet. 2006;367:1173-80 http://www.ncbi.nlm.nih.gov/pubmed/16616560.

[22] Brandt L, Feino Cunha J, Weinreich Olsen A, Chilima B, Hirsch P, Appelberg R, et al. Failure of the Mycobacterium bovis BCG vaccine: some species of environmental mycobacteria block multiplication of BCG and induction of protective immunity to tuberculosis. Infect Immun. 2002;70:672-8 http://www.ncbi.nlm.nih.gov/pubmed/11796598.

[23] Mangtani P, Abubakar I, Ariti C, Beynon R, Pimpin L, Fine PE, et al. Protection by BCG vaccine against tuberculosis: a systematic review of randomized controlled trials. Clin Infect Dis. 2014;58:470-80 http://www.ncbi.nlm.nih.gov/pubmed/24336911.

[24] Setia MS, Steinmaus C, Ho CS, Rutherford GW. The role of BCG in prevention of leprosy: a meta-analysis. Lancet Infect Dis. 2006;6:162-70 http://www.ncbi.nlm.nih.gov/pubmed/16500597.

[25] Roy A, Eisenhut M, Harris RJ, Rodrigues LC, Sridhar S, Habermann S, et al. Effect of BCG vaccination against Mycobacterium tuberculosis infection in children: systematic review and meta-analysis. BMJ. 2014;349:g4643 http://www.ncbi.nlm.nih.gov/pubmed/25097193.

[26] Lalvani A, Millington KA. T cell-based diagnosis of childhood tuberculosis infection. Current opinion in infectious diseases. 2007;20:264-71 http://www.ncbi.nlm.nih.gov/pubmed/17471036.

[27] Koch R. Fortsetzung der mitteilungen über ein heilmittel gegen tuberkulose. Deutsche Medizinische Wochenschrift. 1891;17:101 - 2

[28] Demissie A, Leyten EM, Abebe M, Wassie L, Aseffa A, Abate G, et al. Recognition of stage-specific mycobacterial antigens differentiates between acute and latent infections with Mycobacterium tuberculosis. Clin Vaccine Immunol. 2006;13:179-86 http://www.ncbi.nlm.nih.gov/pubmed/16467323.

[29] Bruffaerts N, Huygen K, Romano M. DNA vaccines against tuberculosis. Expert opinion on biological therapy. 2014;14:1801-13

[30] Cardona PJ. RUTI: a new chance to shorten the treatment of latent tuberculosis infection. Tuberculosis (Edinb). 2006;86:273-89 http://www.ncbi.nlm.nih.gov/pubmed/16545981.

[31] Efremenko YV, Butov DA, Prihoda ND, Zaitzeva SI, Yurchenko LV, Sokolenko NI, et al. Randomized, placebo-controlled phase II trial of heat-killed Mycobacterium vaccae (Longcom batch) formulated as an oral pill (V7). Human vaccines & immunotherapeutics. 2013;9:1852-6 http://www.ncbi.nlm.nih.gov/pubmed/23782489.

[32] Xing Z, McFarland CT, Sallenave JM, Izzo A, Wang J, McMurray DN. Intranasal mucosal boosting with an adenovirus-vectored vaccine markedly enhances the protection of BCG-primed guinea pigs against pulmonary tuberculosis. PLoS One. 2009;4:e5856 http://www.ncbi.nlm.nih.gov/pubmed/19516906.

[33] Leroux-Roels I, Leroux-Roels G, Ofori-Anyinam O, Moris P, De Kock E, Clement F, et al. Evaluation of the safety and immunogenicity of two antigen concentrations of the Mtb72F/AS02(A) candidate tuberculosis vaccine in purified protein derivative-negative adults. Clin Vaccine Immunol. 2010;17:1763-71 http://www.ncbi.nlm.nih.gov/pubmed/20861328.

[34] van Dissel JT, Arend SM, Prins C, Bang P, Tingskov PN, Lingnau K, et al. Ag85B-ESAT-6 adjuvanted with IC31 promotes strong and long-lived Mycobacterium tuberculosis specific T cell responses in naive human volunteers. Vaccine. 2010;28:3571-81 http://www.ncbi.nlm.nih.gov/pubmed/20226890.

[35] Grode L, Seiler P, Baumann S, Hess J, Brinkmann V, Nasser Eddine A, et al. Increased vaccine efficacy against tuberculosis of recombinant Mycobacterium bovis

bacille Calmette-Guerin mutants that secrete listeriolysin. J Clin Invest. 2005;115:2472-9 http://www.ncbi.nlm.nih.gov/pubmed/16110326.

[36] Sun R, Skeiky YA, Izzo A, Dheenadhayalan V, Imam Z, Penn E, et al. Novel recombinant BCG expressing perfringolysin O and the over-expression of key immunodominant antigens; pre-clinical characterization, safety and protection against challenge with Mycobacterium tuberculosis. Vaccine. 2009;27:4412-23 http://www.ncbi.nlm.nih.gov/pubmed/19500523.

[37] Arbues A, Aguilo JI, Gonzalo-Asensio J, Marinova D, Uranga S, Puentes E, et al. Construction, characterization and preclinical evaluation of MTBVAC, the first live-attenuated M. tuberculosis-based vaccine to enter clinical trials. Vaccine. 2013;31:4867-73 http://www.ncbi.nlm.nih.gov/pubmed/23965219.

[38] Smaill F, Xing Z. Human type 5 adenovirus-based tuberculosis vaccine: is the respiratory route of delivery the future? Expert Rev Vaccines. 2014;13:927-30 http://www.ncbi.nlm.nih.gov/pubmed/24935214.

[39] Smaill F, Jeyanathan M, Smieja M, Medina MF, Thanthrige-Don N, Zganiacz A, et al. A human type 5 adenovirus-based tuberculosis vaccine induces robust T cell responses in humans despite preexisting anti-adenovirus immunity. Science translational medicine. 2013;5:205ra134 http://www.ncbi.nlm.nih.gov/pubmed/24089406.

[40] Bertholet S, Ireton GC, Ordway DJ, Windish HP, Pine SO, Kahn M, et al. A defined tuberculosis vaccine candidate boosts BCG and protects against multidrug-resistant Mycobacterium tuberculosis. Science translational medicine. 2010;2:53ra74 http://www.ncbi.nlm.nih.gov/pubmed/20944089.

[41] Hoft DF, Blazevic A, Stanley J, Landry B, Sizemore D, Kpamegan E, et al. A recombinant adenovirus expressing immunodominant TB antigens can significantly enhance BCG-induced human immunity. Vaccine. 2012;30:2098-108 http://www.ncbi.nlm.nih.gov/pubmed/22296955.

[42] Kagina BM, Tameris MD, Geldenhuys H, Hatherill M, Abel B, Hussey GD, et al. The novel tuberculosis vaccine, AERAS-402, is safe in healthy infants previously vaccinated with BCG, and induces dose-dependent CD4 and CD8T cell responses. Vaccine. 2014;32:5908-17 http://www.ncbi.nlm.nih.gov/pubmed/25218194.

[43] Schellack C, Prinz K, Egyed A, Fritz JH, Wittmann B, Ginzler M, et al. IC31, a novel adjuvant signaling via TLR9, induces potent cellular and humoral immune responses. Vaccine. 2006;24:5461-72 http://www.ncbi.nlm.nih.gov/pubmed/16678312.

[44] Betts JC, Lukey PT, Robb LC, McAdam RA, Duncan K. Evaluation of a nutrient starvation model of Mycobacterium tuberculosis persistence by gene and protein expression profiling. Mol Microbiol. 2002;43:717-31 http://www.ncbi.nlm.nih.gov/pubmed/11929527.

[45] Houghton J, Cortes T, Schubert O, Rose G, Rodgers A, De Ste Croix M, et al. A small RNA encoded in the Rv2660c locus of Mycobacterium tuberculosis is induced during

starvation and infection. PLoS One. 2013;8:e80047 http://www.ncbi.nlm.nih.gov/pubmed/24348997.

[46] Aagaard C, Hoang T, Dietrich J, Cardona PJ, Izzo A, Dolganov G, et al. A multistage tuberculosis vaccine that confers efficient protection before and after exposure. Nat Med. 2011;17:189-94 http://www.ncbi.nlm.nih.gov/pubmed/21258338.

[47] Vilaplana C, Montane E, Pinto S, Barriocanal AM, Domenech G, Torres F, et al. Double-blind, randomized, placebo-controlled Phase I Clinical Trial of the therapeutical antituberculous vaccine RUTI. Vaccine. 2010;28:1106-16 http://www.ncbi.nlm.nih.gov/pubmed/19853680.

[48] Nell AS, D'Lom E, Bouic P, Sabate M, Bosser R, Picas J, et al. Safety, tolerability, and immunogenicity of the novel antituberculous vaccine RUTI: randomized, placebo-controlled phase II clinical trial in patients with latent tuberculosis infection. PLoS One. 2014;9:e89612 http://www.ncbi.nlm.nih.gov/pubmed/24586912.

[49] Grode L, Ganoza CA, Brohm C, Weiner J, 3rd, Eisele B, Kaufmann SH. Safety and immunogenicity of the recombinant BCG vaccine VPM1002 in a phase 1 open-label randomized clinical trial. Vaccine. 2013;31:1340-8 http://www.ncbi.nlm.nih.gov/pubmed/23290835.

[50] Idoko OT, Owolabi OA, Owiafe PK, Moris P, Odutola A, Bollaerts A, et al. Safety and immunogenicity of the M72/AS01 candidate tuberculosis vaccine when given as a booster to BCG in Gambian infants: An open-label randomized controlled trial. Tuberculosis (Edinb). 2014 http://www.ncbi.nlm.nih.gov/pubmed/25305000.

[51] Thacher EG, Cavassini M, Audran R, Thierry AC, Bollaerts A, Cohen J, et al. Safety and immunogenicity of the M72/AS01 candidate tuberculosis vaccine in HIV-infected adults on combination antiretroviral therapy: a phase I/II, randomized trial. AIDS. 2014;28:1769-81 http://www.ncbi.nlm.nih.gov/pubmed/24911353.

[52] Montoya J, Solon JA, Cunanan SR, Acosta L, Bollaerts A, Moris P, et al. A randomized, controlled dose-finding Phase II study of the M72/AS01 candidate tuberculosis vaccine in healthy PPD-positive adults. Journal of clinical immunology. 2013;33:1360-75 http://www.ncbi.nlm.nih.gov/pubmed/24142232.

[53] Ndiaye BP, Thienemann F, Ota M, Landry BS, Camara M, Dieye S, et al. Safety, immunogenicity, and efficacy of the candidate tuberculosis vaccine MVA85A in healthy adults infected with HIV-1: a randomised, placebo-controlled, phase 2 trial. The Lancet Respiratory medicine. 2015;3:190-200 http://www.ncbi.nlm.nih.gov/pubmed/25726088.

[54] Stanford J, Stanford C, Grange J. Immunotherapy with Mycobacterium vaccae in the treatment of tuberculosis. Front Biosci. 2004;9:1701-19 http://www.ncbi.nlm.nih.gov/pubmed/14977580.

[55] de Bruyn G, Garner P. Mycobacterium vaccae immunotherapy for treating tuberculosis. The Cochrane database of systematic reviews. 2003:CD001166 http://www.ncbi.nlm.nih.gov/pubmed/12535403.

[56] Ernst JD. The immunological life cycle of tuberculosis. Nat Rev Immunol. 2012;12:581-91 http://www.ncbi.nlm.nih.gov/pubmed/22790178.

5

Molecular Diagnostic Testing on Post Mortem Inspection and Rulings on Bovine Tuberculosis — An Experience Report in Brazil

Ricardo César Tavares Carvalho, Leone Vinícius Furlanetto,
Rafael da Silva Duarte, Luciano Nakazato, Walter Lilenbaum,
Eduardo Eustáquio de Souza Figueiredo and
Vânia Margaret Flosi Paschoalin

1. Introduction

Bovine tuberculosis (BTB) is an infectious disease of chronic evolution and debilitating effects. The etiologic agent of this disease is *Mycobacterium bovis*, which, alongside *M. tuberculosis, M. bovis* BCG, *M. africanum, M. caprae, M. canettii* and *M. microti*, form the *Mycobacterium tuberculosis* complex (MTC) [1]. Members belonging to this complex exhibit high homology between gene sequences present in their genomes. The *M. bovis* genome AF2122/97 (4.345.492-bp) was sequenced in 2003 by Garnier [2], who detected a 99.95% genetic similarity between *M. bovis* and *M. tuberculosis*.

Cattle are the primary hosts for *M. bovis*. Several mammalian species, however, including humans, are also susceptible to this bacillus [3, 4]. This zoonosis is of global importance and shows a high prevalence in developing countries, due to lack of or ineffectiveness of tuberculosis control and eradication programs. BTB can be considered a socioeconomic disease, since it causes decreases in herd productivity, which lead to significant economic losses in the global agriculture industry, estimated at approximately 3 billion dollars a year [5, 6]. Whereas more than 94% of the world population lives in countries where BTB control is limited or absent [7], there is a consensus regarding the imminent risks to human health, especially immunossupressed or convalescent individuals, such as patients infected with the human immunodeficiency virus (HIV) or patients undergoing cancer chemotherapy treatments [8] which present greater risk of infection by BTB [9, 10].

Infection by *M. bovis* in humans is typically caused by the consumption of animal products contaminated with the bovine bacillus, usually unpasteurized milk and milk derivatives [11], leading to disease development in extrapulmonary form [12]. According to the Centers for Disease Control and Prevention (CDC, USA), 35 cases of *M. bovis* infection were reported in the city of New York from 2000 to 2004, and some of these cases were associated with the consumption of cheeses made with unpasteurized milk, imported from countries where BTB is endemic [13]. Another form of *M. bovis* infection in humans is through airborne transmission [14, 15]. Infections caused in this manner are clinically and pathologically indistinguishable from tuberculosis caused *by M. tuberculosis* [5, 12]. It is suspected that infections caused by *M. bovis* are responsible for more than 4000 cases among the 100,000 cases of human tuberculosis described annually in Brazil [10, 16]. However, according to the World Organisation for Animal Health (OIE), the number of human TB cases caused by *M. bovis* in Brazil cannot be estimated [17], since bacteriological culture tests and biochemical identification tests to diagnose whether the infection is caused by *M. bovis* or *M. tuberculosis* are not performed in most tuberculosis cases [18]. The absence of a specific diagnosis to identify the etiological agent of tuberculosis in humans is very detrimental, as patients infected with *M. bovis* require special treatment since the antibiotic pyrazinamide, used as the standard treatment for human tuberculosis, is not effective in infections caused by *M. bovis*. This results in incorrect treatment and subjects resistant to *M. bovis*, that in turn become potential transmitters of resistant strains to other people and animals [19].

Concerning *M. bovis* transmission to cattle, approximately 80-90% of the animals are infected by airborne transmission through inhalation of bacillus-contaminated aerosols [20, 21]. It is important to note that cattle with chronic or recent infections may excrete viable bacilli, thus causing infections in other animals [22]. In calves, airborne transmission of *M. bovis* is also regarded as the most important transmission route [20], although healthy calves can also become infected by ingestion of bacillus-contaminated milk [20, 23]. In countries where no effective measures to control and eradicate the disease exist, the morbidity rates in BTB-infected cattle range at about 8-10%, and fatality rates can reach up to 50% [23, 24]. It should be emphasized that BTB is a disease that mainly affects stabled cattle (dairy cattle), spreading rapidly due to the proximity of the animals to each other. In beef cattle, the opposite occurs, due to the fact that the animals are raised extensively [23, 25].

An important feature of mycobacterial infections is the cell-mediated immune response developed by the infected host, due to the intracellular location of mycobacteria. This leads to the development of granulomatous inflammations in the host, resulting in tuberous lesions [26, 27]. These lesions often occur in organs rich in reticuloendothelial tissue, especially in the head, neck, mediastinal and mesenteric lymph nodes, but also in the lungs, intestines, liver, spleen, pleura and peritoneum [28, 29]. Although tuberous lesions are not considered pathognomonic for BTB in cattle, their presence is closely linked to the appearance of clinical signs of BTB in animals [4, 5].

In developed countries, where TB control programs have been established longer and executed with rigor, BTB control is accomplished through mandatory procedures such as pasteurization of cow milk and its derivatives and sanitary inspection of cattle during slaughter, thereby drastically reducing cases of the disease in humans and animals [30]. Although a tuberculosis control and eradication plan exists in Brazil, illegal sales of meat, milk and dairy products not inspected by sanitary control agents still occur and constitute a risk to public health [19].

The detection of the pathogen responsible for BTB is crucial for the control and eradication of the disease and should be performed as recommended by the OIE [31], by late hypersensitivity reactions in cattle (intradermal tuberculin tests), sanitary inspection in slaughterhouses, tracing the origin of diseased animals and disease sanitation [31].

With the aim of reducing the prevalence and incidence of new BTB outbreaks, the Brazilian national program for control and eradication of brucellosis and tuberculosis (PNCEBT) was instituted in 2001. This program is based on the performance of intradermal tuberculin tests and the slaughter of reactive animals (test and slaughter), associated with the health inspections carried out in slaughterhouses [15]. Although the intradermal tuberculin test is widely used worldwide for BTB diagnosis, this test presents sensitivity and specificity problems, generating false-positive or false-negative results. These flaws are important, since the reference microbiological methods for BTB diagnosis also exhibit low sensitivity and are effective for pathogen detection only when the number of viable bacilli is higher than 100 bacilli/mL. In addition, microbiological testing procedures are laborious and time consuming, taking from 1 to 3 months for bacilli isolation and a further two or three weeks for the biochemical identification of the isolates [32].

Despite the occurrence of BTB, there is no official data on the current prevalence of the disease in Brazil. Data from official reports from 1989-1998 indicate that the national average prevalence was of 1.3% of infected cattle [15]. Since the beginning of the PNCEBT program, however, few studies have been conducted to determine the prevalence of the disease, and estimates vary from 0.7% to 3.3% [33, 34-35, 36]. According to the data obtained by Roxo and Kantor [37, 38], the estimated national prevalence was of 0.83% and the region with the lowest prevalence of BTB was the Brazilian Midwest (0.37 %), where beef cattle in its majority is raised. In studies conducted by Salazar and Furlanetto [6, 39], in slaughterhouses in the state of Mato Grosso, located in the Midwest region of the country, a very low BTB prevalence was detected, of only 0.007%.

One of the main economic activities in the state of Mato Grosso is cattle production. This state is prominently the largest producer of beef cattle, with around 28 million cattle heads, and the second largest beef exporter the country [40], increasing beef exports to EU countries each year. However, countries that buy Brazilian beef are increasing pressure to implant effective, quick and definitive BTB diagnosis methods to identify tuberculosis-suspected lesions. In 2012, the Ministry of Agriculture, Livestock and Supply (MAPA), determined that farms in which suspected cases of BTB had been detected could no longer export beef to the Customs Union of Belarus, Kazakhstan and Russia, and that all lots of animals of the property must be sequestered during slaughter, until confirmation of the diagnosis of the BTB-suspected lesions by official MAPA laboratories [41, 42].

Due to the demands imposed by countries that import Brazilian beef and the difficulties in achieving quick and specific BTB diagnoses, molecular tests based on PCR assays and its variations (*multiplex*-PCR, *nested*-PCR, real-time PCR and *nested* real-time PCR) [42,43 – 44], have been considered the most promising alternatives to accomplish BTB identification quickly and effectively in both live animals [45, 46] and in fragments of tissue samples presenting BTB-suspected lesions [5, 47 – 48, 49, 50], nasal exudates [5, 46 – 51, 52] and milk [53, 54 – 55].

In the present study, different BTB diagnosis tests, used singly or in combination with each other, were evaluated. Different methods, i.e. macroscopic analyses, histopathological examinations and *multiplex*-PCR, were evaluated for the rapid and specific detection of BTB (*M. bovis* and *M. tuberculosis* complex) directly from BTB-suspected lesions, with the aim of accelerating and adding specificity to the diagnosis of the disease, and, consequently, supporting the rulings of the health inspection service (SIF) performed in slaughterhouses, as stipulated by the tuberculosis control and eradication program in Brazil. The apparent prevalence of BTB among animals slaughtered in the state of Mato Grosso was also re-estimated and discussed, due to the great importance that this region has in the production of exported meat to different consumer countries worldwide, including the European Community.

2. Geographic region and study conditions

The study of the prevalence of BTB in animals slaughtered in the state of Mato Grosso, Brazil, was carried out by monitoring cattle slaughter and by *post-mortem* inspection of 41.193 carcasses. The duration of sample collections in each slaughterhouse was of approximately 10 days, between May and October 2009. The inspected carcasses belonged to 492 herds, from 85 (60%) municipalities in the state of Mato Grosso. Most of the slaughtered cattle was male (76.2%), from 1 to 2 years old (2.4%), 2 to 3 (54.2%) and> 3 years old (43.4%). A total of 77.8% (32.048/41.193) of the animals originated form herds monitored by the PNCEBT Program. The sample size (n) was calculated using the standard formula for simple random sampling, considering a degree of confidence of 95%, level of absolute accuracy of ± 0.022% [56] and expected prevalence of 0.05%, considering the results previously described by Salazar [39].

Seven slaughterhouses inspected by the SIF were monitored, located in six different cities in the state of Mato Grosso (Figure 1). As mentioned above, this region is considered the largest producer and second largest beef exporter in the country [40]. For the sampling to be considered representative with regard to cattle herds in this geographical area, slaughterhouses in four areas of Mato Grosso which have significant cattle herd production were selected: Southeast, south central, southwest and north. No sampling was conducted in the northeast area due to the unavailability of establishments with SIF inspection. However, animals from that region were slaughtered at the Paranatinga municipality, an area fortunately covered by this study. The selected sampling sites covered the four Mato Grosso cattle-producing circuits, divided according to Negreiros [57], in: Pantanal-represented by the Cáceres (16º 04' 14" S, 57º 40' 44" W) and Várzea Grande (15º 38' 48" S, 56º 07' 57" W) municipalities; Milk-represented by the Rondonópolis municipality (16º 28' 15" S, 54º 38' 08" W); Fattening-represented by the Paranatinga municipality (14º 25' 54" S, 54º 03' 04" W); and Reproduction-represented by the Juara (11º 15' 18" S, 57º 31' 11" W) and Tangará da Serra (14º 37' 10" S, 57º 29' 09" W) municipalities. Cattle slaughter at Juara was only monitored in two slaughterhouses.

During carcass inspections, all fragments of lesions classified by SIF as lymphadenitis or tuberculosis lesions located in the head, neck, chest cavity or cervical area lymph nodes (areas frequently affected by BTB) were sampled, according to official standards [58]. Once identified, the lesions were photographed, divided into samples and properly packaged. Information on body condition score, age and sex, origin (municipality and property where the cattle were raised) and health status of animals (participation or non-participation in the PNCEBT program), were obtained and recorded during sampling by means of the Animal Traffic Guide (GTA) of each lot.

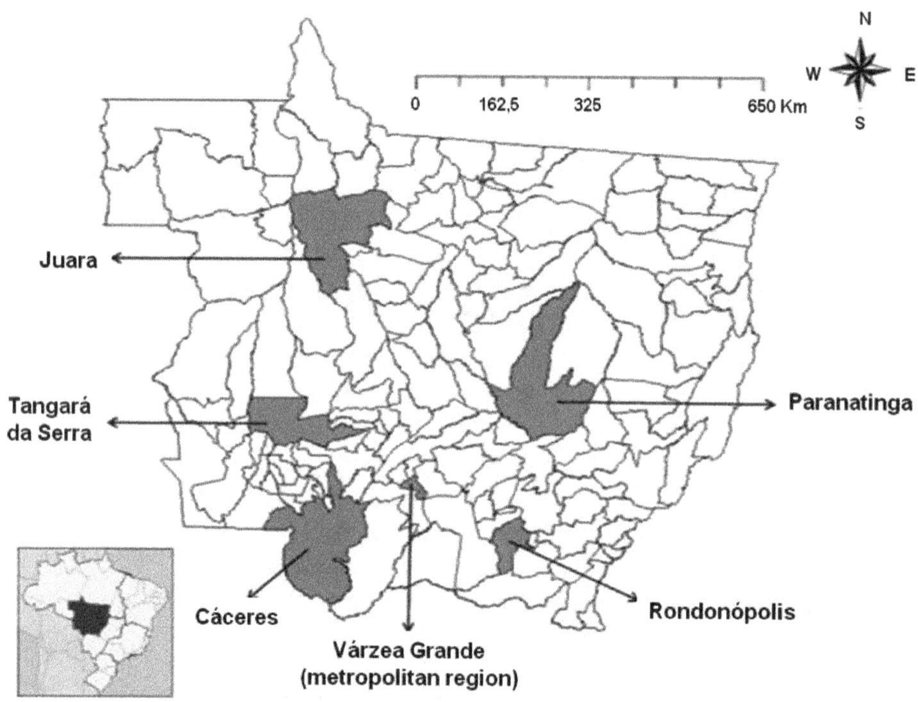

Figure 1. Map of the state of Mato Grosso, Brazil. Municipalities in gray indicate where samplings suggestive of BTB were taken during *post-mortem* inspections carried out in slaughterhouses in the region.

2.1. Prevalence of bovine tuberculosis in herds slaughtered in 2009 in the state of Mato Grosso, Brazil, determined using conventional tests [6]

The inspected carcasses 41.193 carcasses belonged to 492 herds, from 85 (60%) municipalities in the state of Mato Grosso (Figure 2). From the 41.193 carcasses assessed during the *post-*

mortem inspection, 198 (0.48%) showed lesions suggestive of BTB or lymphadenitis located in the front portion of the carcass (BTB-suspected lesions) (Table 1), according to the official standards for *post-mortem* examinations [58]. The decision to sample all lymphadenitis lesions from the head, neck and chest cavity lymph nodes was adopted to avoid losing potentially positive samples due to errors during the evaluations of the macroscopic lesions, since BTB lesions, lymphosarcomas or nonspecific lymphadenitis have very similar features and are difficult to be distinguished by the naked eye [59]. In addition, previous studies report that 86% of BTB lesions are present in the lymph nodes of the head and chest cavity (superior portion of the carcass) [28, 60 – 61].

After the *post-mortem* inspections, the collected lesions were photographed, divided into samples and either preserved in 10% buffered formalin for the histopathology analyses or frozen at-20°C for the bacteriology analyses and subsequent molecular technique applications. All samples fixed in 10% buffered formalin were cleaved so that each fragment of the lesion covered all layers of the granuloma (the necrotic material, capsule and transition area between the lesion and normal tissue). They were then subjected to dehydration techniques, diafanization clarification, embedding in paraffin and microtomizaion of the paraffin block at 4 μm, thus obtaining two histological slides of each sample for hematoxylin and eosin (HE) staining, with the purpose of observing histopathological changes, and Ziehl-Neelsen (ZN) staining, used for the detection of alcohol-acid resistant bacilli (AARB or BAAR) [62].

The HE histopathological examination performed on 198 samples of BTB-suspected lesions, indicated that 83.8% of the lesions were granulomatous, 8.1% were pyogranulomatous, 6.1% were suppurative, and 2.0% were lesions characteristic of interstitial pneumonia. The ZN histopathological examination indicated no AARB in the samples. The absence of AARB in BTB-suspected lesions has been reported by Salazar [39], and may occur due to the low bacilli concentrations in the examined lesions (paucibacillary lesions) [63].

Although granulomas are a classic BTB lesion, they cannot be considered pathognomonic of the disease [20, 32 – 59]. This statement was confirmed in the present study, where 91.9% (182/198) of the samples were granulomatous or piogranulomatose lesions (classic BTB lesions) and only 1.64% (3/182) of the lesions were affected by *M. bovis*. Therefore, the presence of the granulomas observed during the histopathological examinations is not conclusive and cannot be considered a supportive BTB diagnosis.

Samples stored at-20°C were processed for bacteriological analyses within three months after their collection. Approximately 3g of each sample were macerated with ground glass, and subjected to the hexadecylpyridinium chloride (HPC) 0.75% decontamination method and an adapted Petroff method (4% NaOH). The 0.75% HPC decontamination method was performed as described by Ambrosio [64], and the Petroff method [64] was adapted for the simultaneous processing of up to five samples, respecting the collection order and slaughterhouse of origin. When colony growths were observed, samples were reprocessed individually to identify the infected sample. After decontamination, the samples were plated in duplicate in Stonebrink and Lowenstein-Jensen (LJ) culture media, and incubated at 37°C. The samples were observed weekly during the first month and subsequently every two weeks until 90 days of culture. After isolate growth, the samples were stained by ZN to indicate the presence of AARB [62], as recommended in the National Manual of tuberculosis and other mycobacteria laboratory surveillance, by the Ministry of Health [65].

Sampling municipality	Number of slaughtered cattle	Number of carcasses presenting lesions	
		n	%
Cáceres	4,328	77	1.78
Juara	6,591	17	0.26
Paranatinga	8,068	23	0.29
Rondonópolis	5,914	03	0.05
Tangará da Serra	9,689	20	0.21
Várzea Grande	6,603	58	0.80
Total	41,193	198	0.48

Table 1. Occurrence of BTB-suggestive lesions in lymph nodes in the front portion of carcasses during post mortem inspection in 41,193 cattle in slaughterhouses from different municipalities in the state of Mato Grosso, between May and October 2009.

The bacteriology analyses isolated *M. bovis* in three animals from distinct herds, from the cities of Guarantã do Norte and Juína (upstate) and Pontes e Lacerda (southwest region), located in the Mato Grosso cattle reproduction circuit (Figure 2), according to Negreiros [57]. Their lesions were all located in the retropharyngeal lymph nodes and had been classified during HE histopathological examinations as granulomatous or pyogranulomatose.

Because of the characteristics of the present study, in which the purpose was to estimate the prevalence of BTB through animals destined for slaughter without possessing knowledge of the number of cattle specimens from each sampled property, it was not possible to calculate the actual prevalence of BTB in the state. Therefore, we calculated only the simple apparent prevalence of BTB in cattle and herds slaughtered in the state of Mato Grosso under SIF supervision, according to the method described by Martin [66]. BTB prevalence was calculated as 0.007% [CI 95%=-0.001%; 0.016%] for cattle and 0.61% [CI 95%=-0.08%; 1.30%] for herds. These results were similar to those found by Salazar [39], 0.007%, when surveying 57.641 cattle slaughtered in the state of Mato Grosso under supervision of the state sanitary inspection (SSI) service, from November 2004 to August 2005, during the PNCEBT program deployment by bacteriological analyses [15]. Of the total inspected cattle, 0.05% (27/57.641) showed BTB-suggestive lesions according to SISE, with four of these animals (14.8%) confirmed as BTB-positive by the bacteriological analyses. Similar results observed in the present study, four years after the start of the PNCEBT program, indicate a slow progress of the BTB eradication program in Mato Grosso, with the need for greater involvement of all the public and private links involved in this process.

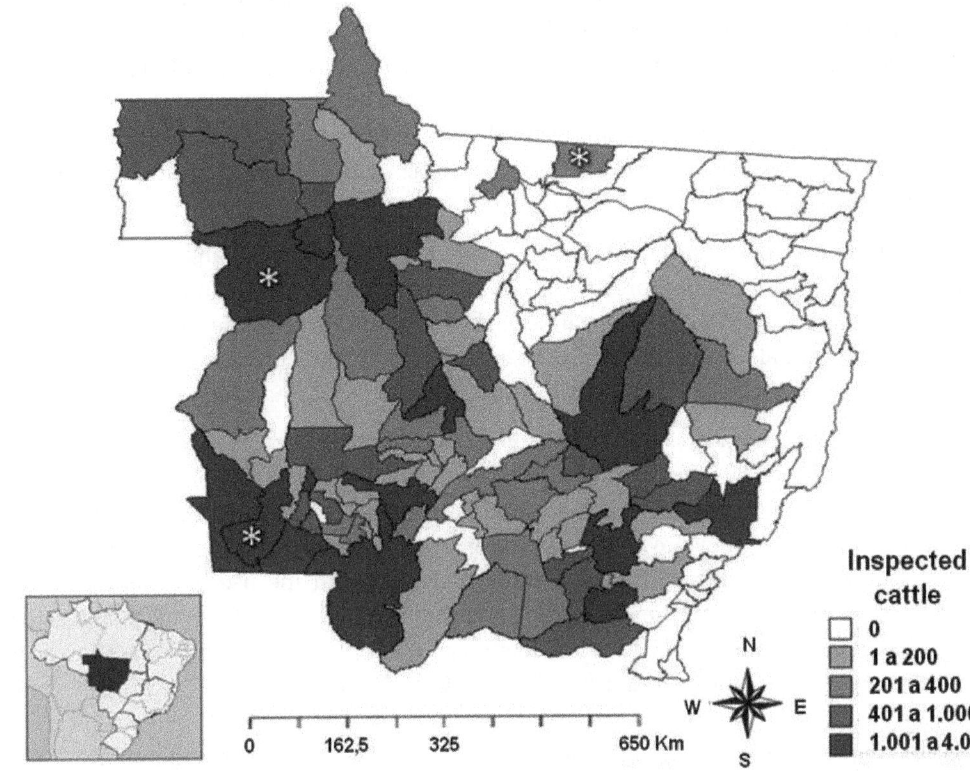

Figure 2. Mato Grosso municipalities, indicating total inspected cattle properties. *Municipalities where 03 animals with BTB were found.

Between 1993 and 1997, the prevalence of BTB in cattle slaughtered at ten slaughterhouses in the state of Minas Gerais (southeastern region) under SIF supervision, was of 0.08%, considering only official macroscopic findings [34]. Meanwhile, estimates on the apparent prevalence of infected animals in the same state, considering the results of the comparative cervical tuberculin test (CTT) (official *in vivo* examination) were 10 times higher (0.8%), according to the 1999 survey conducted on 22.990 animals from 1586 properties [67]. These results confirmed that the estimated prevalence of BTB is higher when applying *in vivo* diagnoses (bovine herds) when compared to *post-mortem* inspection diagnoses. Given this reasoning, it is expected that the prevalence of BTB in cattle herds in the state of Mato Grosso is higher than estimated by the present study, since the macroscopic inspections performed routinely in slaughterhouses are not able to identify all of the infected animals [32]. Other extrinsic factors can also interfere extensively in these estimates, such as the lack of random sampling in the slaughter groups, possible disposal of cattle shipments to state, municipal or clandestine plants, and the elimination of BTB-positive cattle in the breeding areas themselves. Therefore, the low prevalence observed in the present study, should be considered only as an indicative of the real cattle BTB situation in the state of Mato Grosso.

According to Kantor [38], estimates lower than 0.1% suggest areas considered low-prevalence or virtually tuberculosis-free. Therefore, the results of the present study may be underestimating up to 14 times the total number of infected animals and yet, even with this underestimation, Mato Grosso would still be considered a low prevalence or virtually tuberculosis-free area. To provide confirmatory estimates of the disease in Mato Grosso, it would be necessary to conduct a representative BTB sampling survey of the main cattle raising properties in the region [34].

The low prevalence status found in Mato Grosso was expected, since the area presents certain characteristics that hinder the spread of BTB, including a tropical climate, cattle raised predominantly by the extensive system, aimed at beef exports, low pasture stocking, and early slaughter of the animals. Because of this, the animals end up having less contact with each other and, consequently, shorter exposure to possibly infected animals [68].

As a result of the low prevalence status observed in this study, the state of Mato Grosso may advance to the stage of BTB eradication, using strategies such as the implementation of an efficient monitoring system, performed alongside inspection officers and the health defense service, so that, together, they are able to detect remaining BTB foci in the region, the application of *post-mortem* inspection routines in slaughterhouses and the use of additional BTB-diagnostic techniques, such as molecular techniques applied directly to BTB-suggestive lesions. Consequently, these suggested strategies can contribute to accelerate the process of bovine tuberculosis eradication in the state of Mato Grosso, Brazil.

2.2. Use of complementary tests in the *post-mortem* inspection of suspected bovine tuberculosis infections [69]

The association of molecular tests and conventional tests was evaluated to contribute to the choice of additional tests in order to reach the BTB-eradication stage in Mato Grosso, identifying the limitations and benefits of each approach regarding their use in *post-mortem* cattle inspection. The same 198 lymph node samples were evaluated by macroscopic examinations, histopathology and *multiplex*-PCR assay using DNA fragments arrays obtained directly from BTB-suggestive lesions.

DNA extraction was performed using the commercial Qiagen extraction and purification kit (DNeasy® Blood & Tissue kit), with modifications in the protocol as described by Figueiredo [5]. Five microliters of template DNA-about 100 ng-were used for the m-PCR test based on the method described by Figueiredo [50] using a reaction mixture of 5 μL reaction buffer (Invitrogen, USA), 0.2 mM dNTPs (Fermentas, USA), 1.5 U of recombinant Taq polymerase (Platinum® Taq – Invitrogen, USA), 5 mM $MgCl_2$ (Invitrogen, USA) and 20 pmols of each primer (Invitrogen, USA) for the amplification of IS6110 genomic sequences (245 bp) Ixlink: (5′-CGTGAGGGCATCGAGGTGGC-3′) and INS2: (5′-GCGTAGGCGTCGGTGACAAA-3′) [70] present only in MBC members, and *RvD1Rv2031c* (500 pb) Jb21: (5′-TCGTCCGCTGATG-CAAGTGC-3′) and Jb22: (5′-CGTGAACGTAGTCGCCTGC-3′) [71], present only in *M. bovis*, with a final volume of 50 μL. Amplification of the target sequence was performed in a thermocycler GeneAmp 9700 PCR System (Applied Biosystems, USA) according to the following parameters: 94°C for 5 min, followed by 37 1 min cycles at 94°C, 1 min at 68°C and

1 min at 72°C with a final extension at 72°C for 7 min. The resulting PCR products were analyzed by 1.5%, ultrapure agarose gel electrophoresis (Invitrogen, USA) stained with ethidium bromide (10 mg/mL) and visualized/documented in a MiniBIS pro system (DNR Bio-Imaging Systems, USA).

M. bovis was detectable in 7.0% of the samples when performing the m-PCR technique directly on the fragments of BTB-suspicious lesions (Figure 3) (14/198), including lesions from the same three strains in which *M. bovis* was isolated. The results obtained without applying *M. bovis* cultivation and isolation steps, allowed the detection of the pathogen in 14 samples, representing an increment of almost 5 times in method efficiency, consistent with other studies conducted by Meikle, Cardoso and Figueiredo [46, 49-72]. Thus, according to the results, it is suggested that the m-PCR method may be useful in monitoring BTB in slaughterhouses, reducing the diagnosis time from 90 days to only 2 working days in addition to increasing pathogen detection sensitivity.

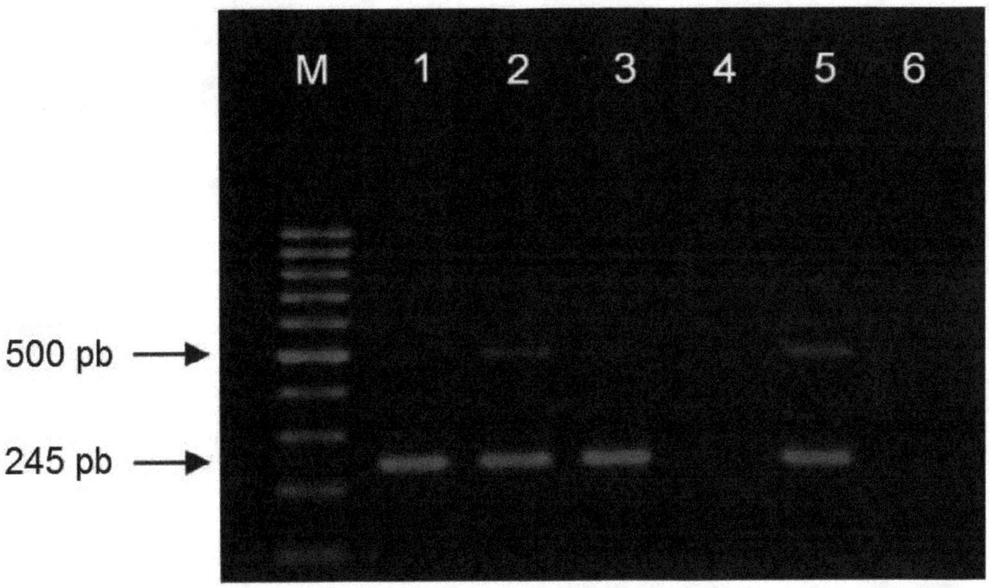

Figure 3. Detection of *M. bovis* directly from fragments of BTB-suspicious lesions using the m-PCR technique. Template DNA extracted directly from the lesions was used to amplify the *RvD1Rv2031c* (500 bp) sequences specific to *M. bovis* and *IS6110* (245 bp) specific to the MTC. Lane M: molecular marker (DNA ladder-100 bp); Lanes 1, 2 and 3: positive reaction to m-PCR, originating from three of the 14 carcasses with BTB-suggestive lesions, inspected in slaughterhouses in the state of Mato Grosso, Brazil.; Lane 4: negative for m-PCR reaction, injury not affected by *M. bovis*; Lane 5: reference strain of *M. bovis* (ATCC 19210), used as positive control reaction; Lane 6: Negative control reaction.

On the revaluation of the macroscopic analyses of the carcasses inspected in the present study, a high incidence of lesions in the pre-scapular and pre-pectoral lymph nodes, of approximately 73.2% (145/198) was observed (Table 2). Despite *M. bovis* having already been detected in these lymph nodes [28, 32], these lesions could be attributed to vaccine reactions (Figure 4A), since the HE histopathological examinations showed that 84.5% (126/145) of the lesions exhibited granulomatous reactivity with intralesional vacuoles (Figure 4B), that indicate the presence of mineral oil drained from the vaccine application site (shoulder or neck), to the cervical lymph nodes (pre-scapular and pre-pectoral lymph nodes), triggering an immunostimulatory effect by vaccine adjuvants [73]. This fact becomes more relevant, since mycobacteria were not isolated from these lesions. Thus, macroscopic findings in these nodes should be considered only alongside the presence of BTB-suggestive lesions in several areas of the carcass and/or in animals from herds showing a history of bovine tuberculosis.

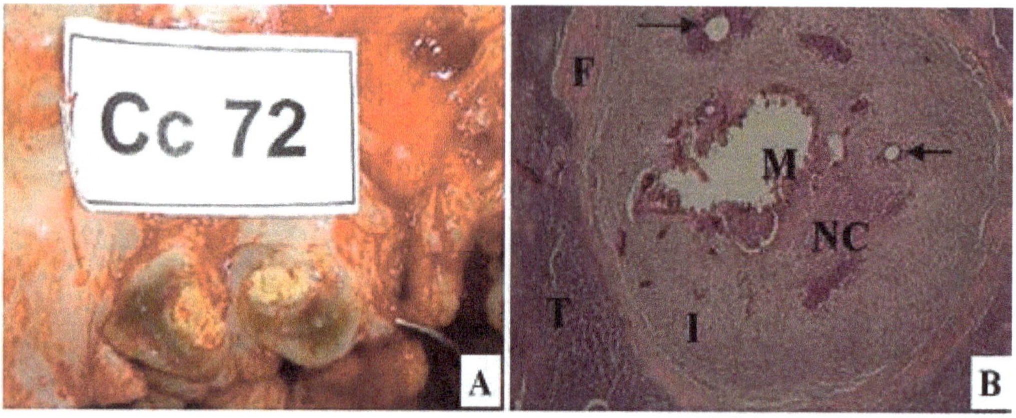

Figure 4. (A). Pre-pectoral lymph node containing a granuloma with a caseous mass of pasty, yellow and calcified consistency surrounded by a capsule of approximately 1 cm of connective tissue; (B). Lesion visualized on a 5X objective during HE histopathological examination, showing a granulomatous reaction characterized by central caseous necrosis (CN) with intense mineralization (M) surrounded by a predominantly mononuclear infiltrate (I), containing occasional intralesional vacuoles (arrow). The lesion is surrounded by fibrous tissue (F) and well-defined when compared to whole tissue (T).

The affected retrofaringeal lymph nodes showed increases in size and number of lesions (Figure 5-A, B and C). However, the lesions were localized (restricted to the retropharyngeal node) with no BTB-suggestive lesions in other areas of the carcasses.

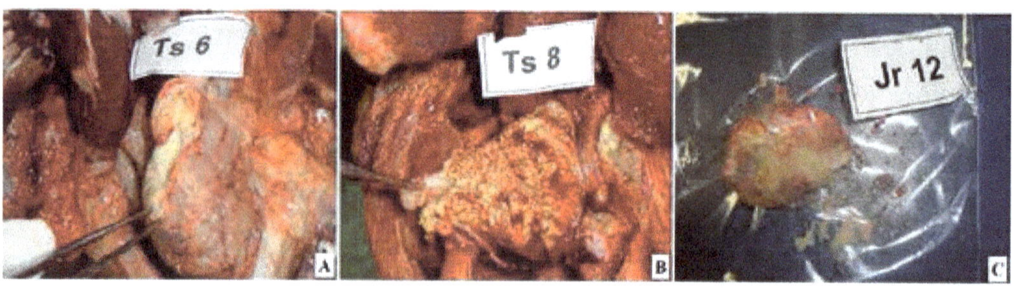

Figure 5. Bovine tuberculosis lesions collected during *post-mortem* examination in slaughterhouses in the state of Mato Grosso, Brazil; (A). retropharyngeal lymph node affected by *M. bovis*, containing purulent exudate; (B-C). retropharyngeal lymph nodes affected by *M. bovis*.

According to these results, it is advisable that *post-mortem* inspections be carried out carefully, especially with regard to the head and thoracic cavity lymph nodes, especially in the retropharyngeal node, since the number of retropharyngeal node samples containing *M. bovis* was higher (Table 2). These results have already been described by other authors, who also found high percentages (22.9 to 49.2%) of BTB lesions in retropharyngeal lymph nodes [28, 74].

	Number and percentage of lesions					
Animal body parts	***Post mortem evaluation***		**Culture**		**m-PCR**	
	N	%	N	%	N	%
Respiratory apparatus	**29**	**14.6**	**0**	**0**	**4**	**2**
Lung	6	3	0	0	1	0.5
Apical lymph node	4	2	0	0	1	0.5
Esophageal lymph node	7	3.5	0	0	0	0
Mediastinal lymph node	4	2	0	0	0	0
Tracheo-bronchial lymph node	6	3	0	0	2	1
Thoracic cavity	2	1	0	0	0	0
Head	**22**	**11.1**	**3**	**1.5**	**5**	**2.5**
Retropharyngeal lymph node	19	9.5	3	1.5	5	2.5
Parotid lymph node	1	0.5	0	0	0	0
Sublingual lymph node	2	1	0	0	0	0
Carcass	**147**	**74.2**	**0**	**0**	**5**	**2.5**
Pre-pectoral lymph node	108	54.5	0	0	4	2
Pre-scapular lymph node	37	18.6	0	0	1	0.5
Ischiatic lymph node	2	1	0	0	0	0
Total	**198**	**100**	**3**	**1.5**	**14**	**7.0**

Table 2. Diagnosis of bovine tuberculosis in samples with BTB-suspected, collected from inspected and slaughtered cattle at slaughterhouses in the state of Mato Grosso, Brazil.

When comparing macroscopic analyses, bacteriological cultures and m-PCR, the results indicate that the macroscopic analyses correctly identified 93% (184/198) of the samples, considering these lesions as common lymphadenitis (non-tuberculosis) samples. However, *M. bovis* was identified in 7.0% (14/198) of samples that were also considered as non-tuberculosis samples. Despite the mistakes made by SIF inspection when ruling positive BTB lesions as common lymphadenitis, the destination of the carcasses adopted by the inspection service (partial condemnation) was consistent with the standards established in Article 196 of the Regulation for Industrial and Sanitary Inspection Products of Animal Origin-RIISPOA [58], with regard to the presence of BTB-suggestive lesions in only one part or area of the carcass.

These mistakes in the rulings of BTB-suspected lesions may be due to the occurrence of, mainly, paucibacillary lesions similar to those observed in the present study, since they did not present classic tuberculosis features, probably because the animals displayed recent infection and were slaughtered early (2-3 years old). This factor can distort BTB estimations in slaughterhouses, and, consequently, hinder the success of the PNCEBT program, making it difficult to eradicate the disease in areas such as in Mato Grosso, where the prevalence of BTB is low. In this case, the Federal Inspection plays a very important role in evaluations of the carcasses in slaughterhouses for BTB diagnoses, assisting in the detection of remaining disease foci and in tracing infected herds. This role is confirmed by the results of disease control programs implemented in high prevalence areas [32, 75]. However, as noted above, as the prevalence decreases, the identification of remaining BTB infected livestock becomes increasingly difficult. Although at present there is no diagnosis method (*ante* or *post* mortem) able to identify all animals infected with *M. bovis*, the detection is more efficient when more than one diagnostic method is used [60]. Thus, in areas where the disease prevalence is very low, such as in the state of Mato Grosso, [6, 39], awareness should be raised regarding the increased difficulty of detecting BTB during *post-mortem* inspections. In addition, the use of complementary tests that result in rapid diagnoses should be adopted, such as the m-PCR in this study, which showed the versatility of combining sensitivity and specificity for rapid diagnoses (approximately 2 working days), since this technique can be used to detect *M. bovis* directly from fragments of BTB-suspected lesions and may contribute to the success of the PNCEBT program with regard to tracking remaining BTB foci.

3. Discussion

The state of Mato Grosso has emerged in the Brazilian national scene as the largest beef cattle producer and second largest beef exporter in the country [40], leading to annual increases in the amount of meat exported to EU countries. Consequently, the pressure on Brazil by countries that buy Brazilian products to implant an effective, rapid and definitive diagnosis of BTB in tuberculosis-suspected lesions has also increased.

In 2012, the Ministry of Agriculture, Livestock and Supply (Ministério da Agricultura, Pecuária e Abastecimento-MAPA) determined that farms where the detection of BTB cases took place can no longer export beef to the Customs Union of Belarus, Kazakhstan and Russia, recalling all lots from these animal farms until the diagnosis of suspicious lesions in samples collected after slaughter could be conducted at an official MAPA laboratory [41, 42].

In view of these commercial and sanitary restrictions, the difficulties in tuberculosis diagnosis must be overcome. Diagnosis alternatives for the quick and specific identification of BTB in clinical samples or isolated colonies have emerged, such as molecular methods based on PCR and its variants (simplex PCR, *multiplex*-PCR, *nested* PCR, real-time PCR and real-time *nested* PCR) [42, 43-44].

In this context, the purpose of the present study was to evaluate the performance of diagnostic tests, such as m-PCR, culture and histopathology, on the detection of MTC species directly from suspected BTB lesions. The apparent prevalence of BTB among animals slaughtered in the state of Mato Grosso was also re-evaluated and discussed, due to the great importance of this geographic region in meat production and export to several consumer countries worldwide, including the European Community.

When comparing macroscopic analyses, bacteriological cultures and m-PCR, the results indicate that the macroscopic analyses correctly identified 93% (184/198) of the samples, categorizing these lesions as common lymphadenitis (non-tuberculosis) samples. However, *M. bovis* was identified by m-PCR tests in 7.0% (14/198) of samples previously considered as non-tuberculosis samples.

As a result of the low prevalence status established in this study, BTB in the state of Mato Grosso may advance to the stage of eradication, using strategies such as the implementation of an efficient monitoring system, performed alongside inspection officers and the health defense service. Alongside the application of *post-mortem* inspection routines in slaughterhouses and the use of additional BTB-diagnostic tests, such as molecular methods applied directly to BTB-suggestive lesions, these strategies should be efficient in detecting any remaining BTB foci in this geographic region, contributing to accelerate the process of bovine tuberculosis eradication in the state of Mato Grosso, Brazil.

Currently, there is no diagnosis test (*ante* or *post* mortem) able to identify all animals infected by *M. bovis*. Detection of contaminated animals is more efficient if two or more diagnostic tests are combined [60]. In geographic regions where the disease shows low prevalence, as the observed in the state of Mato Grosso [6, 39], awareness should be raised regarding the augmented difficulty of detecting BTB during *post-mortem* inspections. The use of complementary tests that result in rapid diagnoses should be adopted, such as the m-PCR described in this study, which demonstrated the versatility of both sensitivity and specificity in the rapid detection of *M. bovis* (approximately 2 working days), directly from fragments of BTB-suspected lesions. The guidelines proposed herein may contribute to the success of the PNCEBT program with regard to tracking remaining BTB foci.

4. Conclusions

The results of the present study indicate that mistakes can occur during rulings of suspected bovine tuberculosis lesions in cattle, particularly those presenting paucibacillary lesions. These mistakes cause a distortion in BTB estimates in slaughterhouses, with harmful consequences to the success of the Brazilian Tuberculosis Control Program (PNCEBT). The results point to the use of complementary molecular assays for rapid diagnoses of lesions situated in frequently BTB-affected carcass areas, thus minimizing mistakes in judging the disease in slaughterhouses. m-PCR was the most sensitive, rapid and specific method among the complementary methods tested in the present study when compared to conventional methods for BTB-diagnosis. It is, therefore, a promising alternative in disease surveillance to be used by the federal inspection service to contribute to the bovine tuberculosis control and eradication program, for disease surveillance in slaughterhouses and for tracking remaining BTB foci in the state of Mato Grosso, as well as in other regions of the country, contributing even further to the success of the PNCEBT program.

Author details

Ricardo César Tavares Carvalho[1], Leone Vinícius Furlanetto[1], Rafael da Silva Duarte[2], Luciano Nakazato[3], Walter Lilenbaum[4], Eduardo Eustáquio de Souza Figueiredo[5] and Vânia Margaret Flosi Paschoalin[1*]

*Address all correspondence to: paschv@iq.ufrj.br

1 Institute of Chemistry, Federal University of Rio de Janeiro, Rio de Janeiro – RJ, Brazil

2 Institute of Microbiology, Federal University of Rio de Janeiro, Rio de Janeiro – RJ, Brazil

3 Laboratory of Molecular Biology, Faculty of Veterinary Medicine, Federal University of Mato Grosso, Cuiabá/MT, Brazil

4 Biomedical Institute, Fluminense Federal University, Niterói – RJ, Brazil

5 Faculty of Nutrition and Food Science and Technology, Federal University of Mato Grosso, Cuiabá/MT, Brazil

References

[1] Huard RC, Lazzarini LC, Butler WR, Van Soolingen D, Ho JL. PCR-based method to differentiate the subspecies of the *Mycobacterium tuberculosis* complex on the basis of genomic deletions. J Clin Microbiol. 2003;41(4):1637-50.

[2] Garnier T, Eiglmeier K, Camus JC, Medina N, Mansoor H, Pryor M, et al. The complete genome sequence of *Mycobacterium bovis*. Proc Natl Acad Sci U S A. 2003;100(13):7877-82.

[3] Romano MI, Alito A, Fisanotti JC, Bigi F, Kantor I, Cicuta ME, et al. Comparison of different genetic markers for molecular epidemiology of bovine tuberculosis. Vet Microbiol. 1996;50(1-2):59-71.

[4] Medeiros LS, Marassi CD, Figueiredo EE, Lilenbaum W. Potential application of new diagnostic methods for controlling bovine tuberculosis in Brazil. Braz J Microbiol. 2010;41(3):531-41.

[5] Figueiredo EES, Conte Júnior CA, Furlanetto LV, Silva FGS, Duarte RS, Silva JT, et al. Molecular techniques for identification of species of the Mycobacterium tuberculosis complex: the use of multiplex PCR and an adapted HPLC method for identification

of *Mycobacterium bovis* and Diagnosis of Bovine Tuberculosis. In: Cardona PJ, editor. Understanding Tuberculosis-Global Experiences and Innovative Approaches to the Diagnosis: InTech; 2012. p. 411-32.

[6] Furlanetto LV, Figueiredo EES, Conte Júnior CA, Silva FGS, Duarte RS, Silva JT, et al. Prevalence of bovine tuberculosis in herds and animals slaughtered in 2009 in the State of Mato Grosso, Brazil. Arq Bras Med Vet Zootec. 2012;64(2):274-80.

[7] Vordermeier HM, Chambers MA, Buddle BM, Pollock JM, Hewinson RG. Progress in the development of vaccines and diagnostic reagents to control tuberculosis in cattle. Vet J. 2006;171(2):229-44.

[8] Mattos IG, Ribeiro MO, Netto IC, d'Azevedo PA. Tuberculosis: a study of 111 cases in an area of high prevalence in the extreme south of Brazil. Braz J Infect Dis. 2006;10(3):194-8.

[9] O'Reilly LM, Daborn CJ. The epidemiology of Mycobacterium bovis infections in animals and man: a review. Tuber Lung Dis. 1995;76 Suppl 1:1-46.

[10] Murakami PS, Fuverki RBN, Nakatani SM, Filho IRB, Biondo AW. Tuberculose Bovina: Saúde Animal e Saúde Pública. Arq Ciênc Vet Zool Unipar. 2009;12(1):67-74.

[11] Acha PN, Szyfres B. Zoonoses and Communicable Diseases Common to Man and Animals. Bacterioses and Mycoses. 3 ed2001. 395 p.

[12] Grange JM. Mycobacterium bovis infection in human beings. Tuberculosis (Edinb). 2001;81(1-2):71-7.

[13] CDC-MMWR. Center for Disease Control and Prevention-Morbidity and Mortality Weekly Report. Human Tuberculosis Caused by Mycobacterium bovis-New York City, 2001-2004. 2005. Available from: http://www.cdc.gov/mmwr/preview/mmwrhtml/mm5424a4.htm. (accessed 20 August 2014).

[14] WHO. World Health Organization. Guidelines for specification withing the Mycobacterium tuberculosis complex. WHO/EMC/ZOO/96.4. Second edition. 1996. Available from: http://whqlibdoc.who.int/hq/1996/who_emc_zoo_96.4.pdf. (accessed 20 August 2014)

[15] Brazil. Ministério da Agricultura, Pecuária e Abastecimento. Secretaria de Defesa Agropecuária-Departamento de Saúde Animal. Programa Nacional de Controle e Erradicação da Brucelose e Tuberculose Animal. Brasília, 2004. Available from: http://www.agricultura.gov.br/arq_editor/file/Aniamal/programa%20nacional%20sanidade%20brucelose/Manual%20do%20PNCEBT%20-%20Original.pdf. (accessed 25 August 2014)

[16] Leite CQ, Anno IS, Leite SR, Roxo E, Morlock GP, Cooksey RC. Isolation and identification of mycobacteria from livestock specimens and milk obtained in Brazil. Mem Inst Oswaldo Cruz. 2003;98(3):319-23.

[17] OIE. World Organisation for Animal Health-WAHID Interface, 2007. Available from: http://www.oie.int/wahid-prod/public.php. (accessed 05 September 2014)

[18] Sequeira MD, Ritacco V, Kantor IN. Mycobacterium bovis Infection in Animals and Humans: Blackwell Publishing, Ames, IA.; 2005.

[19] Abrahão RMCM, Nogueira PA, Malucelli MIC. O comércio clandestino de carne e leite no brasil e o risco da transmissão da tuberculose bovina e de outras doenças ao homem: um problema de saúde pública-Meat and milk black market-Bovine tuberculosis. Arch Vet Scien. 2005;10(2):1-17.

[20] Neill SD, Pollock JM, Bryson DB, Hanna J. Pathogenesis of *Mycobacterium bovis* infection in cattle. Vet Microbiol. 1994;40(1-2):41-52.

[21] Michel AL, Muller B, van Helden PD. *Mycobacterium bovis* at the animal-human interface: a problem, or not? Vet Microbiol. 2010;140(3-4):371-81.

[22] Moda G, Daborn CJ, Grange JM, Cosivi O. The zoonotic importance of *Mycobacterium bovis*. Tuber Lung Dis. 1996;77(2):103-8.

[23] Morris RS, Pfeiffer DU, Jackson R. The epidemiology of *Mycobacterium bovis* infections. Vet Microbiol. 1994;40:153-77.

[24] Pollock JM, Neill SD. *Mycobacterium bovis* infection and tuberculosis in cattle. Vet J. 2002;163(2):115-27.

[25] Menzies FD, Neill SD. Cattle-to-cattle transmission of bovine tuberculosis. Vet J. 2000;160(2):92-106.

[26] Jones TC, Hunt RD, King NW. Patologia Veterinária. 6 ed. ed: Editora Manole Ltda. Bela Vista, São Paulo, SP, Brasil.; 2000.

[27] Neill SD, Bryson DG, Pollock JM. Pathogenesis of tuberculosis in cattle. Tuberculosis (Edinb). 2001;81(1-2):79-86.

[28] Corner L, Melville L, McCubbin K, Small KJ, McCormick BS, Wood PR, et al. Efficiency of inspection procedures for the detection of tuberculous lesions in cattle. Aust Vet J. 1990;67(11):389-92.

[29] Roxo E. *Mycobacteium bovis* como causa de zoonose. Rev Ciênc Farm. 1997;8(1):101-8.

[30] Romero B, Aranaz A, de Juan L, Alvarez J, Bezos J, Mateos A, et al. Molecular epidemiology of multidrug-resistant *Mycobacterium bovis* isolates with the same spoligotyping profile as isolates from animals. J Clin Microbiol. 2006;44(9):3405-8.

[31] OIE. World Organisation for Animal Health-Bovine tuberculosis 2009. Available from: http://www.oie.int/fileadmin/Home/fr/Health_standards/tahm/2.04.07_BOVINE_TB.pdf. (accessed 06 September 2014)

[32] Corner LA. Post mortem diagnosis of *Mycobacterium bovis* infection in cattle. Vet Microbiol. 1994;40(1-2):53-63.

[33] Ribeiro ARP, Lobato FCF, Abreu VLV, Faria ES, Silva JA. Prevalence of bovine tuberculosis and brucellosis in Ilhéus, Bahia-Brazil. Arq Bras Med Vet Zootec. 2003;55(1): 120-2.

[34] Baptista F, Moreira EC, Santos WLM, Naveda LAB. Prevalence of tuberculosis among bovines slaughtered in Minas Gerais, Brazil. Arq Bras Med Vet Zootec. 2004;56(5):577-80.

[35] Poletto R, Kreutz LC, Gonzales JC, Barcellos LJG. Prevalence of tuberculosis, brucelosis and viral infections in dairy cattle from the county of Passo Fundo, RS, Brazil. Cienc Rural. 2004;34(2):595-8.

[36] Oliveira IAS, Melo HPC, Câmara A, Dias RVC, Blanco BS. Prevalência de tuberculose no rebanho bovino de Mossoró, Rio Grande do Norte. Braz J Vet Res Anim Sci. 2007;44(6):395-400.

[37] Roxo E. Situação Atual da Tuberculose Bovina no Brasil. Plano Nacional de Controle e Erradicação da Brucelose e Tuberculose-PNCEBT. Secretaria de Defesa Agropecuária Documento-PNCEBT, São Paulo. 2005:1-5.

[38] Kantor IN, Ritacco V. An update on bovine tuberculosis programmes in Latin American and Caribbean countries. Vet Microbiol. 2006;112(2-4):111-8.

[39] Salazar FHP. Ocorrência de tuberculose causada por Mycobacterium bovis em bovinos abatidos em frigoríficos no Estado de Mato Grosso, Brasil. Universidade Federal de Mato Grosso do Sul, Campo Grande, Brazil.; 2005.

[40] Brazil. Instituto Brasileiro de Geografia e Estatística. Produção Pecuária. Brasília, 2014. Available from: http://www.ibge.gov.br/home/estatistica/indicadores/agropecuaria/producaoagropecuaria/abate-leite-couro-ovos_201401_publ_completa.pdf. (accessed 09 September 2014)

[41] Brazil. Ministério da Agricultura, Pecuária e Abastecimento. Secretaria de Defesa Agropecuária. Norma Interna DAS Nº 02, de 30 de Abril de 2012. Brasília, 2012. Available from: http://www.google.com.br/url?sa=t&rct=j&q=&esrc=s&source=web&cd=1&cad=rja&uact=8&ved=0CBwQFjAA&url=http%3A%2F%2Fwww.dda.agricultura.rs.gov.br%2Fajax%2Fdownload.php%3FqArquivo%3D20130425112834norma_interna_02_sda_2012.pdf&ei=Ml_AU5yBO5OTyATus4LICw&usg=AFQjCNEf8knT1tU9Os9qUReTAKvNHyeyuw. (accessed 09 September 2014)

[42] Araújo CP, Osorio AL, Jorge KS, Ramos CA, Filho AF, Vidal CE, et al. Detection of *Mycobacterium bovis* in bovine and bubaline tissues using nested-PCR for TbD1. PLoS One. 2014;9(3):e91023.

[43] Soini H, Musser JM. Molecular diagnosis of mycobacteria. Clin Chem. 2001;47(5): 809-14.

[44] Araújo CP. Desenvolvimento de nested PCR para a detecção de DNA de membros do complexo *Mycobacterium Tuberculosis* em tecidos de bovinos e bubalinos: Universidade Federal de Mato Grosso do Sul, Campo Grande, Brazil.; 2014.

[45] Serrano-Moreno BA, Romero TA, Arriaga C, Torres RA, Pereira-Suarez AL, Garcia-Salazar JA, et al. High frequency of *Mycobacterium bovis* DNA in colostra from tuberculous cattle detected by nested PCR. Zoonoses Public Health. 2008;55(5):258-66.

[46] Figueiredo EES, Carvalho RCT, Silvestre FG, Lilenbaum W, Fonseca LS, Silva JT, et al. Detection of *Mycobacterium bovis* DNA in nasal swabs from tuberculous cattle by a multiplex PCR. Braz J Microbiol. 2010;41(2):386-90.

[47] Liébana E, Aranaz A, Mateos A, Vilafranca M, Gomez-Mampaso E, Tercero JC, et al. Simple and rapid detection of *Mycobacterium tuberculosis* complex organisms in bovine tissue samples by PCR. J Clin Microbiol. 1995;33(1):33-6.

[48] Zanini MS, Moreira EC, Lopes MT, Oliveira RS, Leao SC, Fioravanti RL, et al. *Mycobacterium bovis*: polymerase chain reaction identification in bovine lymphonode biopsies and genotyping in isolates from Southeast Brazil by spolygotyping and restriction fragment length polymorphism. Mem Inst Oswaldo Cruz. 2001;96(6): 809-13.

[49] Cardoso MA, Cardoso RF, Hirata RD, Hirata MH, Leite CQ, Santos AC, et al. Direct detection of Mycobacterium bovis in bovine lymph nodes by PCR. Zoonoses Public Health. 2009;56(8):465-70.

[50] Figueiredo EES, Silva FGS, Campos WN, Furlanetto LV, Medeiros L, Lilenbaum W, et al. Identification of *Mycobacterium bovis* Isolates by a multiplex PCR. Braz J Microbiol. 2009;40(2):231-3.

[51] Vitale F, Capra G, Maxia L, Reale S, Vesco G, Caracappa S. Detection of *Mycobacterium tuberculosis* Complex in Cattle by PCR Using Milk, Lymph Node Aspirates, and Nasal Swabs. J Clin Microbiol. 1998;36(4):1050-5.

[52] Romero RE, Garzon DL, Mejia GA, Monroy W, Patarroyo ME, Murillo LA. Identification of *Mycobacterium bovis* in bovine clinical samples by PCR species-specific primers. Can J Vet Res. 1999;63(2):101-6.

[53] Zanini MS, Moreira EC, Lopes MT, Mota P, Salas CE. Detection of *Mycobacterium bovis* in milk by polymerase chain reaction. Zentralbl Veterinarmed B. 1998;45(8):473-9.

[54] Zarden CF, Marassi CD, Figueiredo EE, Lilenbaum W. *Mycobacterium bovis* detection from milk of negative skin test cows. Vet Rec. 2013;172(5):130.

[55] Carvalho RCT, Castro VS, Fernandes DVGS, Moura GF, Santos ECC, Figueiredo EES, et al. Use of PCR for detection of bovine tuberculosis bacillus in milk of positive skin test cows. Braz J Vet Res Anim Sci. 2014;51(1):42-8.

[56] Noordhuizen JPTM, Frankena K, Van Der Hoofd CM, E.A.M G. Application of Quantitative Methods in Veterinary Epidemiology. Wageningen Press, The Netherlands1997 Jun. 445 p.

[57] Negreiros RL, Dias RA, Ferreira F, Ferreira Neto JS, Gonçalves VSP, Silva MCP, et al. Epidemiologic situation of bovine brucellosis in the State of Mato Grosso, Brazil. Arq Bras Med Vet Zootec. 2009;61:56-65.

[58] Brazil. Ministério da Agricultura, Pecuária e Abastecimento. Departamento de Inspeção de Produtos de Origem Animal. Divisão de Normas Técnicas-Decreto Nº 30691, de 29 de março de 1952. Regulamento da Inspeção Industrial e Sanitária dos Produtos de Origem Animal. Brasília,1952. Available from: http://www.agricultura.gov.br/arq_editor/file/Desenvolvimento_Sustentavel/Producao-Integrada-Pecuaria/Decreto%2030691%20de%201952.pdf. (accessed 12 September 2014)

[59] Reis DO, Almeida L, Faria AR. Estudo comparativo entre linfossarcoma, tuberculose e linfadenites inespecíficas ocorridas em bovinos abatidos e a confirmação histológica. Hig Alim. 1995;35:28-30.

[60] Whipple DL, Bolin CA, Miller JM. Distribution of lesions in cattle infected with *Mycobacterium bovis*. J Vet Diagn Invest. 1996;8(3):351-4.

[61] Asseged B, Woldesenbet Z, Yimer E, Lemma E. Evaluation of abattoir inspection for the diagnosis of *Mycobacterium bovis* infection in cattle at Addis Ababa abattoir. Trop Anim Health Prod. 2004;36(6):537-46.

[62] Prophet EB, B. M, J.B. A, Sobin LH. Laboratory methods in histotechnology. Armed Forces Institute of Pathology, Washington, D.C.: Armed Forces Institute of Pathology, Washington, D.C.; 1992.

[63] Andrade GB, Riet-correa F, Mielke PV, Méndez MDC, Schild AL. Estudo histológico e isolamento de micobactérias de lesöes similares à tuberculose em bovinos no Rio Grande do Sul. Pesq Vet Bras. 1991;11(3):81-6.

[64] Ambrosio SR, Oliveira EMD, Rodriguez CA, Ferreira Neto JS, Amaku M. Comparison of three decontamination methods for *Mycobacterium bovis* isolation. Braz J Microbiol. 2008;39(2):241-4.

[65] Brazil. Ministério da Saúde. Secretaria de Vigilância em Saúde-Departamento de Vigilância Epidemiológica. Manual nacional de vigilância laboratorial da tuberculose e outras micobactérias. Brasília, 2008. Available from: http://bvsms.saude.gov.br/bvs/publicacoes/manual_vigilancia_laboratorial_tuberculose.pdf. (accessed 05 September 2014)

[66] Martin SW, Meek AH, Willeberg P. Veterinary epidemiology : principles and methods. 1 ed. ed. Ames : Iowa State University Press: Ames : Iowa State University Press; 1987.

[67] Belchior APC. Prevalência, distribuição regional e fatores de risco da tuberculose bovina em Minas Gerais: Universidade Federal de Minas Gerais, Belo Horizonte; 2000.

[68] Abrahão RMCM. Tuberculose humana causada pelo *Mycobacterium bovis*: considerações gerais e a importância dos reservatórios animais. 1999;4:5-15.

[69] Furlanetto LV, Figueiredo EES, Conte Júnior CA, Carvalho RCT, Silva FGS, Silva JT, et al. Use of complementary methods in *post-mortem* inspection of carcasses with suspected bovine tuberculosis. Pesq Vet Bras. 2012;32(11):1138-44.

[70] Hermans PW, Van Soolingen D, Dale JW, Schuitema AR, McAdam RA, Catty D, et al. Insertion element *IS986* from *Mycobacterium tuberculosis*: a useful tool for diagnosis and epidemiology of tuberculosis. J Clin Microbiol. 1990;28(9):2051-8.

[71] Rodriguez JG, Fissanoti JC, Del Portillo P, Patarroyo ME, Romano MI, Cataldi A. Amplification of a 500-base-pair fragment from cultured isolates of *Mycobacterium bovis*. J Clin Microbiol. 1999;37(7):2330-2.

[72] Meikle V, Schneider M, Azenzo G, Zumarraga M, Magnano G, Cataldi A. Individual animals of a cattle herd infected with the same *Mycobacterium bovis* genotype shows important variations in bacteriological, histopathological and immune response parameters. Zoonoses Public Health. 2007;54(2):86-93.

[73] Cox JC, Coulter AR. Adjuvants--a classification and review of their modes of action. Vaccine. 1997;15(3):248-56.

[74] Milian-Suazo F, Salman MD, Ramirez C, Payeur JB, Rhyan JC, Santillan M. Identification of tuberculosis in cattle slaughtered in Mexico. Am J Vet Res. 2000;61(1):86-9.

[75] Latini O, Canal AM, Ferrara ME, Sequeira MD, Sequeira G, Bagnaroli R, et al. Confiabilidad en la determinación de prevalencia de infección por *Mycobacterium bovis* en ganado bovino por decomisos en frigoríficos. Arch med vet. 1997;29(2):197-204.

6

Early Exposure of Human Neutrophils to Mycobacteria Triggers Cell Damage and Pro-Inhibitory Molecules, but not Activation

M. Orozco-Uribe, L. Donis-Maturano, J. Calderón-Amador, R. Chacón-Salinas, J. Castañeda-Casimiro, S. Estrada-Parra, I. Estrada-García and L. Flores-Romo

1. Introduction

Mycobacterium tuberculosis (Mtb) is responsible for causing tuberculosis (TB) [1], a chronic re-emerging infectious disease with a major impact on public health worldwide [2]. Primary TB occurs by inhalation of microdroplets containing Mtb bacilli [3]. If the innate immune response is not efficient to control and eliminate the mycobacteria, then adaptive T cell responses might contain the bacteria resolving the infection [3-5].

Being TB a long-lasting affliction, most research on the immune responses to TB has addressed the chronic stages. In contrast, the earliest contacts of bacilli with cells responsible of the first defenses have been rather neglected, until recent years. Neutrophils (PMNs) are short-lived leukocytes, functioning as the primary defense against microorganisms [6, 7], with special ability to kill pathogens by phagocytosis, degranulation and the formation of extracellular traps [8-11]. The activation of neutrophils is associated with changes in the spatial and temporal expression of certain molecules [12, 13] such as CD16b, CD11b and CD66b, molecules responsible for adhesion, degranulation and migration, and are therefore well established as neutrophil activation markers [13-19]. On the other hand, it is documented that intracellular pathogens causing chronic infections can co-opt the pathway of a pair of molecules, PD-1 and its ligand PD-L1, involved in decreasing crucial T cell responses, provoking a phenomenon called "T cell exhaustion" [20]. In physiological conditions, this pathway is important for peripheral tolerance and the control of adaptive immune responses [21], but it has been barely explored in TB.

In this work we wanted to assess the phenotype of neutrophils during the very early interactions with three different strains from the *Mycobacterium tuberculosis*-complex.

2. Materials and methods

2.1. Ethics

This research was performed on healthy competent volunteers in accordance with the Declaration of Helsinki of the world Medical Association, and the Mexican General Health Law regarding research. The ethics committee of the National School of Biological Sciences ENCB-IPN approved this study (permission number: "Protocolo #CEI-ENCB 011/2013") and informed written consent was obtained from donors.

2.2. Bacterial strains and cultures

Mycobacterium tuberculosis H37Rv, *Mycobacterium canetti* and *Mycobacterium bovis* Bacillus Calmette-Guérin (BCG) strains were grown in Middlebrook 7H9 broth (Difco, Detroit, MI, USA. Cat. 271310), enriched with 10% OADC (Oleic, Albumin, Dextrose, Catalase) (Becton, Dickinson, USA. Cat. 211886) at 37°C until exponential growth phase. Bacteria were diluted in D-MEM (Dulbecco's modified Eagle's medium) (Invitrogen, Grand Island, NY, USA. Cat. 12430) supplemented with 10% FBS (fetal bovine sera) (Invitrogen, Grand Island, NY, USA. Cat. 16000). Mycobacteria were quantified prior to use.

2.3. Isolation of human neutrophils

Human blood neutrophils were isolated from healthy donors using two gradients: Histopaque 1119 (Sigma-Aldrich, St. Louis, MO, USA. Cat. 11191) for 20 min at 800g and Percoll (GE Healthcare Bio-sciences AB, Uppsala, Sweden. Cat. 17-0891-01) at the densities indicated next: 1105 g/mL (85%), 1100 g/mL (80%), 1093 g/mL (75%), 1087 g/mL (70%) y 1081 g/mL (65%), for 20 min at 800g.

2.4. Stimulation and staining of neutrophils

10^6 healthy neutrophils/mL of RPMI-1640 medium supplemented with 5% fetal bovine serum (FBS) were used either unstimulated or stimulated with 10 nM Phorbol 12-Myristate 13-Acetate (PMA) (Sigma-Aldrich, St. Louis, MO, USA. Cat. P-81-39), 5 μg/mL LPS (Sigma-Aldrich, St. Louis, MO, USA. Cat. L-3755), *Mycobacterium bovis* BCG, *Mycobacterium canetti* or *Mycobacterium tuberculosis* H37Rv at 37°C in 5% CO_2 atmosphere for 15, 30 and 60 min. Subsequently, cells were treated 5 min with universal blocking reagent (Biogenex¸ cat HK085-5K) and stained with different combinations of purified fluorochrome-conjugated antibodies: anti-human CD16b-APC (R&D Systems, Minneapolis, MN, USA. Cat. FAB2546A), CD66b-FITC (AbD Serotec, Kidlington, UK. Cat. MCA216F) and CD11b-PE (BD Pharmingen, San Jose, CA, USA. Cat. 340712). To evaluate the pro-inhibitory phenotype we used anti-human PD-1-FITC (BioLegend, San Diego, CA, USA. Cat. 329903) and anti-human PD-L1-PE (BioLegend, San

Diego, CA, USA. Cat. 329705). After this, cells were washed with 2 mL of FACS solution (PBS 1X, BSA 1%, Sodium azide 0.01%) and the events were acquired in FACS CyAn™ ADP (Beckman Coulter, Inc). FACS data were analyzed using FlowJo X 10.0.7r2 software (Tree Star Inc.)

2.5. Statistics

Statistics were performed with Two-way ANOVA using Bonferroni *t*-test for all multiple pairwise comparisons using GraphPad Prism 5 project (©2013 GraphPad Software).

3. Results

3.1. Neutrophils purity

Blood neutrophils from healthy donors were enriched to about 90% purity, which was checked through staining with Hematoxylin and Eosin (H&E) as well as by flow cytometry parameters such as cell size (FSC) vs. granularity/internal complexity (SSC) (Figure 1 A, B). PMNs were incubated either with culture medium alone, LPS, PMA or the various mycobacteria at two different multiplicity of infection (MOI: 0.1, 1) of *Mycobacterium bovis* BCG, *Mycobacterium canetti* and *Mycobacterium tuberculosis* H37Rv. To corroborate that isolated neutrophils were not contaminated with other leukocyte subpopulations, by means of Fluorescence Activated Cell Sorter (FACS) we evaluated the presence of T lymphocytes (Lc), B Lc and macrophages (Mfs) using specific antibodies to CD3, CD19 and CD14 (Figure 1 B right panel).

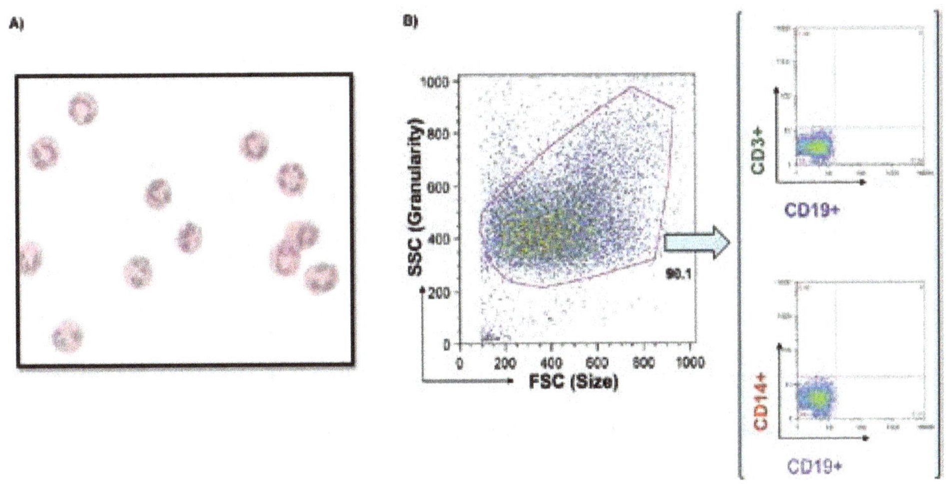

Figure 1. Analysis of peripheral blood neutrophils isolated from healthy donors. Enriched Neutrophils were analyzed both by staining with H&E (A) and by flow cytometry (B). By flow cytometry (B) we evaluated the Size and Granularity (left panel) of the isolated PMNs. The purity of the PMN-enriched cell suspensions was also verified by using markers both for T and B cells (right top panel) and macrophages (right bottom panel).

3.2. *Mycobacterium* affects neutrophils integrity at early times of interactions

By means of flow cytometry we analyzed the neutrophils incubated either with culture medium alone, LPS, PMA, *Mycobacterium bovis* BCG, *Mycobacterium canetti* or *Mycobacterium tuberculosis* H37Rv. We observed an increase in neutrophils autofluorescence, i.e., those that were incubated only with mycobacteria but that were not labeled with any fluorescent reagent at all. Autofluorescence was analyzed in a free channel or filter without staining (FL-6=405 nm) (figure 2). In flow cytometry it has long been described that autofluorescence indicates (membrane) cell damage or even cell death [22-27]. In this case, the neutrophils incubated with BCG or with Mtb H37Rv increased their autofluorescence emission since early times of exposure to mycobacteria. At 15 min of incubation (figure 2B, D) approximately 60-80% of PMNs were autofluorescent, while for neutrophils interacting with *Mycobacterium canetti* the autofluorescence increased approx. 15% at 30 minutes (figure 2G). In contrast, neutrophils incubated with culture medium alone showed basal levels, approximately 10% of autofluorescence (figure 2 A, E, I)

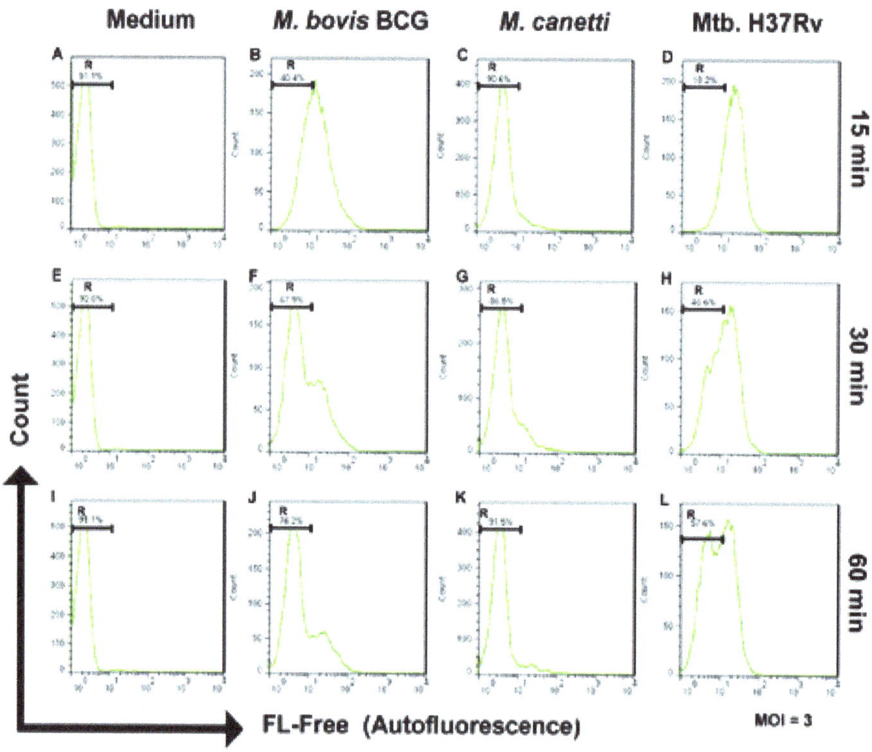

Figure 2. Mycobacteria of different virulence can induce damage to neutrophils at early exposure times, as determined by autofluorescence using flow cytometry. Healthy volunteers' neutrophils were incubated 15, 30 and 60 min with either culture medium alone (Medium), *Mycobacterium bovis* (BCG), *Mycobacterium canetti* or *Mycobacterium tuberculosis* H37Rv. Histograms show the autofluorescence emitted by neutrophils in a free channel (FL-6=405 nm) when using bacilli at a multiplicity of infection (MOI) of 3:1 for each mycobacterial strain.

3.3. Mycobacteria do not activate neutrophils at early times of interaction

Blood neutrophils incubated separately with three different strains of Mycobacteria (BCG, Canetti and Mtb) were evaluated for the expression of CD16b (Figure 3), CD11b and CD66b (Figure 4), at 15, 30 and 60 min incubation. Although these molecules are constitutively expressed on neutrophils, it is well documented that neutrophils modify the expression of these markers upon activation [13, 15, 17, 19, 28-30].

Neutrophils incubated with mycobacteria did not display changes in the percentages of expression of CD16b (Figure 3A), CD11b, CD66b (Figure 4A, C) at the 3 time-points evaluated. There was, however, a decreased in the *median fluorescence intensity* (MFI) for CD16b (figure 3B) and CD66b (figure 4D) and an increment for CD11b (Figure 4B) with Mtb at 15 min incubation, compared with neutrophils in culture medium alone. Short incubation periods with the microbial product LPS or with PMA (both used as positive controls) increased the expression of CD11b (figure 4B) and CD66b (figure 4C), i.e., since 15 min of exposure.

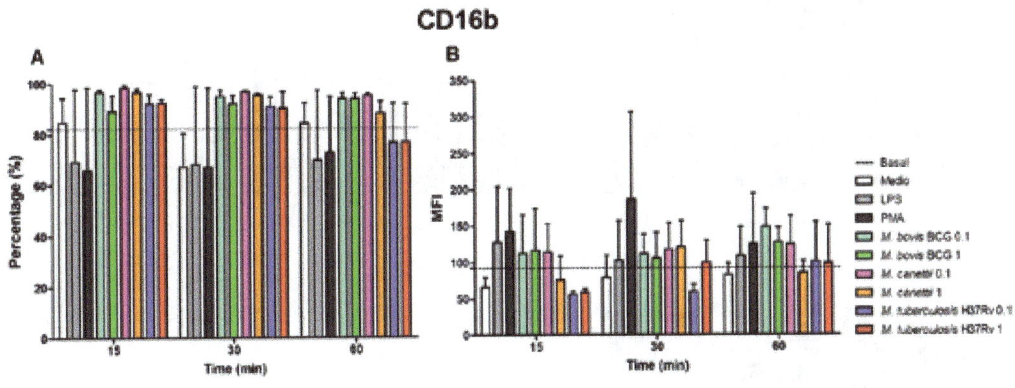

Figure 3. FcγRIIIb-expression in neutrophils exposed to different Mycobacteria. Healthy donor neutrophils were incubated with medium alone (white bars), LPS (gray bars), PMA (black bars), *Mycobacterium bovis* (BCG) MOI 0.1 (aqua bars) and 1 (green bars), *Mycobacterium canetti* MOI 0.1 (pink bars) and 1 (orange bars) and *Mycobacterium tuberculosis* H37Rv MOI 0.1 (blue violet bars) and 1 (red bars). Percentage (A) and MFI (B) of neutrophils labeled for CD16b evaluated at 15, 30 and 60 min incubation with mycobacteria of different virulence. Error bars denote the s.e.m. and dotted lines represent the basal level of CD16b expression (A, B). s.e.m: standard error mean, MFI: Median fluorescence intensity, MOI: Multiplicity of infection, M: *Mycobacterium.*

3.4. Mycobacteria rapidly induce pro-inhibitory molecules on neutrophils

Mycobacteria have evolved diverse mechanisms to escape, divert or even subvert the immune responses [4, 31]. The molecular pair PD1-PD-L1 has been recently shown to induce a phenomenon called T cell exhaustion, and the expression of these two molecules has been shown manipulated by certain pathogens for their advantage [32, 33]. The percentage of PD1 expression in neutrophils incubated with mycobacteria increased only with Mtb H37Rv (figure 5A, black arrows) since 15 min, compared with basal expression levels. In contrast, PMNs interacting with the other mycobacterial strains did not modify the percentage of PD-1 expression (Figure 5A). Regarding MFI we observed a decrease in PD-1 intensity in neutrophils incubated with Mtb H37Rv MOI:1 at 15 and 30 min, but an increase at 60 min (figure 5B, black arrow). With respect to PD-1 Ligand (PD-L1), the percentage increased in neutrophils incubated with BCG and *Mycobacterium canetti* at 15 min, compared with basal controls (Figure 5C). Neutrophils incubated with Mtb H37Rv show a tendency to increase the MFI of PD-L1 at 15 and 60 min of incubation (figure 5D, blue arrow), this increase was more clear after 60 min, compared with basal intensity and with the other mycobacterial strains tested.

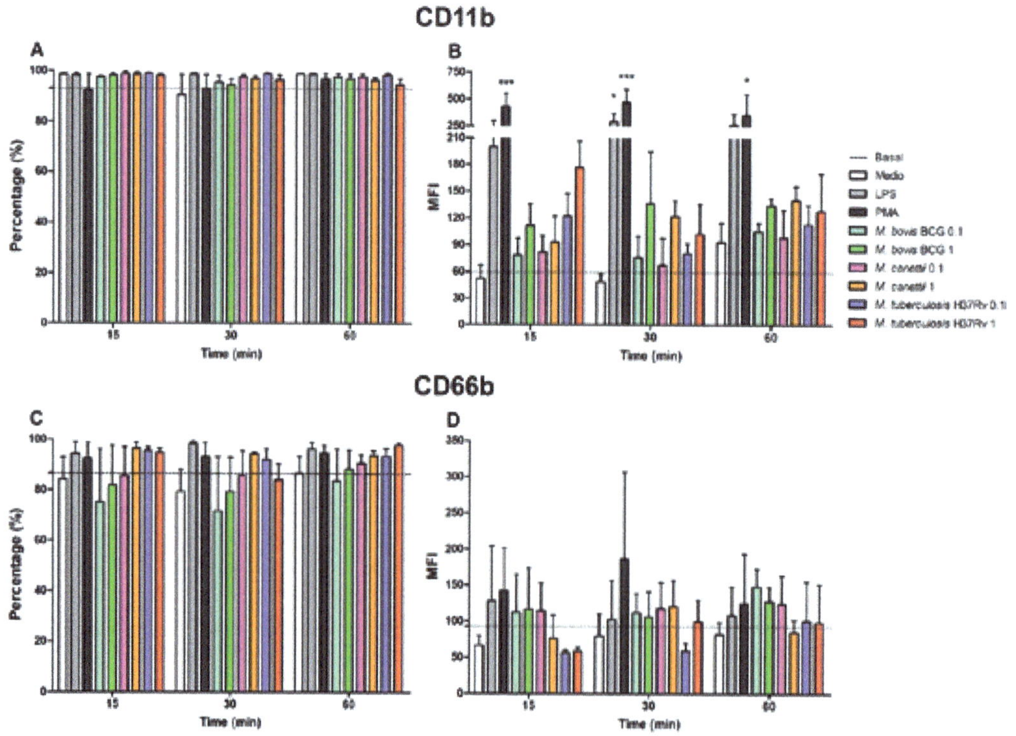

Figure 4. Activation kinetics of human neutrophils exposed to different Mycobacteria. Healthy donor neutrophils were incubated with culture medium alone (white bars), LPS (gray bars), PMA (black bars), *Mycobacterium bovis* (BCG) MOI 0.1 (aqua bars) and 1 (green bars), *Mycobacterium canetti* MOI 0.1 (pink bars) and 1 (orange bars) and *Mycobacterium tuberculosis* H37Rv MOI 0.1 (blue violet bars) and 1 (red bars). Percentage (A, C) and MFI (B, D) of neutrophils labeled for CD11b and CD66b evaluated at 15, 30 and 60 min incubation with different bacilli. Error bars denote the s.e.m. and dotted lines represent CD11b (A,B) and CD66b (C,D) basal expression. *P=0.01; ***P < 0.0001, one-way ANOVA, s.e.m: standard error mean, MFI: Median fluorescence intensity, MOI: Multiplicity of infection, M: *Mycobacterium*.

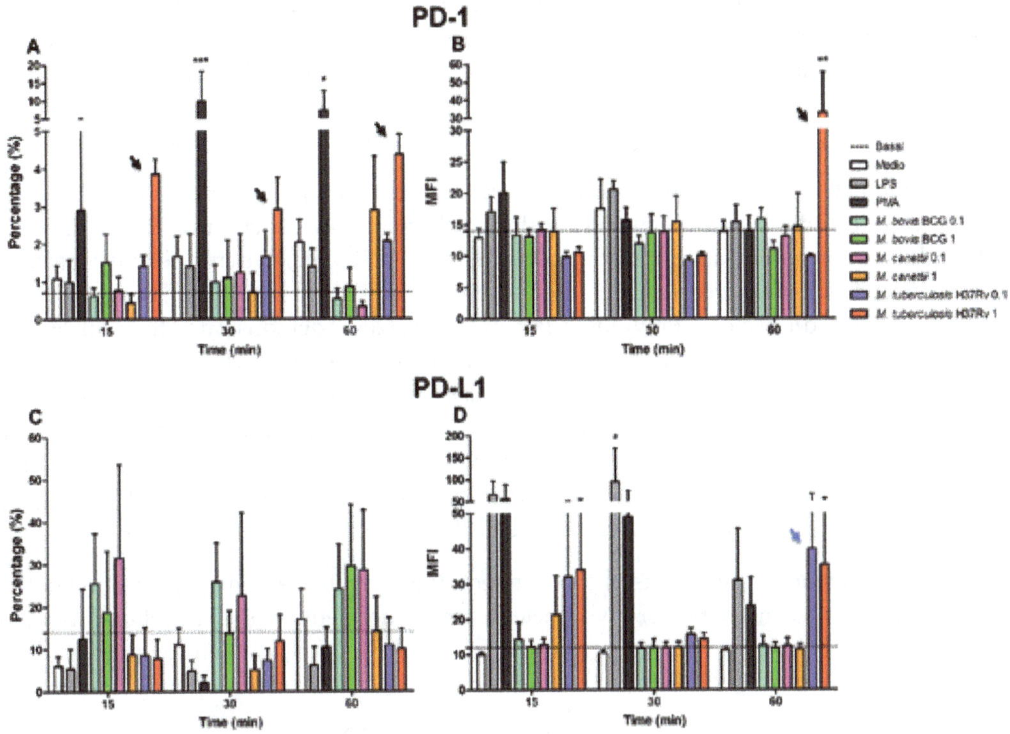

Figure 5. Kinetics of expression of pro-inhibitory molecules in neutrophils exposed to Mycobacteria at early time points. Healthy donor neutrophils were incubated with medium alone (white bars), LPS (gray bars), PMA (black bars), *Mycobacterium bovis* (BCG) MOI 0.1 (aqua bars) and 1 (green bars), *Mycobacterium canetti* MOI 0.1 (pink bars) and 1 (orange bars) and *Mycobacterium tuberculosis* (Mtb) H37Rv MOI 0.1 (blue violet bars) and 1 (red bars). Percentage (A, C) and MFI (B, D) of neutrophils labeled for PD-1 and PD-L1 evaluated at 15, 30 and 60 min incubation with different mycobacteria. Error bars denote the s.e.m. and dotted lines represent the basal levels for PD-1 (A, B) and PD-L1 (C, D). *P=0.01; **P=0.001; ***P < 0.0001, one-way ANOVA, s.e.m: standard error mean, MFI: Median fluorescence intensity, MOI: Multiplicity of infection, M: *Mycobacterium.*

4. Discussion

Mycobacterium tuberculosis is the causative agent of tuberculosis (TB) [1]. According to the World Health Organization (WHO), TB caused the death of 1.3 million people worldwide in 2012 [2]. Despite the vast amount of TB research in more than 100 years, there are still many aspects of the disease that remain poorly known, for instance the host's innate response during the earliest stages of the infection. The involvement of neutrophils in the immune response against Mtb has been rather neglected until recently. Conceivably, this might be due to the short life span of these cells, the quickness of their mechanisms of action and also to the chronicity of TB.

We aimed at assessing activation as well as pro-inhibitory molecules on neutrophils from healthy donors using flow cytometry, thus PMNs were incubated for short periods with three different strains of mycobacteria. As positive controls for PMN activation at the time points evaluated, we used two standard components, a microbial one such as lipopolysaccharide (LPS), and a chemical one such as phorbol myristate acetate (PMA). At least two main FACS criteria were evaluated, the percentage of cells and the median fluorescence intensity (MFI). The latter directly reflects the intensity of expression of a given molecule in the cells evaluated.

In flow cytometry the emission of autofluorescence in both animal and plants cells has been indicative of cell damage or even cell death. In addition, the reduction of NADH induces intracellular fluorescence, also indicating cell damage [22-27]. When we cultured mycobacteria with neutrophils, these increased their autofluorescence emission since 15 min, compared with neutrophils in medium alone. Previously, Perskvist *et al.* (2002) demonstrated that Mtb H37Rv induced apoptosis in neutrophils, but this was evaluated at 5h of interaction [34, 35]. However other studies of neutrophils with *Leishmania major* showed increased IL-8 production and inhibition of apoptosis at 24h [36]. Corleis *et al.* (2012) described that at 20 min, neutrophils can kill *Mycobacterium smegmatis* but not *Mycobacterium tuberculosis* [37]. In addition, Ramos-Kichik *et al.* (2009) showed that Mtb induced neutrophil extracellular traps (NETs) at 180 min [38], compared with other microorganisms such as *C. albicans* that do it in shorter time [39].

Few and recent studies have focused on the effects that mycobacteria might have on neutrophils [40-42], for instance whether mycobacteria can induce neutrophil extracellular traps, as seen when PMNs interact with other microorganisms [38]. Of note, even the phenotype of neutrophils during and after their interaction with mycobacteria remains poorly addressed.

From the set of molecules that we measured, some (CD16b, CD11b, CD66b) are well established neutrophil activation markers, while the others (PD1/PD1-L) are very important pro-inhibitory molecules. Interestingly, however, even at the longest time of incubation with mycobacteria (60 min), we did not observe statistically significant differences in the percentages of PMNs expressing CD16b, CD11b or CD66b, compared to neutrophils incubated with the control substances LPS, PMA or with culture medium alone. In contrast, it is known that certain components from microorganisms such as *E. coli, S. thyphimurium. S. flexneri* and *Y. enterocolitica* induce activation of neutrophils at early times (30 min) of exposure [43]. Interestingly, even at 15 min incubation the percentage and the MFI of CD11b, CD66b, CD18 or CD62L increased in human healthy neutrophils incubated with DNA of E. coli, LPS, fMLP, C5a and three different strains of *Staphylococcus aureus* [19, 44].

On the other hand, decrease in surface CD16b in neutrophils is also related to the activation of these cells [29, 30]. When we analyzed the median fluorescence intensity (MFI) of CD16b on mycobacteria-incubated neutrophils, we did not find significant differences compared to the controls, although there was a slight decrease at 15 minutes in cells incubated with Mtb H37Rv compared to freshly isolated neutrophils. Regarding the expression of CD11b and CD66b, both LPS and PMA (used as positive controls for stimulation), increased the expression of these two markers since 15 minutes compared to neutrophils in medium alone, indicative of the intact capacity of neutrophils to respond. Although there was a subtle decrease in CD66b expression at 15 minutes of incubation with bacilli, compared to freshly isolated neutrophils.

Previous studies have evaluated the expression of CD16b and CD66b as activation markers in neutrophils from patients with active TB [45]. Likewise, in healthy neutrophils incubated with clinical isolates of Mtb, the expression of CD16, CD69 and CXCR2 was evaluated, but only at 3 and 18 h [46]. Hilda *et al.* in 2012 demonstrated that the virulent strain Mtb H37Rv can modulate the expression of FcγRII (CD32), FcγRI (CD64), TLR-4 and CXCR3 in neutrophils, while BCG increased CD32 expression only, and a vaccine strain, *Mycobacterium indicus pranii,* did not produce any apparent effect with MOI: 3, all at 4h of incubation [47]. We did not see differences in neutrophil activation in response to the three strains of mycobacteria, regardless of their different virulence.

The PD-1/PD-L1 pathway is important for the establishment and maintenance of peripheral tolerance as well as to modulate immune and inflammatory responses to pathogens [21, 48]. This pathway has been found altered during chronic viral [49, 50], parasitic [51], fungal [52] and bacterial [32] infections, provoking a phenomenon known as "exhaustion" in CD8+T cells, exerting an inhibitory effect related to pathogens evasion of immune responses [20]. Apparently, Mtb H37Rv can also modulate and manipulate the PD/PD-L1 path not only in T cells, but also in antigen presenting cells and even in elements of the innate immune response, such as NK cells [53]. However, this pair of molecules has been poorly explored in neutrophils, especially in the interplay with microorganisms. Therefore, we sought to evaluate also the neutrophils expression of PD-1 and PD-L1 in the early response to mycobacteria. There was an apparent increase in the proportion of neutrophils expressing surface PD-1 following incubation with Mtb H37Rv (MOI 1), which was more evident at 60 minutes; although not statistically significant. These results are interesting and opposed to data by Yao *et al.* (2009) where they reported that neither NK cells, macrophages nor neutrophils express PD-1 during infection with *Listeria monocytogenes* [54]. On the other hand, we did not observe changes in the proportion of neutrophils expressing PD-L1 after incubation with the different mycobacteria strains at the time points we evaluated. Regarding the mean fluorescence intensity (MFI) of PD-1, we observed that at 15 and 30 min there were no differences in its expression in neutrophils incubated with mycobacteria. However, at 60 min the expression of PD-1 increased importantly in neutrophils but only with Mtb H37Rv at MOI 1. When evaluating the MFI for PD-L1 we did not find significant differences among neutrophils incubated with mycobacteria or with culture medium alone. McNab *et al.* (2011) also evaluated these pro-inhibitory molecules but at the mRNA level in the blood from tuberculosis patients [55]. They found that the polymorphonuclear population overexpressed the PD-1 ligand in patients with active TB, in comparison to patients with latent TB and healthy donors.

Our results indicate that, while neutrophils are readily stimulated upon short time of incubation with either LPS or PMA, they do not get activated during early interactions with three mycobacteria of different virulence. This is revealed by the PMNs inability to modify activation molecules which are involved in crucial processes such as migration, adhesion, phagocytosis and degranulation. However, at these early times of interactions with mycobacteria, there are indeed alterations occurring in other important molecules in PMNs, such as PD1/PD1-L.

It is conceivable that early during a mycobacterial infection neutrophils might encounter and interact with other recruited cells of the immune system while still expressing inhibitory molecules such as PD-1 or PD-L1, thus limiting the intensity of the response at the site of infection. The fact that neutrophils infected with Mtb express both the receptor and the ligand of PD-1 could be related to an autocrine regulation of this population. Further experiments are required to understand the role of the early innate immune response against *Mycobacterium tuberculosis*. Since there are few studies focused on the neutrophils phenotype during the very early interactions with mycobacteria, we consider our results of interest and we expect that this work will instigate more research on the participation of neutrophils during the early stages of mycobacterial infection.

List of abbreviations

BCG: Bacillus Calmette-Guérin

FACS: Fluorescence Activated Cell Sorter

MFI: Median fluorescence intensity

Mfs: Macrophages

MOI: Multiplicity of infection

Mtb: *Mycobacterium tuberculosis*

PMN: Polymorfonuclear leukocytes or Neutrophils

TB: Tuberculosis

Acknowledgements

I Estrada-García, S Estrada-Parra, R Chacon-Salinas, J Calderon-Amador and L Flores-Romo are members of the National System of Researchers (SNI) from Mexico. I Estrada-García (Conacyt project 221002), S Estrada-Parra, R Chacon-Salinas are fellow-holders from EDI and COFAA. M Orozco-Uribe, J Castañeda-Casimiro and L Donis-Maturano were fellow-holders from the National Council for Science and Technology, Conacyt. LDM was a postdoctoral fellow from Conacyt. Authors acknowledge the help from V Rosales at the FACS facilities.

Author details

M. Orozco-Uribe[1], L. Donis-Maturano[1], J. Calderón-Amador[1], R. Chacón-Salinas[2], J. Castañeda-Casimiro[2], S. Estrada-Parra[2], I. Estrada-García[2] and L. Flores-Romo[1*]

*Address all correspondence to: lefloresromo@gmail.com

1 Department of Cell Biology, CINVESTAV-IPN, Zacatenco, México City, Mexico

2 Department of Immunology, ENCB-IPN, México City, Mexico

References

[1] Maartens, G. and R.J. Wilkinson, *Tuberculosis.* Lancet, 2007. 370(9604): p. 2030-43.

[2] (WHO), W.H.O., *Global Tuberculosis Report 2013.* 2013.

[3] Martineau, A.R., et al., *Neutrophil-mediated innate immune resistance to mycobacteria.* J Clin Invest, 2007. 117(7): p. 1988-94.

[4] Gupta, A., et al., *Mycobacterium tuberculosis: immune evasion, latency and reactivation.* Immunobiology, 2012. 217(3): p. 363-74.

[5] Zuniga, J., et al., *Cellular and humoral mechanisms involved in the control of tuberculosis.* Clin Dev Immunol, 2012. 2012: p. 193923.

[6] Zychlinsky, A., Y. Weinrauch, and J. Weiss, *Introduction: Forum in immunology on neutrophils.* Microbes Infect, 2003. 5(14): p. 1289-91.

[7] Pruchniak, M.P., M. Arazna, and U. Demkow, *Life of neutrophil: From stem cell to neutrophil extracellular trap.* Respir Physiol Neurobiol, 2013. 187(1): p. 68-73.

[8] Brinkmann, V., et al., *Neutrophil extracellular traps kill bacteria.* Science, 2004. 303(5663): p. 1532-5.

[9] Simon, H.U., *Neutrophil apoptosis pathways and their modifications in inflammation.* Immunol Rev, 2003. 193: p. 101-10.

[10] Zakhireh, B., L.H. Block, and R.K. Root, *Neutrophil function and host resistance.* Infection, 1979. 7(2): p. 88-98.

[11] Fox, S., et al., *Neutrophil apoptosis: relevance to the innate immune response and inflammatory disease.* J Innate Immun, 2010. 2(3): p. 216-27.

[12] Smith, J.A., *Neutrophils, host defense, and inflammation: a double-edged sword.* J Leukoc Biol, 1994. 56(6): p. 672-86.

[13] Nair, K.S. and S.M. Zingde, *Adhesion of neutrophils to fibronectin: role of the cd66 antigens.* Cell Immunol, 2001. 208(2): p. 96-106.

[14] Witko-Sarsat, V., et al., *Neutrophils: molecules, functions and pathophysiological aspects.* Lab Invest, 2000. 80(5): p. 617-53.

[15] David, A., et al., *Interaction of proteinase 3 with CD11b/CD18 (beta2 integrin) on the cell membrane of human neutrophils.* J Leukoc Biol, 2003. 74(4): p. 551-7.

[16] Schroder, A.K., et al., *Crosslinking of CD66B on peripheral blood neutrophils mediates the release of interleukin-8 from intracellular storage.* Hum Immunol, 2006. 67(9): p. 676-82.

[17] Feuk-Lagerstedt, E., et al., *Identification of CD66a and CD66b as the major galectin-3 receptor candidates in human neutrophils.* J Immunol, 1999. 163(10): p. 5592-8.

[18] Skubitz, K.M., K.D. Campbell, and A.P. Skubitz, *CD66a, CD66b, CD66c, and CD66d each independently stimulate neutrophils.* J Leukoc Biol, 1996. 60(1): p. 106-17.

[19] Schmidt, T., et al., *CD66b overexpression and homotypic aggregation of human peripheral blood neutrophils after activation by a gram-positive stimulus.* J Leukoc Biol, 2012. 91(5): p. 791-802.

[20] Hofmeyer, K.A., H. Jeon, and X. Zang, *The PD-1/PD-L1 (B7-H1) pathway in chronic infection-induced cytotoxic T lymphocyte exhaustion.* J Biomed Biotechnol, 2011. 2011: p. 451694.

[21] Folkl, A. and D. Bienzle, *Structure and function of programmed death (PD) molecules.* Vet Immunol Immunopathol, 2010. 134(1-2): p. 33-8.

[22] Barenboim GM, D.A., Turoverov KK (Eds.), *Luminescence of Biopolymers and Cells.* 1969, New York: Plenum Press.

[23] Chance, B. and B. Thorell, *Localization and kinetics of reduced pyridine nucleotide in living cells by microfluorometry.* J Biol Chem, 1959. 234: p. 3044-50.

[24] Davis, R.P. and M. Canessa-Fischer, *Spectrofluorometric Identification of Reduced Pyridine Nucleotide in the Intact Isolated Urinary Bladder of the Toad.* Anal Biochem, 1965. 10: p. 325-43.

[25] Haitinger, M., *Fluoresenz-Mikroskopie.* 1959, Leipzig: Academie-Verlag.

[26] Pearse, A., *Histochemistry: Theoretical and Applied.* 1972, London: churchill Livingstone Co.

[27] Udenfriend, S., *Fluorescence Assay in Biology and Medicine.* 1969, New York: Academic Press.

[28] Silveira, A.A., et al., *Simvastatin abrogates inflamed neutrophil adhesive properties, in association with the inhibition of Mac-1 integrin expression and modulation of Rho kinase activity.* Inflamm Res, 2013. 62(2): p. 127-32.

[29] Leino, L. and E.M. Lilius, *The up-and down-modulation of immunoglobulin G Fc receptors and complement receptors on activated human neutrophils depends on the nature of activator.* J Leukoc Biol, 1992. 51(2): p. 157-63.

[30] Nagarajan, S., N.H. Fifadara, and P. Selvaraj, *Signal-specific activation and regulation of human neutrophil Fc gamma receptors.* J Immunol, 2005. 174(9): p. 5423-32.

[31] Meena, L.S. and Rajni, *Survival mechanisms of pathogenic Mycobacterium tuberculosis H37Rv.* FEBS J, 2010. 277(11): p. 2416-27.

[32] Jurado, J.O., et al., *Programmed death (PD)-1:PD-ligand 1/PD-ligand 2 pathway inhibits T cell effector functions during human tuberculosis.* J Immunol, 2008. 181(1): p. 116-25.

[33] Donis-Maturano, L., *Caracterización fenotípica de las subpoblaciones de linfocitos T en parénquima pulmonar murino durante la infección con Mycobacterium tuberculosis,* in *Depar-*

*tamento de Inmunología*2006, Escuela Nacional de Ciencias Biológicas (ENCB)-IPN: México, D.F.

[34] Perskvist, N., et al., *Mycobacterium tuberculosis promotes apoptosis in human neutrophils by activating caspase-3 and altering expression of Bax/Bcl-xL via an oxygen-dependent pathway.* J Immunol, 2002. 168(12): p. 6358-65.

[35] Blomgran, R., et al., *Mycobacterium tuberculosis inhibits neutrophil apoptosis, leading to delayed activation of naive CD4 T cells.* Cell Host Microbe, 2012. 11(1): p. 81-90.

[36] Aga, E., et al., *Inhibition of the spontaneous apoptosis of neutrophil granulocytes by the intracellular parasite Leishmania major.* J Immunol, 2002. 169(2): p. 898-905.

[37] Corleis, B., et al., *Escape of Mycobacterium tuberculosis from oxidative killing by neutrophils.* Cell Microbiol, 2012. 14(7): p. 1109-21.

[38] Ramos-Kichik, V., et al., *Neutrophil extracellular traps are induced by Mycobacterium tuberculosis.* Tuberculosis (Edinb), 2009. 89(1): p. 29-37.

[39] Urban, C.F., et al., *Neutrophil extracellular traps capture and kill Candida albicans yeast and hyphal forms.* Cell Microbiol, 2006. 8(4): p. 668-76.

[40] Pedrosa, J., et al., *Neutrophils play a protective nonphagocytic role in systemic Mycobacterium tuberculosis infection of mice.* Infect Immun, 2000. 68(2): p. 577-83.

[41] Kisich, K.O., et al., *Tumor necrosis factor alpha stimulates killing of Mycobacterium tuberculosis by human neutrophils.* Infect Immun, 2002. 70(8): p. 4591-9.

[42] Persson, A., et al., *Induction of apoptosis in human neutrophils by Mycobacterium tuberculosis is dependent on mature bacterial lipoproteins.* Microb Pathog, 2009. 47(3): p. 143-50.

[43] Soler-Rodriguez, A.M., et al., *Neutrophil activation by bacterial lipoprotein versus lipopolysaccharide: differential requirements for serum and CD14.* J Immunol, 2000. 164(5): p. 2674-83.

[44] Alvarez, M.E., et al., *Neutrophil signaling pathways activated by bacterial DNA stimulation.* J Immunol, 2006. 177(6): p. 4037-46.

[45] Aleman, M., et al., *Activation of peripheral blood neutrophils from patients with active advanced tuberculosis.* Clin Immunol, 2001. 100(1): p. 87-95.

[46] Pokkali, S., et al., *Phenotypic modulation in Mycobacterium tuberculosis infected neutrophil during tuberculosis.* Indian J Med Res, 2009. 130(2): p. 185-92.

[47] Hilda, J.N., A. Selvaraj, and S.D. Das, *Mycobacterium tuberculosis H37Rv is more effective compared to vaccine strains in modulating neutrophil functions: an in vitro study.* FEMS Immunol Med Microbiol, 2012. 66(3): p. 372-81.

[48] Odorizzi, P.M. and E.J. Wherry, *Inhibitory receptors on lymphocytes: insights from infections.* J Immunol, 2012. 188(7): p. 2957-65.

[49] Barber, D.L., et al., *Restoring function in exhausted CD8 T cells during chronic viral infection.* Nature, 2006. 439(7077): p. 682-7.

[50] Freeman, G.J., et al., *Reinvigorating exhausted HIV-specific T cells via PD-1-PD-1 ligand blockade.* J Exp Med, 2006. 203(10): p. 2223-7.

[51] Gutierrez, F.R., et al., *Regulation of Trypanosoma cruzi-induced myocarditis by programmed death cell receptor 1.* Infect Immun, 2011. 79(5): p. 1873-81.

[52] Lazar-Molnar, E., et al., *The PD-1/PD-L costimulatory pathway critically affects host resistance to the pathogenic fungus Histoplasma capsulatum.* Proc Natl Acad Sci U S A, 2008. 105(7): p. 2658-63.

[53] Alvarez, I.B., et al., *Role played by the programmed death-1-programmed death ligand pathway during innate immunity against Mycobacterium tuberculosis.* J Infect Dis, 2010. 202(4): p. 524-32.

[54] Yao, S., et al., *PD-1 on dendritic cells impedes innate immunity against bacterial infection.* Blood, 2009. 113(23): p. 5811-8.

[55] McNab, F.W., et al., *Programmed death ligand 1 is over-expressed* by neutrophils in the blood of patients with active tuberculosis. Eur J Immunol, 2011. 41(7): p. 1941-7.

7

ENT Manifestations in Tuberculosis

Luiz Alberto Alves Mota,
Paula Cristina Alves Leitão and
Ana Maria dos Anjos Carneiro-Leão

1. Introduction

Tuberculosis (TB) is one of the oldest diseases that afflicts mankind, and has re-emerged as a significant cause of morbidity and mortality in several countries [1]. It is an infectious and contagious disease caused by a bacterium, *Mycobacterium tuberculosis,* also called Koch's Bacillus (KB) [2]. According to the location of the outbreak, it can be classified as pulmonary TB, primary TB, TB reactivation and extrapulmonary TB [3].

2. Epidemiology

According to the World Health Organization (WHO), there were nearly nine million new cases in 2011, and about 1.4 million TB deaths (990,000 among Human Immunodeficiency Virus (HIV) negative people and 430,000 TB deaths associated with HIV). TB is also more common in men than in women, affecting in particular adults in economically productive age groups [

Figure 1 shows the estimated number of TB cases and deaths [4]. 4].

The estimates show that most cases have occurred in Asia (59%) and Africa (26%). Smaller proportions of the global total have occurred in the Eastern Mediterranean Region (7.7%), Europe (4.3%) and the Americas (3%) [4].

Figure 2 shows the estimated incidence rates of TB in each country [4].

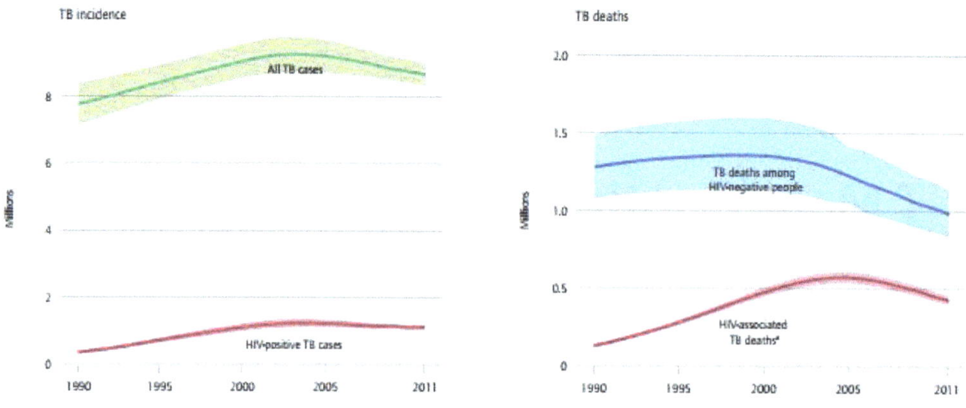

Figure 1. Estimated absolute numbers of TB cases and deaths (in millions), 1990–2011.

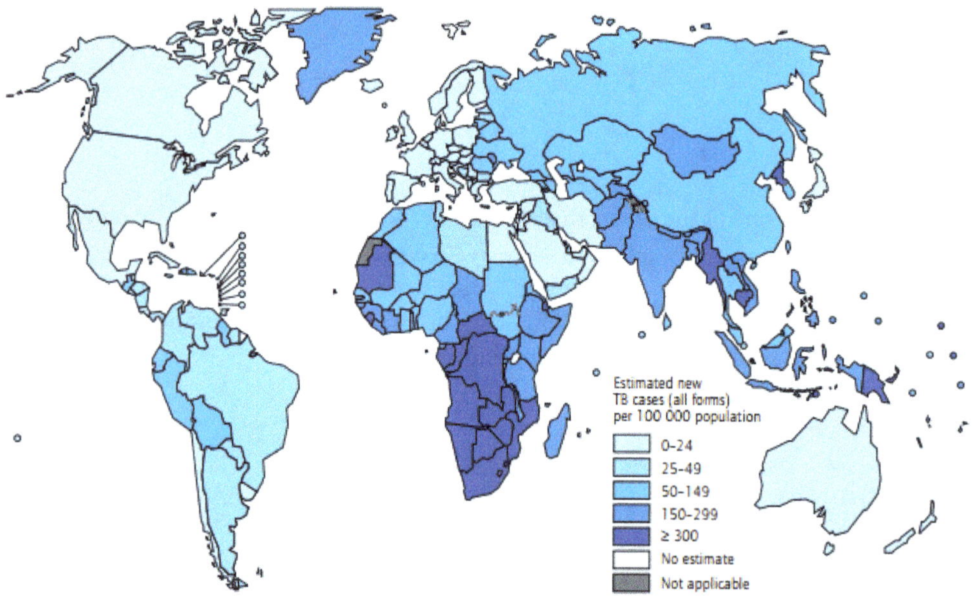

Figure 2. Estimated TB incidence rates, 2011.

In Brazil, TB is still a serious health problem. Each year, approximately 70,000 new cases are reported and 4,600 deaths occur due to the disease [5]. In Pernambuco in 2012, the incidence rate of TB was 52.21 per 100 thousand inhabitants with 3,879 new cases of pulmonary TB reported, of which 2,657 were in the metropolitan region of Recife [6].

3. Transmission

Transmission usually occurs through direct contact of the patient with a healthy person. Indirect contagion by handling contaminated material and animals can take place, but this is exceptional. When one coughs, sneezes or talks, Flügge droplets are exhaled, which can lead to contagion in a healthy individual. The gateway in about 90% of cases is the airway. Therefore, pulmonary TB is the dominant form. Other pathways, may, however, be conduits, such as the digestive system, skin, tonsils, eye and others that might have direct contact with the aggressor agent [7].

4. Clinical manifestations

Manifestations of TB in cervico-cephalic regions are among the most frequent, and have attracted interest mainly because of the changes in the pattern of attack of the disease. This is because it is currently uncommon to find acute or rapidly progressive forms, it being more frequent to find forms that evolve with a subclinical pattern [8].

In the region of the head and neck, TB manifests itself predominantly in the larynx; less frequently, it is found in the middle and external ear, tonsils, cervical lymph nodes, pharynx, oral cavity, and salivary glands [9].

4.1. Laryngeal TB

One of the organs that can be secondarily affected by TB is the larynx, even although in some cases, laryngeal TB may have a primary involvement [7].

There are two theories that attempt to explain its pathogenesis: bronchogenic theory, which is the most accepted, says bronchogenic secretions are responsible for contaminating the larynx through the direct contact of the secretions with the laryngeal mucosa; and hematogenous theory, which says that *Mycobacterium tuberculosis* reaches the blood and lymph vessels and thus affects the larynx, it being possible for there not to be any pulmonary damage [10].

Before the use of antibiotic therapy, laryngeal TB was considered one of the most serious complications of pulmonary TB and was often fatal. In the 1940s, after the development of various treatment regimens, the incidence of pulmonary TB decreased and pharyngolaryngeal involvement became less frequent. However, in the last two decades due to the decline in the quality of treatment and supervision worldwide, and as a consequence of the emergence of AIDS as a global epidemic and the development of multidrug-resistant strains of TB, the number of cases of the disease has been increasing progressively [11].

In the clinical framework of laryngeal TB, the most common symptom is dysphonia, which is present in 100% of patients in many studies, and this can progress to aphonia. In addition, other important manifestations include dysphagia due to ulceration of the laryngeal vestibule or perichondritis of the cricoid cartilage; cough and hemoptysis because of the affect on the lungs; dyspnea due to edema or laryngeal granulomas that may obstruct light from the larynx [12].

In laryngeal TB, the most commonly affected site is the region of the vocal folds, followed by the vestibular folds and may involve the epiglottis, the aryepiglottic fold, the arytenoids, the posterior commissure and the subglottis [10]. Figure 3 shows a lesion in the posterior third of the left vocal fold [7].

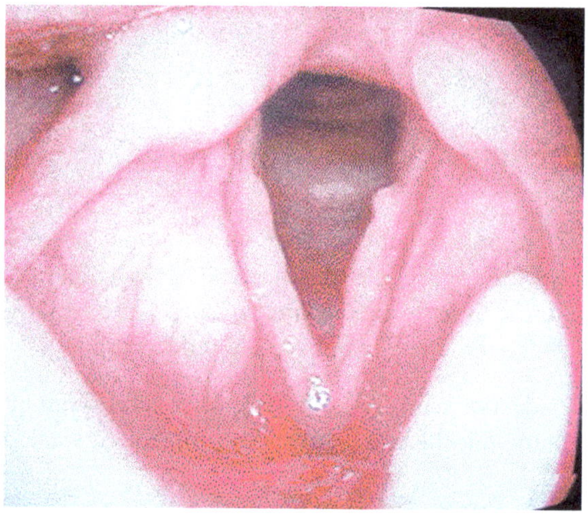

Figure 3. A lesion in the posterior third of the left vocal fold.

4.2. TB of cervical lymph nodes

Lymph node TB may result from dissemination via the blood stream, of bacillary pulmonary foci [13], as well as from the bacilli gaining entrance via the tonsils, dental or pharyngeal foci [14]. It is located most frequently in the cervical, supraclavicular and hilar and mediastinal regions. However, any lymph node may be affected [13].

It is one of the most prevalent forms of TB in the head and neck. In general, it presents itself insidiously with a gradual increase in the lymph node and evolution to caseification [14].

No gender difference was found among those suffering from TB in cervical lymph nodes. However, what was verified is that there was greater prevalence in the 35-44 year-old age group [15].

4.3. TB of the ear

TB located in the middle ear as the primary focus is uncommon. Classically it affects children more than adults [9].

Several theories attempt to explain the infection of the middle ear by TB, but its pathogenesis is still controversial. It is suggested that routes may be through the bloodstream by direct extension from the nasopharynx through the Eustachian tube via the lymphatic system; externally, by perforation of the tympanic membrane; by direct extension from adjacent structures, the central nervous system, congenital infection (via the placenta) or during passage through the birth canal [9].

Classically it is presented as the triad: painless otorrhea, multiple perforation of the tympanic membrane, and peripheral facial palsy; but currently its presentation has become polymorphic. Among its complications are the following: peripheral facial paralysis, retro-auricular fistula, labyrinthitis, meningitis, tuberculous osteomyelitis of the petrous pyramid, subperiosteal, cerebral or cerebellar abscess, acute mastoiditis and cellulites [9].

4.4. Nasal TB

Nasal TB is an extremely rare form [16]. Butt in his review of nasal TB in the 20th century identified only 35 reported cases, 12 of which were of the primary form. The most common symptoms were nasal obstruction and aqueous secretions [17].

Less common symptoms include nasal discomfort, presence of a mass, epistaxis, crusting, lachrymation, postnasal drip, recurrent polyps, and nasal ulcer [17]. The most common site is the anterior-inferior portion of the nasal septum, in the region of greatest arteriovenous confluence called the Kiesselbach zone. In anterior rhinoscopy, a pale, torpid mucosa is observed and can present with perforation of the nasal septum [14].

Figure 4 shows an image of nasal TB lesions. Figure 5 gives the histopathological assessment which revealed a caseous granulomatous reaction, epithelioid cells lymphatics, and some giant cells [18].

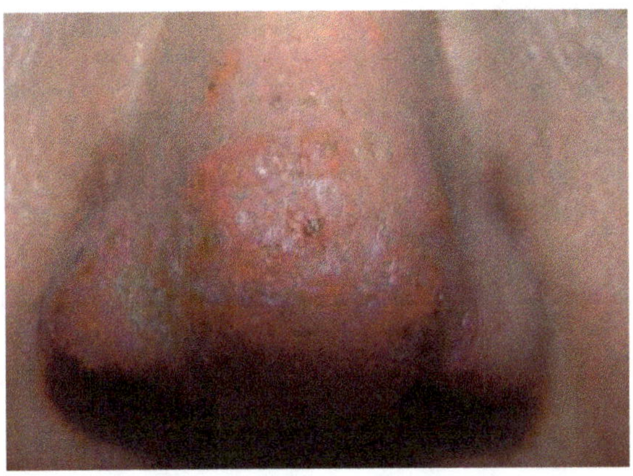

Figure 4. Reddish ulcerative lesion on the nose and in the internal mucosal layer.

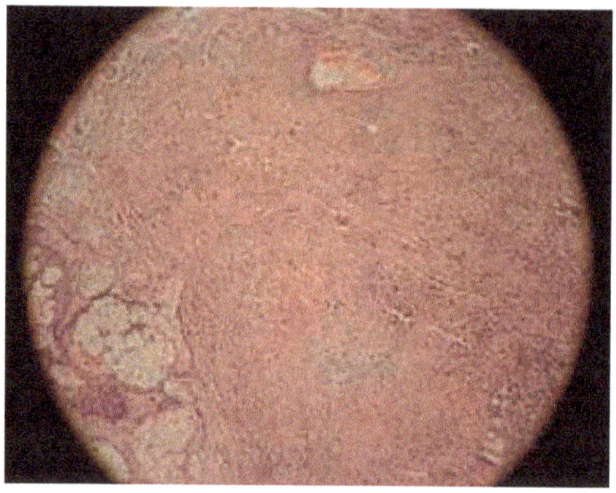

Figure 5. Caseating granulomatous reaction, epithelioid cells, lymphocytes, and a few giant cells.

4.5. TB in the oral cavity

Oral TB is a rare form representing 0.1-5% of the total of TB infections. *Mycobacterium tuberculosis* can infect all parts of the mouth, such as gums, hard and soft palate, lips, maxilla and mandible [19]. It is more frequent in men than in women appearing mainly in the form of ulcerative lesions [20]. The tongue is the most common site of TB oral [19].

The integrity of the oral mucosa, the cleaning action of the saliva, the presence of oral saprophytes and submucosal antibodies represent a natural resistance to the invasion of *Mycobacterium tuberculosis* [19]. Oral trauma, tooth extraction, inflammatory conditions and poor hygiene represent gateways [20].

Its presentation occurred as a secondary infection in 58% of patients and as a primary infection in 42%. Carcinomas have been found coexisting in the same site of the lesion in 3% of patients. In approximately 50%, the oral manifestation of TB led to the diagnosis of systemic infection [20].

4.6. TB in the tonsils

Primary tuberculosis in tonsils, in the absence of active pulmonary disease is rare [21]. In a study by Ricciardiello [8] et al., 0.62% of the sample was found to have this form of TB.

It may result from contact with materials containing bacilli. In the secondary form, it may be due to the contact of sputum containing bacilli from a pulmonary focus. What favors this site being affected are factors such as alcoholism, HIV and infection [22].

Its clinical features are nonspecific; sometimes it can simulate chronic tonsillitis [23]. The oral examination may show hypertrophy of the tonsils, bulging in the oropharynx with edema and erythema, as well as yellow platelets on its surface [24].

4.7. TB in the salivary glands

Primary TB is a relatively common cause of granulomatous disease of the salivary glands. Generally it affects one side, and the usual target is the parotid gland. The primary form can occur in two ways: as an acute inflammatory lesion mimicking an acute suppurative sialadenitis, or as a chronic tumor [25].

As to secondary tuberculosis, unlike the primary form, this more often involves the submandibular and the sublingual glands than it does the parotid one [25].

TB of the salivary gland is more common in immune-depressed patients, and it is difficult to distinguish it clinically from other diffuse diseases of this site [26].

Figure 6 shows a patient who has TB of the submandibular gland [26].

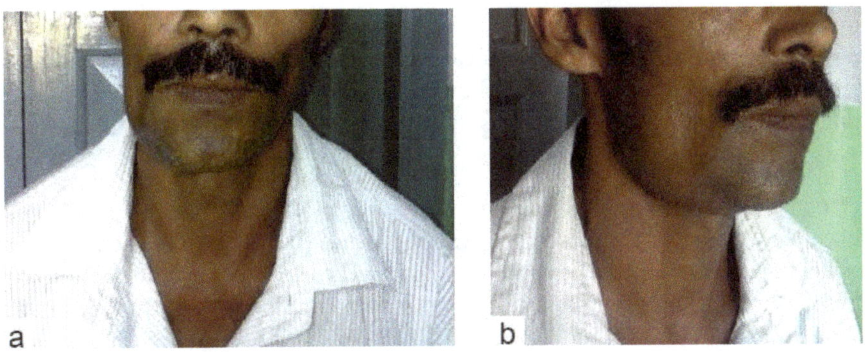

Figure 6. Photograph of the patient showing right submandibular swelling (a) Frontal view. (b) Right lateral view. Source: Tauro, 2011, p.83.

5. Diagnosis

The forms of extrapulmonary TB can be challenging to diagnose because bacteriological confirmation can only be obtained in about a quarter of cases. The reasons for this difficulty include difficult access to some lesions and the fact they are usually paucibacillary. Moreover, the histopathological findings of granulomatous reaction do not rule out the possibility of other diseases. Imaging studies can provide important information, although there are no specific standards for the sites affected [27].

In laryngeal TB, diagnosis may be obtained from the isolation and culture of *Mycobacterium tuberculosis*, but this diagnosis only emerges after about four weeks of cultivation. The best material for culture is obtained by biopsy, but this is positive in only 40% of cases. A biopsy can also be used to check if there is concomitance with cancer of the larynx [28]- [30].

Some authors consider the anatomatopathological exam as the "gold standard" for the diagnosis of laryngeal TB [7]. By using microscopy, we observe inflammatory, granulomatous reactions. The granulomas consist of giant cells, and central caseous necrosis can occur, which aids a positive diagnosis to be made before receiving a positive culture of *Mycobacterium tuberculosis* [29]. Since most patients have a concomitant pulmonary problem, chest radiography can assist in this diagnosis [7], [12].

The Mantoux or intradermal test is often used. Its positivity is given by a 10mm diameter wheal after up to 48 hours or 5mm in immune-compromised patients. This positive test only indicates infection [7], [12]. The PCR is a test that can amplify amounts of specific segments of deoxyribonucleic acid from microorganisms such as *Mycobacterium tuberculosis* present in a sample [12]. Chest X-ray, the Mantoux test and PCR tests are examinations that are sensitive to the presence of *Mycobacterium tuberculosis*. However, they are not specific to laryngeal disease.

We stress the importance of taking care over recording the patient´s medical history and conducting an ENT examination accurately, with emphasis being given to indirect laryngoscopy and videolaryngoscopy [28].

In the form of TB affecting lymph nodes, diagnosis can be made by aspirative punction. The smear material is positive in 10% to 25% of cases as is culture, in 50% to 85% of them. A biopsy of the lymph node is often inconclusive, showing granuloma with caseous necrosis in 91% to 96% of patients. Usually, the tuberculin test is a strong reactor, except in immumo-suppressed individuals [27].

In suspected cases of tuberculosis of the middle ear, the following tests are important: Gram stain and culture of the middle ear secretion, specific for AFB (acid fast bacilli); biopsy of polyp or mucosa of the middle ear and histopathological studies with tissue culture; tuberculin skin test (Mantoux); chest X-ray. Other tests may clarify some details: a radiological and tomographic study of the mastoids; audiogram [31].

In TB of the middle ear, the histopathological examination of the granulation tissue (when it is abundant), is still the most reliable diagnostic method, but very often the biopsy needs to be repeated for confirmation. The method is used to demonstrate caseous necrosis and specific granulation with epithelioid and giant Langerhans cells [10].

Audiometric tests detect precocious hipoacusia and out of proportion to the apparent degree of development of the disease seen at otoscopy. Radiographic studies of the middle ear and mastoid do not reveal specific features, but the detection of well-pneumatized mastoid in patients with chronic otorrhea may suggest the possibility of hypocausia [31].

The diagnosis of nasal TB can be established by smear (using nasal exudate) and the biopsy of the lesion [14]. The diagnosis of tonsillar TB is also based on histopathological findings and on identifying the bacillus [21].

6. Differential diagnosis

In laryngeal TB, differential diagnosis with inflammatory diseases and with laryngeal carcinoma should be conducted [7]. Similarly, in TB which affects the ear, differential diagnosis may reveal other diseases with chronic suppuration which do not improve with conventional treatment, such as cholesteatoma, syphilis, Wegener's granulomatosis, fungal infection, eosinophilic granulomatosis and sarcoidosis [9].

Traumatic ulcers, aphthous ulcers, blood disorders, actinomycosis, syphilis, midline granuloma, Wegener's disease and cancer are differential diagnoses of oral tuberculosis [21]. In nasal TB, differential diagnosis should include looking for inflammatory processes, as well as other diseases that can manifest themselves with similar lesions, such as herpes simplex, leishmaniasis, syphilis and some fungal infections [16].

TB of lymph nodes can be determined by making a differential diagnosis with diseases such as lymphomas and atypical mycobacterioses [13].

7. Tuberculosis and HIV

Individuals who live with HIV and who are also infected with TB are more likely to develop the disease of TB than those who are HIV negative. From the 80s, the HIV epidemic has led to a large increase in TB cases and TB mortality in several countries [4].

In 2011, 1.1 million (13%) of the 8.7 million people who had developed tuberculosis worldwide were HIV positive. In the same year, there were an estimated 0.4 million deaths from HIV-associated tuberculosis in the world [4].

HIV has been pointed out as being one of the factors for the resurgence of TB, as well as having an impact on its epidemiology, natural history and clinical evolution. This is also related to the reactivation of latent infections of TB [32]. HIV infection also modifies the clinical presentation of TB, the duration of treatment, tolerance to antituberculosis and resistance to the drugs available [33].

8. Treatment

TB is a serious but curable disease in almost 100% of new cases, as long as the principles of chemotherapy are followed [34]. However, in the absence of beginning treatment, it is estimated that 60-70% of patients with pulmonary TB without co-infection by HIV progress to death [35].

Treatment of active baciliferous TB is the priority activity of TB control, since this allows the greatest sources of infection to be annulled. Tubercle bacilli practically lose their virulence, a few days after the start of chemotherapy [34].

The drugs used are: isoniazid, rifampicin, pyrazinamide and ethambutol. The inclusion of ethambutol in Brazil, was authorized in 2008 and is indicated for adults and adolescents (> 10 years old), in the first-line treatment of TB in Brazil. Thus, the use of rifampicin, isoniazid, pyrazinamide and ethambutol in the first phase of treatment is recommended for two months followed by rifampicin and isoniazid for four months, thus maintaining the short duration regime of 6 months. For children, this continues with three drugs in the first phase [34].

This scheme is used in Brazil for the treatment of all forms of pulmonary and extrapulmonary TB (except meningoencephalitis) in new cases of patients whether or not they are infected by HIV [34].

9. Prevention

The best way to prevent TB is to diagnose and isolate infectious cases quickly by administering treatment appropriately until the patient is no longer infectious the disease is cured [36].

BCG vaccination and the treatment of individuals with latent TB infection, who are at high risk of developing the disease are other strategies that can be used [36].

10. Final remarks

TB is a disease with a very long history and one which has sprung up again and been affecting various countries. Among the factors responsible for this resurgence, HIV should be mentioned. HIV has been regarded as responsible for changing the characteristics of TB, such as its epidemiology, natural history, clinical presentation, and resistance to drugs.

The manifestations of TB in cervico-cephalic regions are frequent and have aroused interest, mainly because of changes in the pattern of how the disease is caught. These forms can also be challenging to diagnose.

Provided appropriate treatment is begun promptly, TB is a curable disease, and doing so for infectious cases is moreover a form of prevention.

In this context, public policies are needed that encourage not only the adoption of preventive measures, but also aid early diagnosis and seek to ensure adherence to TB treatment. This is because the earlier that treatment is started and is done so appropriately, the more likely that the patient will suffer from fewer sequelae and deformities.

Author details

Luiz Alberto Alves Mota[1,2,3*], Paula Cristina Alves Leitão[1] and
Ana Maria dos Anjos Carneiro-Leão[4]

*Address all correspondence to: luizmota10@hotmail.com

1 Faculty of Medical Sciences, Universidade de Pernambuco, Brazil

2 Hospital Universitário Oswaldo Cruz, Brazil

3 Rede Nordeste de Biotecnologia (RENORBIO), , Brazil

4 Department of Animal Morphology and Physiology - Universidade Federal Rural de Pernambuco, Brazil, Brazil

References

[1] Prado TN, Caus AL, Marques M, Maciel EL, Golub JE, Miranda AE. Perfil epidemiológico de pacientes adultos com tuberculose e AIDS no estado do Espírito Santo, Brasil: relacionamento dos bancos de dados de tuberculose e AIDS. J. bras. pneumol. 2011; 37 (1):93-99.

[2] Ministério da Saúde (Brasil). Cadernos de Atenção Básica/ Vigilância em saúde: dengue, esquistossomose, hanseníase, malária, tracoma e tuberculose. 2º Edição- revisada: 2008, Brasília/DF.

[3] Antunes AA, Antunes AA, Antunes AP. Tuberculose da laringe: estudo retrospectivo e revisão de literatura. Rev. Bras de Cirurgia de Cabeça e Pescoço. 2001; 25(1-2): 19-22.

[4] World Health Organization. Global Tuberculosis Control Report 2012. Available at: http://apps.who.int/iris/bitstream/10665/75938/1/9789241564502_eng.pdf (accessed on 18 June 2014).

[5] Portal saúde. Available at: http://portalsaude.saude.gov.br/, accessed on 19/09/2014.

[6] Ministério da Saúde (Brasil), DATASUS. Available at: http://tabnet.datasus.gov.br/cgi/deftohtm.exe?idb2012/d0202.def/. (accessed on 18 June 2014).

[7] Garcia RID, Cecatto SB, Mendonça RR, Barcelos CEM, Santos RO, Rapoport PB. Tuberculose e blastomicose laríngeas: relato de três casos e revisão de literatura. Rev Bras Otorrinolaringol. 2004; 70(2):255-9.

[8] Ricciardiello F, Martufi S, Cardone M, Cavaliere M, D'errico P, Iengo M. Otorhinolaryngology-related tuberculosis. Acta Otorhinolaryngol Ital. 2006; 26: 38-42.

[9] Sens PM, Almeida CIR,Valle LO, Costa LHC, Angeli MLS. Tuberculose de orelha, doença profissional? Rev Bras Otorrinolaringol. 2008;74(4):621-7.

[10] Fagundes RCF, Cury RI, Anelli-Bastos W, Silva L, Duprat A. Tuberculose laríngea: proposta de intervenção fonoaudiológica nas sequelas de voz após o tratamento farmacológico. Rev Soc Bras Fonoaudiol. 2011; 16(1):99-103

[11] Sá LCB, Meirelles RC, Atherino CCT, Fernandes JRC, Ferraz FR. Tuberculose faringolaríngea. Rev Bras Otorrinolaringol 2007; 73(6):862-6.

[12] Yencha MW, Linfesty R, Blackmon A. Laryngeal Tuberculosis. Am J Otolaryngol. 2000; 21(2): 122-126.

[13] Landim MHC. Disseminated lynphonodal tuberculosis with no onset of peripheral lynphonodes. Rev Med Minas Gerais. 2009; 19(1): 67-70

[14] Sousa RT, Briglia MFS, Lima LCN, Teixeira LM, Marcião AHR, et al. Frequency of Otorhinolaryngologies' Manifestations in Patients with Pulmonary Tuberculosis. Int. Arch. Otorhinolaryngol. 2010;14(2): 156-62.

[15] Abebe, G; Deribew, A; Apers, L; Abdissa, A; Deribie, F; Woldemichael, K; et al. Tuberculosis lymphadenitis in Southwest Ethiopia: a community based cross-sectional study. 2012; 12(1):1-7.

[16] Moon SY, Lee JA, Joung MK, Chung DR, Song JH, Peck KR. Nasal Deformity Due to Tuberculous Chondritis. 2014; 7(3): 229-31.

[17] Butt AA. Nasal tuberculosis in the 20th century. Am J Med Sci. 1997;313(6):332-5.

[18] Alavi SM, Nashibi R.Nasal tuberculosis in a 56 year old woman. Caspian J Intern Med. 2014; 5(1): 49-51

[19] Assante LR, Barra E, Bocchino ML, Zuccarini G, Ferrara G, Sanduzzi A. Tuberculosis of the tongue in a patient with rheumatoid arthritis treated with methotrexate and adalimumab. Le Infezioni in Medicina. 2014; 2: 144-8.

[20] Kakisi OK, Kechagia AS, Kakisis IK, Rafailidis PI, Falagas ME. Tuberculosis of the oral cavity: a systematic review. Eur J Oral Sci. 2010; 118: 103–109.

[21] Kant S, Verma SK, Sanjay. Isolated tonsil tuberculosis. Lung India. 2008; 25(4): 163–4.

[22] Santosh UP, Vinay B. Tuberculosis of tonsil associated with pulmonary foci. J. Otolaryngol. Head Neck Surg.2008; 60:263–5.

[23] Amine C, Amal H, Nawar O, Abdelatif O, Nouredine EA. La tuberculose des amygdales palatines. Pan African Medical Journal. 2010; 4(1):1-5.

[24] Gupta KB, Tandon S, Jaswal TS, Singh S. Tuberculosis of tonsil with unusual presentation. The Indian Journal of Tuberculosis. 2001; 48(4): 223-4.

[25] Dadwal M. Primary Submandibular Tuberculosis: An Unusual Cause of Submandibular Salivary Gland Enlargement. Indian J Otolaryngol Head Neck Surg. 2011; 63(3): 298–9.

[26] Tauro LF, George C, Kamath A, Swethadri GK, Gatty R. Primary Tuberculosis of Submandibular Salivary Gland. J Glob Infect Dis. 2011; (1): 82–5.

[27] Lopes AJ, Capone D, Mogami R, Tessarollo B, Cunha DL, Capone RB, et al. Extrapulmonary tuberculosis: clinics and image aspects. Pulmão RJ. 2006; 15(4):253-61.

[28] Mota LAA, Sefer MPC. Tuberculose laríngea: relato de caso. Rev Bras de Cirurgia de Cabeça e Pescoço. 2003; 32(3):7-8.

[29] Martins AG, Marques MPC, Ferreira NGM, Valete CM, Tomita S, Kós AOA. Manifestações otorrinolaringológicas da tuberculose. Rev Bras Otorrinolaringol. 2000, 66(6):666-71.

[30] Bailey BJ, Calhoun KH, Friedman N, Newlands SD, Vrabec JT. Head & Neck Surgery- Otolaryngology. Second edition. Lippincott - Raven; 1998.

[31] Pinho MM, Kós AOA.Otite média tuberculosa. Rev Bras Otorrinolaringol. 2003; 69(6) 829-37.

[32] Guimarães RM, Lobo AP, Siqueira EA, Borges TFF, Melo SCC. Tuberculosis, HIV, and poverty: temporal trends in Brazil, the Americas, and worldwide. J Bras Pneumol. 2012;38(4):511-7.

[33] Neto MS, Silva FL, Sousa KR, Yamamura M, Popolin MP, Arcêncio RA. Clinical and epidemiological profile and prevalence of tuberculosis/HIV co-infection in a regional health district in the state of Maranhão, Brazil. J Bras Pneumol. 2012;38(6):724-32.

[34] Brasil. Ministério da Saúde. Guia de vigilância epidemiológica. 7º edição. Brasília: Ministério da Saúde, 2009.

[35] Borgdorff MW, Floyd K, Broekmans JF. Interventions to reduce tuberculosis mortality and transmission in low- and middle-income countries. Bull World Health Organ. 2002;80(3):217-27.

[36] Harrison. Medicina Interna. 17º edição. Rio de Janeiro: McGraw-Hill Interamericana do Brasil, 2008.

8

Molecular Epidemiology of Tuberculosis

Magda Lorena Orduz and Wellman Ribón

1. Introduction

Tuberculosis (TB) is one of the infections with major impact worldwide and it is produced by members of the *Mycobacterium tuberculosis* complex, this bacteria mainly affects the lungs. The TB is considered the second cause of death for an infectious disease after of the Human Immunodeficiency Virus(HIV)in the world [1]. It is one of the oldest diseases and has accompanied mankind during its evolution. Evidence of the etiologic agent for the disease was found in skeletons 4000 years old in Europe and the Middle East [2].According to the Global Tuberculosis Report 2013 of the World Health Organization, in the 2012, an estimated 8.6 million new cases of diseased and 1.3 million deaths from this cause occurred. This data shows that despite the many efforts of government organizations to control the disease, it remains an important public health public worldwide.

In the last years the biology molecular methodologies have led many advances which allow the analyses of genetic material of different microorganisms such as *M. tuberculosis*, with the analysis of the Insertion element IS6110, the polymorphism within the direct repeat (DR) locus and analysis using mycobacterial interspersed repetitive units, this methodologies allow the molecular typing of the mycobacteria and the knowledge of the different lineages of *M. tuberculosis*, contributing to the development of the molecular epidemiology and the control politics of the disease in the different cities and countries.

2. General aspects of disease and etiologic agent

2.1. Epidemiology

TB is a global disease. In 2012, the World Health Organization(WHO) estimated in its annual report about 8.6 million new cases of the disease (100,000 less than in 2011) which represents an incidence rate of 122 cases per 100,000 inhabitants in average worldwide: 5.7 million cases were diagnosed as new cases, and it is estimated that 1.1 million of the total cases showed co-infection infection with HIV; and 450,000 cases of multi-drug-resistant tuberculosis (MDR-TB), being South East Asia, Africa, and the Pacific region the most affected areas. Additionally, an estimate of 1.3 million deaths were caused by the disease, and despite of noticing a reduction in the mortality rate, the increase of deaths in populations such as children and women is remarkable.

On the other hand, approximately 2.9 million cases were lost, that is to say, they were not diagnosed or they were not notified to the national tuberculosis programmes. Regarding treatment, 56 million people were successfully treated from 1995 to 2012, saving 22 million lives among the countries which adopted the Directly Observed Treatment, Short-course (DOTS) strategy, proposed by the WHO.

According to the WHO report, the Americas and the Western Pacific regions are the only ones, out of the six regions, which have achieved goals with regards to the decrease of mortality, prevalence, and incidence by the year 2015.Prevalence of the disease was approximately 31 – 41 cases and incidence was 27 – 31 cases per 100,000 inhabitants in the Americas. Out of the 280,000 incident cases, about 31,000 showed co-infection with HIV; however only 219,349 cases were reported. Mortality of the disease reached a rate of 1.9 deaths per 100,000 inhabitants, that is to say 20,000 deaths among people suffering the disease.

In Colombia, 11990 confirmed cases of tuberculosis in all of its forms were confirmed for the same period. Out of these, 10956 corresponded to new cases for an incidence of 23.5 cases per 100,000 inhabitants. According to the clinical presentation of the disease, 80.4% of cases were pulmonary tuberculosis and 19.6% were extra pulmonary TB [3].

The departments with the largest number of cases in Colombia correspond to Antioquia, Cundinamarca concentrating its high number of cases in the city of Bogota, Valle del Cauca, Atlántico, Risaralda, and Santander.

2.2. Clinical forms

2.2.1. Pulmonary tuberculosis

It is the most common type since it is the manner in which the disease can be spread to other persons. The disease is directly transmitted from person to person; when a diseased person coughs, sneezes, or spits, bacilli are expelled to the air and they will be inhaled by people around the patient [4].

It is estimated that one third of the world population has latent TB; that is to say, they are infected by the bacillus but they have not gotten sick, nor they can spread the infection. People infected with the tuberculosis bacillus have a 10% risk of getting TB throughout their lives. However, this risk is higher for people who have a deficiency or compromise of their immune system, as in cases of infection with the human immunodeficiency virus (HIV), malnutrition, diabetes, or tobacco users [5].

When the disease appears, the symptoms (coughing, fever, night sweats, and weight loss, among others) may be mild for several months. As a result, patients delay seeking medical attention and they transmit the bacteria to other people. During one year, a tuberculosis diseased may infect approximately 10 to 15 people by close contact. Up to two thirds of tuberculosis patients die if they do not receive appropriate treatment [6].

2.2.2. Extra pulmonary tuberculosis

Even though it represents only a small proportion of TB cases, approximately 10 – 15%, patients develop the most severe forms of the disease. Since the disease may affect any organ, the diagnosis is often more difficult and delayed [7]. Populations most affected by extra pulmonary TB are children and persons with immunosuppression, such as those who have leukemia, diabetes and living with HIV.

In accordance with the WHO criteria, the forms of extra pulmonary TB are classified into severe and less severe. Meningitis, milliary, pericarditis, peritonitis, extensive or bilateral pleural, intestinal, spinal, genital urinary are considered to be severe forms. TB of lymph nodes, unilateral pleural, bones (except for the spine), and skin are considered to be the less severe [8].

2.3. Etiologic agent

The *Mycobacterium* genus is taxonomically located in the *Mycobacteriacea* family (table 1) and comprises 150 species [9], among which there are species of the *M. tuberculosis* complex, made up of *M. tuberculosis, M. bovis, M bovis BCG, M. africanum, M microtti, M caprae, M. pinipedii, M. canetti, M. mungi, M. orygis* [10].

Kingdom	*Bacteria*
Phylum	*Actinobacteria*
Class	*Actinobacteria*
Subclass	*Actinobacteridae*
Order	*Actinomycetales*
Suborder	*Corynebacterineae*
Family	*Mycobacteriaceae*
Genus	*Mycobacterium*

Table 1. Taxonomic classification

2.3.1. Microscopic characteristics

The dimensions of the bacillus are approximately 1-10 μm long (usually 3-5 μm) and 0.2 – 0.6μm wide (Figure 1) [11]. It has a complex cellular envelope composed of a cellular membrane and cellular wall; the latter provides mechanical support for the bacteria and gives its characteristic in acid-fast staining due to the large content of lipids [12]. The morphologic feature of presence of cord in the Zielh Neelsen staining is presumptive of mycobacteria of the *M. tuberculosis* complex; formation of the cord is attributed to the trehalose glycolipid 6, 6-dimycolate or cord factor composed of mycolic acids molecules [13].

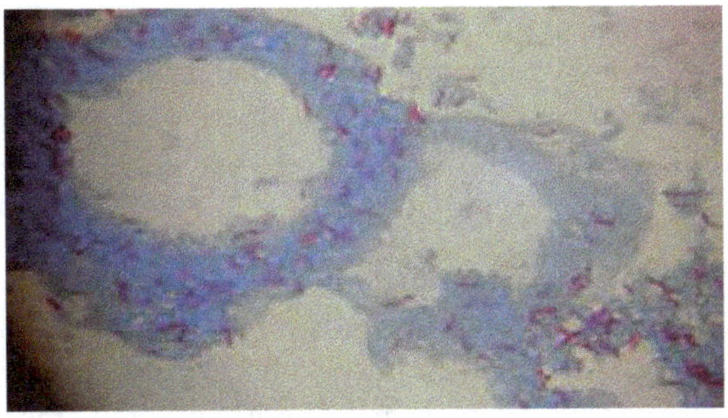

Figure 1. Acid-fast bacilli in a bacilloscopy.

2.3.2. *Morphologic characteristics in culture*

M. tuberculosis is characterized by having slow growth in synthetic media since its generation time ranges from 18 to 24 hours. Low growth rate is associated to the wall permeability which limits the entry of nutrients [14] and additionally, it has been observed that one or two operons rm are found in the mycobacteria managed by the P1 and P2 promoters. The rmA operon located in the *mur*A gene is found in all of the species, including *M. tuberculosis* and *M. leprae.* Nevertheless, in some species such as the fast-growth ones, an additional *rm*B operon is found, located in the *tyr*S gene [15, 16]

Synthetic media use for the isolation of *M. tuberculosis* contain nutrients such as glycerol, carbon source, asparagine, and ammonia ions as source of nitrogen and micronutrients besides albumin incorporated in the culture media with the aggregate of hen eggs or bovine seroalbumin. Colonies characteristic of *M. tuberculosis* developed in a solid medium based on eggs are often rough, without pigment, and dry (Figure 2) [17]

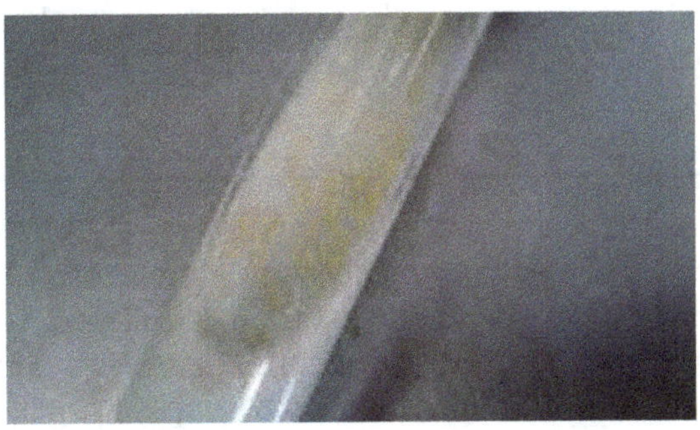

Figure 2. *M. tuberculosis* culture

3. Genome of *Mycobacterium tuberculosis*

With the complete genome sequencing of *M. tuberculosis*, H37Rv strain, more genetic information of the bacterium was generated. In total, a sequence of 4,411,539 pairs of bases which contain about 4000 genes and a high content of guanine + cytosine (G+C) of 65.6%. The point for the beginning of numbering was the initiation codon for the dnaA gene, a marker for the origin of replication oriC. The G+C content is relatively constant and several regions showing larger content of G+C were detected, corresponding to sequences that belong to a large family of genes which include the polymorphic GC-rich repetitive sequence (PGRS) [18].

Genome is rich in repetitive DNA, particularly in insertion sequences and in new multigene families; an example of these is the presence and distribution of insertion sequences (IS). IS6110, a sequence of the IS3 family, is of particular interest. It is widely used for typing of strains and molecular epidemiology due to its variation in the insertion site and the number of copies [19]. In the H37Rv *M. tuberculosis* genome, sixteen copies of IS6110 were identified; some sites of these copies were grouped in sites with the insertion name of hot spots[20].

Recently another repetitive region highly preserved within the chromosome of *M. tuberculosis* was described: the DR locus [21] [22], which is a member of the Clustered Regularly Interspersed Palindromic Repeats – CRISP sequences [23]. After the discovery of the DR region, the variable number of tandem repetitions (VNTR) was found [24], subsequently, the mycobacterial intergenic repetition units (MIRU) were identified [25] that are also listed as VNTR multiple locus analysis. Multilocus sequences typing (MLST) was introduced as an alternative method [26]; and recently, the single nucleotide polymorphism (SNP) was described [27] followed by large sequence polymorphism (LSP). The latter is carried out either by micro arrangements or polymerase chain reaction (PCR) in real time [28]

4. Molecular markers of *M. tuberculosis* genotyping

4.1. IS6110

Insertion element found within species of the *M. tuberculosis* complex, and was shown to be related to the IS3 family of insertion sequences which were discovered in members of the family Enterobacteriaceae [29].

IS6110 is 1,361 bp long and contains 28-bp, imperfect inverted repeats at its extremities with three mismatches and 3-bp direct repeats that probably result from repetition of the target sequence [30] are present in different copy numbers and are integrated at various chromosomal site [31]. The number of IS6110 copies present in the genome is species- and strain-dependent. Most strains of *M. tuberculosis* carry between eight to 15 copies in different positions of the genome although single copy strains are common. [32]The polymorphism of restriction fragments generated by breaking the IS6110 fragment with the PvuII enzyme, has been used as a method for genotyping of *M. tuberculosis* complex species

4.2. IS1081, direct repeat and major polymorphic tandem repeat

It is a 1324-bp insertion sequence found in *M. tuberculosis* complex. It has a lower degree of polymorphism than IS6110 because of its low transpositional activity [33, 34]

4.3. Polymorphic GC-rich repetitive sequence

It has numerous copies [35- 37] and consists of many tandem repeats of a 96 bp GC rich consensus sequence. PGRS elements are present in 26 sites of *M. tuberculosis* chromosomes [38] and have been detected in mycobacteria not belonging to the *M. tuberculosis* complex [39].

4.4. DR locus

It contains multiple repeated DR regions of 36 pb, interspersed with non-repetitive spacer sequences of 34 to 41 pb which constitute DVR (Figure 3); the size of the DR locus varies from 6 DVR (06 kb) to 56 DVR (6 KB), and both the DR region and the spacers have shown little variation in the order of presentation among strains.

The DR region has been identified as an integration hot-spot of the IS6110 insertion element [40].

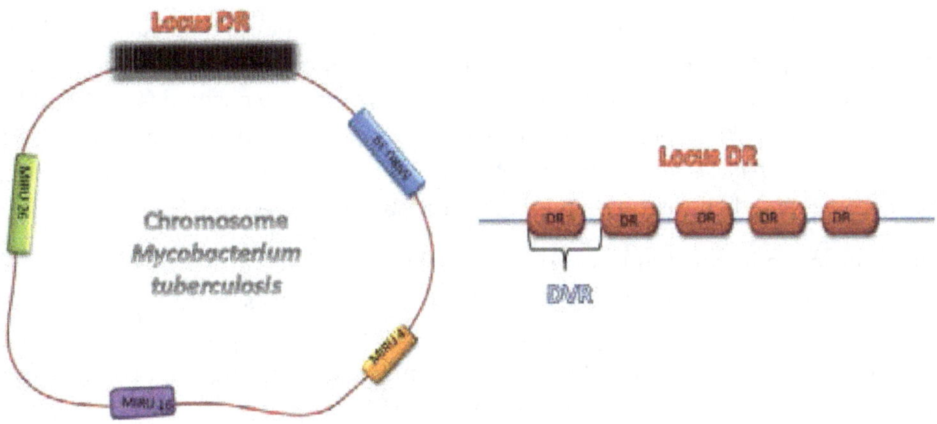

Figure 3. DR locus

Deletion of one or more DVR [41] and duplication of DVR are the mechanisms which generate the variation among different strains. These deletions and duplications are likely to be mediated by the homologous recombination among neighboring or distant DRs, or by Splicing processes during DNA replication [42]. Nevertheless, the process in which the deletion of a DR occurs due to transposition of the IS6110 has also been described [43]. All of these changes generated in the DR locus are the foundation for the development of the Spoligotyping methodology [44].

4.5. VNTR

DNA segments containing "tandem repeated" sequences in which the number of copies of the repeated sequence varies among strains. Variable Number Tandem Repeat (VNTR) sequences have emerged as valuable markers for genotyping. MIRUs are a class oftandem repeated sequences. There are a total of 41 MIRU loci[45].

5. Genotyping methodologies

The following are the genotyping methodologies based on repetitive regions of the *M. tuberculosis* chromosome mostly used worldwide:

- IS6110-based restriction fragment length polymorphism (RFLP) analysis.
- Spoligotyping.
- Mycobacterial interspersed repetitive units (MIRU) analysis

5.1. IS6110-RFLP methodology

Identification of IS6110 was a great break through for epidemiology of tuberculosis [46]. IS6110 is an insertion sequence made up by 1361 bp, capable of making copies of themselves and then inserting the copies in a genome locus in a process known as transposition [47]. IS6110-based restriction fragment length polymorphism analysis has been considered the golden standard method for *M. tuberculosis* genotyping [48-49]. Strains of *M. tuberculosis* differ in the number of IS6110 copies and their distribution is highly variable in the genome [50].

The first step in conducting RFLP is purification of DNA from a culture of *M. tuberculosis*; then the *Pvu*II restriction enzyme cuts the DNA on specific sequences in hundreds of different fragments. The fragments are separated per size in an agarose gel and transferred to a membrane. A probe is used in order to detect fragments containing IS6110; the picture is caught on a film, and each IS6110 copy produces a band. RFLP patterns with seven or more bands provide more specificity for discrimination of isolations, contrary to strains with patterns of six or less bands in which there is lower discrimination. Usually, there are eight to 18 copies per strains, but the number may vary from zero to 25 [51].

There is a small number of *M. tuberculosis* strain that do not contain the IS6110 sequence, so a print without bands will be obtained in the analysis, or those which contain a low number of copies will show less polymorphism than the ones containing a large number of copies. The main disadvantages of this methodology is the complexity of the procedure which has a length of approximately five days, and the amount of DNA necessary for the digestion with restriction enzymes; this requires obtaining cultures with sufficient growth in order to perform DNA extraction unlike PCR based methods such as MIRU and spoligotyping [52].

5.2. Spoligotyping

It is a PCR-based method for detection and typing of the *M. tuberculosis* complex using a single chromosome locus with high polymorphism, the direct repeated region DR. It consists on a sequence of 36 pb which are separated by 43 non-repeated spacers, each of which contains 36 to 41 pairs of bases [53].

The amplification of the DR locus is carried out by means of PCR, using primers, one of which is marked with biotin. The PCR products are hybridized perpendicularly to the membrane that contains 43 oligonucleotides of known sequence. The membrane is incubated with streptavidine-peroxydase conjugate which links to biotin of the PCR products. The detection of hybridization signals is made by means of a chemiluminiscence system (ECL). When DR regions of several strains are compared, the order of the spacers is almost the same in all of the strains, but deletions of the spacers may be found which generate the differences among each one of the strains [54].

In order to compare the patterns obtained with the results published, it is necessary to make the conversion of the obtained bands pattern. Each one of the 43 spacers produces either a dark box (indicating the presence of the spacer) or a clear box (indicating the absence of the spacer), and a binary numeric code 1 -0 is assigned respectively.

To simplify this numbering, the 43-digit binary code is converted to a 15-digit octal code (i.e. digits 0 to 7). Each 3-digit binary set is converted to its octal equivalent, and ultimately the remaining digit shall be either 1 or 0. The translation of the binary numbers to octal numbers is as follows: 000 = 0; 001 = 1; 010 = 2; 011 = 3; 100 = 4; 001 = 5; 110 = 6; 111 = 7. Each octal designation is unique, thus representing a specific brands pattern [55]. Finally, this code is entered in the SITVIT WEB international database which presents information on the diverse lineages and its world distribution. It contains information about the genetic diversity of the *M. tuberculosis* complex based on 62,582 clinical isolates from 153 countries [56].

Spoligotyping offers great advantages such as its usefulness in genotyping strains of *M. tuberculosis* that contain little IS6110 sequences [57]; the use of the methodology directly on clinical samples [58] which would allow simultaneous diagnosis and typing of *M. tuberculosis, M. bovis,* and differentiation of species comprising the *M. tuberculosis* complex. Studies conducted with clinical samples showed unique hybridization pattern, whereas strains of an outbreak shared the same pattern. Patterns obtained from direct examination of the clinical samples were identical to the ones obtained by means of using DNA from cultures of these samples [59].The use of a second generation spoligotyping membrane was proposed with the aim of increasing the test´s power of discrimination using 51 oligonucleotides of spacers [60].

By using spoligotyping, species and subspecies comprising the *M. tuberculosis* complex can be classified based on the patterns obtained on hybridization, and at the same time the diverse lineages of the *M. tuberculosis* species [61].

5.3. MIRU-VNTR methodology

Mycobacterial interspersed repetitive units are loci in the genome of *M. tuberculosis* containing a number of variable tandem repetitions [62]. The length of MIRU is in the range of 50 – 100 pb and belong to the category of VNTR "mini satellites" [63]. Forty-one loci of this type have been identified in *M. tuberculosis,* among them, 12 loci have shown that they vary in the number of tandem repetitions and most of them among the repeating units.

It is a PCR-based method that uses these 12 different interspersed units for genotyping. The estimation to determine the number of repetitions is based on the size of the amplicon. The results are reported as 12 numbers, each one corresponding to the number of repetitions. The power of discrimination of the 12 MIRU-VNTR regions is much greater than the one of spoligotyping and close to IS6110 RFLP for typing of *M. tuberculosis* strains. Recently a system was proposed which includes typing of 24-loci MIRU-VNTR combining multiplex PCR analysis or a DNA analyzer based on fluorescence with the computer automation of genotyping was proposed [64].

6. Species and lineages of *M. tuberculosis*

6.1. *M. tuberculosis*

It was the first member of the complex to be described by Doctor Robert Koch in 1882. It is the species most frequently involved in the development of pulmonary TB in humans [65].*M. tuberculosisis* by far the most important pathogen of the complex in terms of the number of infected hosts and its public health implications.

6.2. *M. bovis*

It causes TB in a wide range of wild and domestic animals. *M. bovis* is naturally resistant to pyrazinamide, a first-line anti TB drugs[66]. Its epidemiologic importance lies in the zoonotic transmission of *M. bovis* to humans due to contact with infected animals, or to consumption of products from these animals.

6.3. *M. africanum*

It is the species that causes more TB in humans in Western Africa [67]. There are two large variants of *M. africanum*: the African Variation I, isolated in the east of Africa, and variant II, to the west [68]. Besides, M. africanum type I has been recently subdivided into *M. africanum* type I, eastern African I (MAF1), prevalent around the Gulf of Guinea; and *M. africanum* type I, eastern African 2 (MAF2), prevalent in southeast Africa. *M. africanum* type II has been reclassified into *M. tuberculosis* and indicated as the "Uganda" genotype [46].

6.4. *M. bovis* BCG or Bacillus Calmette-Guerin (BCG)

It is the vaccine's strain, and it is a live attenuated variant of *M. bovis*. Its spoligotype is characterized by the absence of spacers 3, 10, 17, 22, and 39 to 43 [47].The efficacy of this vaccine varies in different populations, with a consistently low efficacy in many tropical regions of the world [48], [49]. High efficacy when BCG is used to vaccinate newborns. Neonatal vaccination with BCG imparts protection against the childhood manifestations of TB (in particular, meningitis) [50], [51].

6.5. *M. microti*

It causes the disease in voles,wood mice and shrews. Its isolation is rare in human clinical samples, but recently, isolations from humans have been characterized. The spoligotypes analysis in isolates reveals the single presence of spacers 37 and 38 [53].

6.6. *M. canetti*

It was added to the list of *M. tuberculosis* complex in 1997. It isolated in 1993 from a 2-year-old Somali child with lymphadenitis, this isolate exhibited an unusually smooth and glossy colony morphology. To this date there have been few reports of TB cases due to this subspecies, and it is thought that animals are natural hosts of the bacterium [52].

6.7. *M. caprae*

This subspecies has been isolated mainly from goats in Spain [44], but it has also been found in boars, pigs, and in some cases of persons related to goat breeding [54]. The genetic footprint obtained by spoligotyping is characterized by the absence of spacers 1, 3 to 16, 10 to 33, and 39 to 43 [54].

6.8. *M. pinnipedii*

It was originally isolated from TB cases in pinnipeds such as sea lions and seals. Recently, cases have been described in terrestrial animals such as the Brazilian tapir. Its spoligotype has only the spacers 25 to 38 [55].

6.9. *M. mungi*

Identified in 2010 as a pathogen of the *M. tuberculosis* complex as TB causal agent in banded mongooses that live close to humans in the district of Chobe, Botswana, because these animals live in human-made structures and scavenge human waste, including feces.TB has been identified in only humans and mongooses. Strain assessment of human TB has not been conducted; the full host spectrum and transmission dynamics of this pathogen, currently unknown [56].

The spoligotype pattern of *M. mungi* isolates is characterized by absence of spacers 3, 7, 9, 12 to 36, and 39. It was determined that this pattern is preserved in the described isolates, but it is not included yet in international databases [56].

6.10. *M. orygis*

Species described in 2012 by Van Ingen and collaborators. It has been isolated from members of the Bovidae family such as oryx, gazelles, antelopes, cows, rhesus monkeys and waterbucks, although their exact host range remains unsettled, however cases have been described in humans [57]. Its spoligotype pattern is characterized by the absence of spacers 4-9, 14-24. 35, 36, and 39.The most common spoligotype (ST587) is present in the SITVIT WEB database and labeled *M. africanum* [58].

6.11. *M. tuberculosis* lineages (Fig. 4)

The lineages of *M. tuberculosis* are distributive a worldwide.

6.12. Haarlem (H)

Characterized by a pattern with absence of spacer 31 and the presence of at least one spacer between 1 and 30. It is highly prevalent in Northern Europe, while it is less extended in the Caribbean and Central Africa, where it is thought to be introduced by the European colonization [59].

6.13. Latin America and Mediterranean (LAM)

Characterized by the absence of spacers 21 to 24, 33 to 36, and the presence of at least one spacer between 1 and 30. It is frequent in Mediterranean and Latin American countries. Some genotypes have shown strong geographic associations, for instance LAM10-Cameroon or LAM7-Turkey which were initially catalogued as LAM although there has not been phylogenetic association with other spoligotypes [60, 61].

6.14. T Lineage

Comprised by modern strains of TB. This lineage is characterized "by default" and it includes strains which are difficult to classify into other groups [11] It has absence of spacers 33 to 36 and presence of at least one spacer between 1 to 30 besides the presence of the spacers 9 or 10, and 31; there is also presence of one spacer between 21 to 24 [62].

6.15. X lineage

Its pattern has absence of spacers 18 and 33 to 36. It was identified in Anglo-Saxon cities, and it is highly prevalent in South Africa, less in Latin America. However, there is high presence of this genotype in Mexico, which can be explained by its closeness to the United States. The X lineage was the first group identified in Guadeloupe [63] and the French Polynesia [64].

6.16. East African-Indian (EAI)

Absence of spacers 29 to 32 and 34; and presence of at least one spacer between 1 and 30. It is frequent in South East Asia, India, and Western Africa [62].

6.17. Central Asian (CAS)

Absence of spacers 4 to 27, and 23 to 34. It is highly prevalent in sub-Saharan countries and Pakistan. This linage has also proved to be endemic in Sudan, sub-Saharan countries, and Pakistan. This spoligotype has numerous variants and subgroups such as CAS1-Kili (Kilimanjaro), CAS-Dar (Dar-es-Salaam), and CAS-Delhi [62].

6.18. Beijing

This genotype has absence of spacers 1 to 33 and presence of spacers 34 to 43; in terms of public health it continues to be a serious problem for TB control due to its high virulence and association with multi-drug resistance [11].

6.19. MANU

It may be the ancestral clone of the strains in genetic group 1. It was subdivided into Manu 1 (absence of spacer 34), Manu 2 (absence of spacers 33-34), and Manu 3 (absence of spacers 34 to 36). It is a new family from India [62].

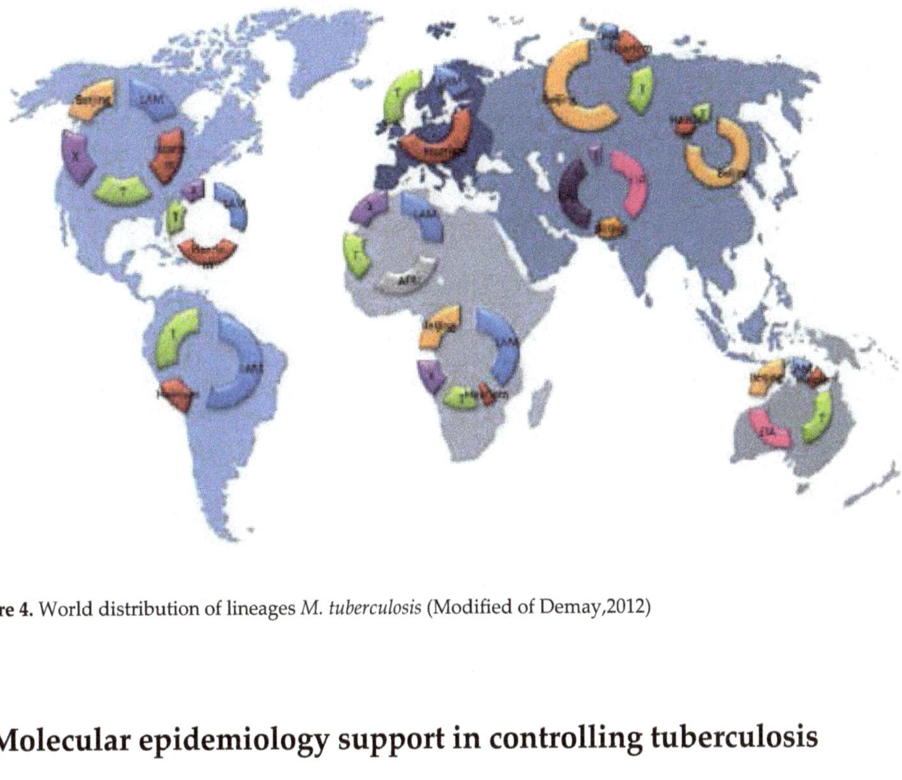

Figure 4. World distribution of lineages *M. tuberculosis* (Modified of Demay,2012)

7. Molecular epidemiology support in controlling tuberculosis

Molecular epidemiology has become in recent years an essential tool in the study of cases of tuberculosis, together with classical epidemiology, thus making the analysis of situations such as:

- Early detection and rapid control of outbreaks.
- Set transmission cases restricted communities
- Establish the geographic origin of the strains
- Monitoring of cross-contamination in the laboratories of TB

- Detection of genotypes associated with drug resistance
- Differentiation of cases of relapse and reinfection

In the analysis of data obtained by molecular epidemiology is essential to know definitions created from the development of molecular epidemiology, as they are

Cluster: A genotyping cluster is two or more *M. tuberculosis* isolates that share matching genotypes or the same DNA fingerprinting. An epidemiologic cluster is two or more persons with TB who share known epidemiologic links [38].

Matching genotypes: two or more *M. tuberculosis* isolates that share the same genotype.

Nonmatching genotype: an isolate that has a unique genotype (i.e., a genotype pattern that does not match the pattern of any other isolate in a TB program's database) [38].

7.1. Early detection of outbreaks

Analysis of clinical isolates of certain areas can help determine if isolates share the same genotype, and they form a cluster. But additionally be analyzed factors such as place of residence, work and time spent on them [38].

Genotypic guide Atlanta CDC studies raises three criteria for an outbreak [38].

1. An increase in the expected number of TB cases.
2. Transmission continues despite adequate control efforts by the TB program.
3. The contact investigation has grown to a size that requires additional outside help.

7.2. Transmission between cases of restricted communities

In conducting the study epidemiologically linked contacts and TB patients can be established [38]:

- Epidemiologic links between two TB cases that were identified during contact investigations and later confirmed by subsequent cluster investigations.
- New epidemiologic links that were identified during cluster investigations but not discovered during previous contact investigations.

7.3. Establishment of the geographical origin of the isolates

The analysis of several clinical isolates obtained worldwide, has established partnerships lineages with specific geographical areas, and in the case of LAM lineage or Latin American and Mediterranean, which as its name suggests occurs at high frequency in these geographic areas. The EIA or East African Indian [41].

7.4. Detecting genotypes associated drug resistance

The main genotype associated with drug resistance is the Beijing genotype, these strains exhibit high virulence and ease of propagation, but additionally the majority of clinical isolates belonging to this lineage with mutations that confer drug resistance, so its eradication much more difficult in the population, was first identified in China in 1995 [65], but has quickly spread to other countries, and has been responsible for outbreaks of MDR-TB [66, 67]:

7.5. Differentiation of relapses and reinfections

Initially, we must take into account in terms of TB programs, it only considers the situation of relapse which is defined as a patient previously treated for TB who has been declared cured or completed treatment and is newly diagnosed with bacteriologically positive tuberculosis. But the genotypic analysis classifies this situation relapse and reinfection, which are defined as, a case of relapsed TB represents a worsening of an infection after a period of improvement and is caused by the same strain of *M. tuberculosis*. TB that represents a reinfection is caused by a second infection with a strain that is different from the strain that caused the initial infection [38].

7.6. Cross contamination in the laboratories of TB

With the genotypic analysis of clinical isolates processed in a laboratory during the same time period can be set if cross-contamination occurred between crops.

Genotyping can help identify instances of incorrect TB diagnoses that are based on false positive cultures. Incorrect diagnoses can result from laboratory cross-contamination of cultures during batch processing, pipetting, transfer of bacilli from a broth-culture system, work in a faulty exhaust hood, and species-identification procedures, mislabeling of patient specimens, clinical equipment contaminated [38].

The identification of cross-contamination in a laboratory setting allows control measures to prevent patients are misdiagnosed.

7.7. Incorporating genotyping methodologies in TB diagnostic laboratories

Since the development of the genotyping methodologies, especially those that are based on nucleic acid amplification, it has been observed their advantage for use with isolated genetic material directly from clinical samples. Examples of these methodologies is spoligotyping, described by Kameberck, which allows simultaneous detection and typing of *M. tuberculosis*. Rapid identification and genotyping of *M. tuberculosis* families through the methodology implemented in multibacillary cases of TB, causing the rapid spread of the disease in community, reduce the time between suspicion of disease and treatment. Additionally, the application of the methodology of Spoligotyping in paucibacillary cases allows for quick diagnosis in cases of extrapulmonary tuberculosis, and rapid identification of *M. tuberculosis* complex species involved in the infection, supporting the clinician in addressing treatment.

8. Conclusion

The methods most commonly used in developing countries via bacteriological diagnoses were smear and culture show the presence of the causative agent of the disease. Currently being implemented new, more sensitive diagnostic technologies based on the detection of deoxyribonucleic acid (DNA) mycobacterial [68] and with which results are obtained in less time. Some of these methods provide the additional advantage of performing genotyping processes allowing the identification of family or families of *M. tuberculosis* present in the region, some of these methods are the analysis of the insertion sequence IS6110, polymorphism of the spacer sequences of Direct repeat region DR and analysis of the intergenic repeat units mycobacterial MIRU, and thus support the strategies of disease control with the detection of cases, relapse, and reinfection of new strain circulation, thus contributing to the development of molecular epidemiology.

9. Application exercise

9.1. Exercise 1: analyses of cases

Case 1

Patient presented an episode of TB in 2010, he completed his treatment but with some disruption, then in 2013, he presents a new case of TB. The following are spoligotypes patterns identified for Spoligotyping in each of the isolated (table 2).

2010	■■■■■■■■■■■■■■■■■■■■□□□□■■■■■■■■□□□□■■■■■■■	LAM9
2013	■■■■■■■■■■■■■■■■■■■■□□□□■■■■■■■■□□□□■■■■■■■	LAM9

Table 2. Spoligotypes case 1

Case 2

Patient presented an episode of TB in 2012, he completed his treatment in June of this year. In October 10th 2013, the patient was diagnosed with TB. The analyses for spoligotyping of the strains showed the following patterns (table 3).

2012	■■■■■■■■■■■■■■■■■■■■■■■■■■■■■■■■□□□□■■■■■■■	T1
2013	■■□■■■■■■■■■□■■■■■■■□□□□■■■■■■■■□□□□■■■■■■■	LAM2

Table 3. Spoligotypes case 2

Questions

1. Define the situation of each case, justified your response
2. Which other diagnosis methodologies you can use for confirmation the case.

9.2. Exercise 2

Complete the gaps on the table 4

Number	Binary code	Octal code	SIT	Lineage
001	1101111111101111111000011111111100001111111			
002	1111111111111111111111111111111100001111111			
003	1111111111111111111100001111111100001111111			
004			273	
005	1111111111111111111111111000000100001110111	777777774020731	62	
006			91	
007	1111111111111111111100001111111100001111111			
008	1111111111111111111111111000000100001110111			
009		777777777720771		
010	0000000000000000000000000000000000111111111	000000000003771	1	
011	1111111111111111111111111111111010000111111			
012			447	
013	1111111111111111111111101111111100001111111			
014	1111111111111111111111111111111100001111111			
015	1101111111101111111000011111111100001111111			
016	1110000111111111111111000000000000111111111			
017	1001111111111111111111111111100001011000111		11	
018		777777607760771		
019	1111111111111011111111111111111100001111111			
020	1111111111111111111100001111111100001111111			
021			373	
022			42	
023			64	
024		777777477760771		
025	1111111100111111111111111000000000000110111			
026	0000111111111111111100000111101110000111011			
027	1111111111111111111101111111111100001110111			
028	1111111111111111111100001111111100001111111			
029			33	
030			53	

Table 4. Exercise 2

Author details

Magda Lorena Orduz and Wellman Ribón

Universidad Industrial de Santander, Bucaramanga, Colombia

References

[1] Ministerio de la Protección Social. Guía de atención de la tuberculosis pulmonar y extrapulmonar. Guía 11 Guías de promoción de la salud y prevención de enfermedades en la salud pública. Programa de Apoyo a la Reforma de Salud/PARS.2007. http://www.nacer.udea.edu.co/pdf/libros/guiamps/guias11.pdf

[2] Jordao L, Vieira O. Tuberculosis: New Aspects of an Old Disease.International Journal of Cell Biology, 2011. Article ID 403623. doi:10.1155/2011/403623

[3] INSTITUTO NACIONAL DE SALUD. Informe de evento tuberculosis, hasta el periodo epidemiológico 13 del año 2012. 2012

[4] World Health Organization. WHO Global tuberculosis report 2012. ISBN 978 92 4 156450 2. http://www.who.int/tb/publications/global_report/gtbr12_main.pdf

[5] Ministerio de la Protección Social. Guía de atención de la tuberculosis pulmonar y extrapulmonar. Guía 11 Guías de promoción de la salud y prevención de enfermedades en la salud pública. Programa de Apoyo a la Reforma de Salud/PARS.2007. http://www.nacer.udea.edu.co/pdf/libros/guiamps/guias11.pdf

[6] Solovic I, Jonsson J, Korzeniewska- Koseła M, Chiotan D, Pace-Asciak A., Slump E. *et al*. Challenges in diagnosing extrapulmonary tuberculosis in the European Union, 2011. Euro Surveill. 2013; 18(12): pii=20432. http://www.eurosurveillance.org/ViewArticle.aspx?ArticleId=20432

[7] World Health Organization. Treatment of tuberculosis: Guidelines for national programmes. Third edition. Geneva 2003

[8] Dai J, Chen Y, Lauzardo M. Web-Accessible Database of *hsp65* Sequences from *Mycobacterium* Reference Strains. J Clin Microbiol, 2011; 49: 2296–2303

[9] Jordao L, Vieira O. Tuberculosis: New Aspects of an Old Disease. International Journal of Cell Biology, 2011. Article ID 403623. doi:10.1155/2011/403623

[10] Cole S, Brosch R, Parkhill J. et al. Deciphering the biology of *Mycobacterium tuberculosis* from the complete genome sequence. Nature, 1998; 393: 537-44.

[11] Palomino J, Leão S, Ritacco V. Tuberculosis 2007: From basic science to patient care. First Edition. 2007. http://www.TuberculosisTextbook.com

[12] Ribon W. Biochemical Isolation and Identification of Mycobacteria. Biochemical testing. Rijeka: Intech; 2012. pag 21-52.Available fromhttp://cdn.intechopen.com/pdfs-wm/30397.pdf

[13] Palomino J, Leão S, Ritacco V. Tuberculosis 2007: From basic science to patient care. First Edition. 2007. http://www.TuberculosisTextbook.com

[14] Arnvig K, Gopal B, Papavinasasundaram K, Cox R , Colston J. The mechanism of upstream activation in the rrnB operon of *Mycobacterium smegmatis* is different from the Escherichia coli paradigm Microbiology, 2005; 151: 467–473

[15] Verma A, Avinash K, Wami J. *Mycobacterium tuberculosis rrn* Promoters: Differential Usage and Growth Rate-Dependent Control. Journal of Bacteriology, 1999; 181(4): 4326–4333

[16] Organización Panamericana de la Salud. Manual para el diagnóstico Bacteriológico de la tuberculosis. Normas y Guía Técnica. Parte I baciloscopia. 2008. Disponible en http://files.sld.cu/tuberculosis/files/2009/12/tb-labs-baciloscopia1.pd

[17] van Embden J, Cave M, Crawford J, Dale J, Eisenach K, Gicquel B, Hermans P, Martin C, Mcadam R, Shinnick T, et al. Strain identification of *Mycobacterium tuberculosis* by DNA fingerprinting: recommendations for a standardized methodology. J. Clin. Microbiol. 1993; 31: 406–409.

[18] Groenen P, Bunschoten A, Van Soolingen D, Van Embden J. Nature of DNA polymorphism in the direct repeat cluster of *Mycobacterium tuberculosis*: application for strain differentiation by a novel typing method. Mol. Microbiol, 1993; 10:1057–1085

[19] Kamerbeek J, Schouls L, Kolk A, Van Agterveld M, Van Soolingen D, Kuijper S, Bunschoten A, Molhuizen, H, Shaw R, Goyal M, Van Embden J. Simultaneous detection and strain differentiation of *Mycobacterium tuberculosis* for diagnosis and epidemiology. J. Clin. Microbiol, 1997; 35: 907–914.

[20] Frothingham R, Meeker-O'Connell W. Genetic diversity in the *Mycobacterium tuberculosis* complex based on variable numbers of tandem DNA repeats. Microbiology, 1998; 144: 1189-96.

[21] Supply P, Mazars E, Lesjean S, Vincent V, Gicquel B, Locht C. Variable human minisatellite-like regions in the *Mycobacterium tuberculosis* genome. Mol. Microbiol, 2000; 36: 762–771.

[22] Baker L, Brown T, Maiden M, Drobniewski F. Silent nucleotide polymorphisms and a phylogeny for *Mycobacterium tuberculosis*. Emerg Infect Dis, 2004; 10: 1568-77.

[23] Filliol I, Motiwala A, Cavatore M. et al. Global phylogeny of *Mycobacterium tuberculosis* based on single nucleotide polymorphism (SNP) analysis: insights into tuberculosis evolution, phylogenetic accuracy of other DNA fingerprinting systems, and recommendations for a minimal standard SNP set. J Bacteriol, 2006; 188: 759

[24] Mostowy S, Inwald J, Gordon S. et al. Revisiting the evolution of *Mycobacterium bovis*. J Bacteriol, 2005; 187: 6386-95.

[25] McAdam, R. A., P. W. M. Hermans, D. van Soolingen, Z. F. Zainuddin, D. Catty, J. D. A. van Embden, and J. W. Dale. 1990. Characterization of a Mycobacterium tuberculosis insertion sequence belonging to the IS3 family. Mol. Microbiol. 4:1607-1613.

[26] Thierry D, Brisson-Noel A, Vincent-Levy-Frebault V, Nguyen S, Guesdon J, Gicquel B. Characterization of a *Mycobacterium tuberculosis* insertion sequence, IS6110, and its application in diagnosis. J. Clin. Microbiol, 1990; 28: 2668–2673.

[27] van Soolingen D, Hermans P, De Haas P, Soll D, Van Embden J. Occurrence and stability of insertion sequences in *Mycobacterium tuberculosis* complex strains: evaluation of an insertion sequence-dependent DNA polymorphism as a tool in the epidemiology of tuberculosis. J. Clin. Microbiol, 1991;29: 2578–2

[28] Kanduma E, Mchugh T, Gillespie S. Molecular methods for *Mycobacterium tuberculosis* strain typing: a user guide. Journal of Applied Microbiology, 2003; 94: 781–791

[29] Van Soolingen, D., Hermans, P.W., De Haas, P.E. and Van Embden, J.D. (1992) Insertion element IS1081-associated restriction fragment length polymorphism in *M. tuberculosis* complex species: a reliabletool for recognizing Mycobacterium bovis BCG. Journal of Clinical Microbiology 30, 1772–1777.

[30] Van Soolingen, D., De Haas, P.E., Hermans, P.W., Groenen, P.M., and Van Embden, J.D. Comparison of various repetitive DNA elements as genetic markers for strain differentiation and epidemiology *of M. tuberculosis* Journal of Clinical Microbiology . 1993; 31, 1987–1995

[31] De Wit D, Steyn S, Shoemaker S, Sogin M. (1990) Direct detection of *M. tuberculosis* in clinical specimens by DNA amplification. Journal of Clinical Microbiology 28, 2437–2441

[32] Poulet S, Cole S. (1994) Characterization of the polymorphic GC-rich repetitive sequence (PGRS) present in *M. tuberculosis*. Archives of Microbiology 163, 87–95.

[33] Ross B, Raios K, Jackson K, Dwyer B. (1992) Molecular cloning of a highly repeated DNA element from *M. tuberculosis* and its use as an epidemiological tool. Journal of Clinical Microbiology 30, 942–946.

[34] Poulet S, Cole S. (1995) Characterization of the highly abundant polymorphic GC-rich-repetitive sequence (PGRS) present in *M. tuberculosis*. Archives of Microbiology 16, 87–95.

[35] Fang Z, Morrison N, Watt B, Doig C, Forbes K. IS6110 transposition and evolutionary scenario of the direct repeat locus in a group of closely related *Mycobacterium tuberculosis*strains. J. Bacteriol, 1998; 180:2102– 2109.

[36] van Embden J, Van Gorkom T, Kremer K, Jansen R, Van Der Zeijst B, Schouls L. Genetic Variation and Evolutionary Origin of the Direct Repeat Locus of *Mycobacterium*

tuberculosis Complex Bacteria. J. Bacteriol, 2000; 182(9): 2393. DOI: 10.1128/JB.182.9.2393-2401.2000

[37] Legrand E, Filliol I, Sola C, Rastogi N. Use of Spoligotyping to Study the Evolution of the Direct Repeat Locus by IS*6110* Transposition in *Mycobacterium tuberculosis. J. Clin. Microbiol,* 2001; 39 (4):1595. DOI: 10.1128/JCM.39.4.1595- 1599.2001.

[38] National Tuberculosis Controllers Association /Centers for Disease Control and Prevention Advisory Group on Tuberculosis Genotyping. Guide to the Application of Genotyping to Tuberculosis Prevention and Control Handbook for TB controllers, Epidemiologists, Laboratorians, and Other Program Staff June 2004. Disponible en: http://www.cdc.gov/tb/programs/genotyping/images/TBGenotyping-Guide_June2004.pdf

[39] Burgos M, Méndez J, Ribon W. Molecular epidemiology of tuberculosis: methodology and applications. Biomedica, 2004; 24(Supl.): 188-201

[40] Bauer J, Andersen A, Kremer K, Miorner H. Usefulness of spoligotyping to discriminate IS6110 low-copy-number *Mycobacterium tuberculosis* complex strains cultured in Denmark. J. Clin. Microbiol, 1999; 37: 2602–2606.

[41] Demay C, Liens B, Burguière T, Hill V, Couvin D, Miller J, Mokrousov I, Sola C, Zozio T, Rastogi N. SITVITWEB – A publicly available international multimarker database for studying *Mycobacterium tuberculosis* genetic diversity and molecular epidemiology. Infection, Genetics and Evolution, 2012; 12: 755–766

[42] van der Zanden A, Kremer K, Schouls L, Caimi K, Cataldi A, Hulleman A, Nagelkerke N, Van Soolingen D. Improvement of differentiation and interpretability of spoligotyping for *Mycobacterium tuberculosis* complex isolates by introduction of new spacer oligonucleotides. J. Clin. Microbiol. 2002; 40: 4628–4639.

[43] Supply P, Allix C, Lesjean S, Cardoso-Oelemann M, Rusch-Gerdes S, Willery E, *et al.* Proposal for standardization of optimized mycobacterial interspersed repetitive unit-variable number tandem repeat typing of *Mycobacterium tuberculosis.* J. Clin. Microbiol, 2006; 44: 4498–4510

[44] Leao S, Martin A, Mejia G, Palomino J, Robledo J, Da Silva Telles M, Portaels, F. Practical handbook for the phenotypic and genotypic identification of mycobacteria.2004

[45] Vasconcellos S, Huard R, Niemann S, Kremer K , Santos A, Suffys P, Ho J. Distinct genotypic profiles of the two major clades of *Mycobacterium africanum.* BMC Infectious Diseases 2010, 10:80 http://www.biomedcentral.com/1471-2334/10/80

[46] de Jong B, Antonio M, Gagneux S. *Mycobacterium africanum*—Review of an Important Cause of Human Tuberculosis in West Africa. PLoS Negl Trop Dis, 2010; 4(9): e744. doi:10.1371/journal.pntd.0000744

[47] Brandt L, Feino J, Weinreich A, Chilima B, Irsch P, Appelberg R, Andersen P. Failure of the *Mycobacterium bovis* BCG Vaccine: Some Species of Environmental Mycobacte-

ria Block Multiplication of BCG and Induction of Protective Immunity to Tuberculosis. Infection and immunity, 2002; 70(2): 672–678

[48] Fine,P. The BCG story: lessons from the past and implications for the future. Rev. Infect. Dis. 1989; 11(Suppl. 2):S353–S359.

[49] Fine, P. Variation in protection by BCG: implications of and for heterologous immunity. Lancet 1995; 346:1339–1345.

[50] Al-Kassimi F, Al-Hajjaj M, Al-Orainey I, Bamgboye E.. Does the protective effect of neonatal BCG correlate with vaccineinduced tuberculin reaction? Am. J. Respir. Crit. Care Med. 1995; 152:1575–1578.

[51] Colditz, G. A., C. S. Berkey, F. Mosteller, T. F. Brewer, M. E. Wilson, E. Burdick, and H. V. Fineberg. The efficacy of bacillus Calmette-Guerin vaccination of newborns and infants in the prevention of tuberculosis: metaanalyses of the published literature. Pediatrics 1995; 96:29–35.

[52] Van Soolingen D, Hoogenboezem T, De Haas Pe, Hermans P, Koedam M, Teppema K. et al. A Novel Pathogenic Taxon of the *Mycobacterium tuberculosis* Complex, Canetti: Characterization of an Exceptional Isolate from Africa. International Union of Microbiological Societies, 1997; 47(4): 1236-1245

[53] Cavanagh R, Begon M, Bennett M, Ergon T, Graham I, De Haas P, Hart C, et al. *Mycobacterium microti* Infection (Vole Tuberculosis) in Wild Rodent Populations. J Clin Microbiol, 2002;40(9): 3281–3285.

[54] Aranaz A, Cousins D, Mateos A, Domínguez L. Elevation of *Mycobacterium tuberculosissubsp. caprae* Aranaz et al. 1999 to species rank as *Mycobacterium caprae* comb. nov., sp. nov. International Journal of Systematic and Evolutionary Microbiology, 2003; 53: 1785–1789

[55] Cousins D, Bastida R, Cataldi A, Quse V, Redrobe S, Dow S *et al.* Tuberculosis in seals caused by a novel member of the *Mycobacterium* tuberculosis complex: *Mycobacterium pinnipedii* sp. nov. International Journal of Systematic and Evolutionary Microbiology, 2003; 53: 1305–1314

[56] Alexander K, Laver P, Michel A, Williams M, Van Helden P, Warren R, Gey Van Pittius N. Novel *Mycobacterium tuberculosis* Complex Pathogen, *M. mungi*. Emerging Infectious Diseases, 2010; 16(8). DOI: 10.3201/eid1608.100314

[57] Kara L. Dawson,a Anita Bell,b R. Pamela Kawakami,c Kathryn Coley,b Gary Yates,c and Desmond M. Collins. Transmission of *Mycobacterium orygis* (*M. tuberculosis* Complex Species) from a Tuberculosis Patient to a Dairy Cow in New Zealand. Journal of Clinical Microbiology p. 3136–3138 September 2012 Volume 50 Number 9

[58] van Ingen J, Rahim Z, Mulder A, Boeree M, Simeone R, Brosch R, van Soolingen D. Characterization of *Mycobacterium orygis* as *M. tuberculosis* Complex Subspecies.

Emerging Infectious Diseases, 2012; 18(4). DOI: http://dx.doi.org/10.3201/eid1804.110888

[59] Filliol I, Driscoll J, Van Soolingen D, et al. Snapshot of moving and expanding clones of *Mycobacterium tuberculosis* and their global distribution assessed by spoligotyping in an international study. J Clin Microbiol 2003; 41: 1963-70.

[60] Niobe-Eyangoh Sn, Kuaban C, Sorlin P., et al. Genetic biodiversity of *Mycobacterium tuberculosis* complex strains from patients with pulmonary tuberculosis in Cameroon. J Clin Microbiol, 2003; 41: 2547-53.

[61] Zozio T, Allix C, Gunal S, et al. Genotyping of *Mycobacterium tuberculosis* clinical isolates in two cities of Turkey: description of a new family of genotypes that is phylogeographically specific for Asia Minor. BMC Microbiol, 2005; 5: 44.

[62] Brudey K, Driscoll J, Rigouts L, et al. *Mycobacterium tuberculosis* complex genetic diversity: mining the fourth international spoligotyping database (SpolDB4) for classification, population genetics and epidemiology. BMC Microbiol, 2006; 6: 23

[63] Sola C, Horgen L, Goh K, Rastogi N. Molecular fingerprinting of *Mycobacterium tuberculosis* on a Caribbean island with IS*6110* and DRr probes. J Clin Microbiol, 1997; 35:843-6.

[64] Torrea G, Levee G, Grimont P, Martin C, Chanteau S, Gicquel B. Chromosomal DNA fingerprinting analysis using the insertion sequence IS*6110* and the repetitive element DR as strain-specific markers for epidemiological study of tuberculosis in French Polynesia. J Clin Microbiol, 1995; 33: 1899-904.

[65] van Soolingen D, Qian L, de Haas P E, et al. Predominance of a single genotype of *Mycobacterium tuberculosis* in countries of East Asia. J Clin Microbiol 1995; 33: 3234–3238.

[66] Bifani P J, Mathema B, Kurepina N E, Kreiswirth B N. Global dissemination of the *Mycobacterium tuberculosis* W-Beijing family strains. Trends in Microbiol 2001; 10: 45–52.

[67] Moss A R, Alland D, Telzak E, et al. A city-wide outbreak of a multiple drug-resistant strain of *Mycobacterium tuberculosis* in New York. Int J Tuberc Lung Dis 1997; 1: 115–121

[68] Neonakis I, Gitti Z, Krambovitis E, Spandidos D. Molecular diagnostic tools in mycobacteriology. Journal of Microbiological Methods, 2008; 75: 1–11

9

Pathophysiological Implications of Cell Envelope Structure in *Mycobacterium tuberculosis* and Related Taxa

David E. Minnikin, Oona Y-C Lee, Houdini H.T. Wu, Vijayashankar Nataraj, Helen D. Donoghue, Malin Ridell, Motoko Watanabe, Luke Alderwick, Apoorva Bhatt and Gurdyal S. Besra

1. Introduction

Members of the *Mycobacterium tuberculosis* complex are successful pathogens due in a large part to the complex interactions of an array of very special lipid molecular classes and associated macromolecules that have been known for many years [1-6]. The cooperative assembly of these components results in the presence of very robust cell envelopes. In particular there is a specialised outer membrane; this can be termed a "mycomembrane", but in this review the abbreviation, MOM, for "mycobacterial outer membrane" will be used. Subtle structural variations in mycobacterial lipid components point to important roles in the integrity and function of the mycobacterial cell envelope. Over three decades ago, an attempt was made to rationalise the role of the known constituent molecules with a proposal for a "chemical" model of the cell envelope [4]. This general model has been supported in subsequent studies but a wealth of new knowledge suggests that a significant upgrade is needed. Each class of cell envelope structural units will be introduced, reasons for "why" such structures are produced will be explored and an updated cell envelope model presented as a working hypothesis. Close comparisons of the cell envelope compositions of *M. tuberculosis* and related taxa will be interpreted in terms of evolution and pathogenicity. In various diseases, the term "pathophysiology" is usually used to describe physiological changes in affected hosts; here its meaning is turned around to explore the impact of aspects of mycobacterial cell physiology in pathogenic members of the *M. tuberculosis* complex.

Precise structures of the lipid moieties displayed in members of the *M. tuberculosis* complex have become established during the past five decades, so it is now possible to explore the significance of structure in the pathophysiological role of such lipids. Attention will focus on lipids, whose regular occurrence in significant proportions indicates that they are integral structural members of the mycobacterial cell envelope. Details of general biosynthetic pathways will not be considered, nor will particular biological effects of individual lipid classes. Recent cryo-electron microscopy studies have allowed the absolute dimensions of the mycobacterial cell envelope to be estimated [7-9] so all components must adopt conformations that allow their integration into an effective organelle. Tubercle bacilli also have a less clearly defined capsule external to the more coherent cell envelope [10,11]; a detailed discussion of this important region will not be attempted here. Similarly, a detailed exploration of protein content is not given, even for structurally vital proteins such as well-characterised porins [12]. The main chemical structures that must be accommodated in the cell envelope of *M. tuberculosis* are considered in the following sections, commencing with the long-chain mycolic acids that are mycobacterial signature components [4,13-18].

2. Mycolic acids

The 70 to 90 carbon mycolic acids (MAs) are very characteristic chemical components in the genus *Mycobacterium*. Members of the *M. tuberculosis* complex have three classes, the so-called α-mycolates, methoxymycolates and ketomycolates (Figure 1) [4,13-18]. The latter two varieties (Figure 1B) are comprised of subclasses having either *cis*-cyclopropane rings or *trans*-cyclopropane rings with an adjacent methyl branch. In the case of the α-mycolates (Figure 1A), representative C_{80} mycolates from *Mycobacterium kansasii* and the *M. tuberculosis* complex are compared to highlight the importance of key structural differences, whose importance will be discussed later. All these MA classes occur naturally with at least five homologues and variations in the numbers of carbons between the various functional groups. The majority of MAs are covalently bound to arabinose termini of a mycoloylarabinogalactan-peptidoglycan (mAGP) macromolecule to form a lipid monolayer inner leaflet of the MOM [4,19], as will be described in detail later.

Recent physiochemical investigations have clearly demonstrated that mycolic acids characteristically adopt distinctly different folded conformations depending on structural niceties [20-24]. Ketomycolates in *M. tuberculosis* predominately fold to yield a compact "W" conformation, with four chains in parallel [20,21,23,24]. Such tight packing can provide the foundation for an effective hydrophobic permeability barrier in the inner leaflet of the MOM. In contrast, α- and methoxymycolates can form W-conformations but also more readily inhabit a range of more extended conformations [20-23], some of which can be visualised as "U" or "Z" shaped [24]. The α-mycolates tend towards an open fully extended U-conformation with the two distal chains extended and methoxymycolates show intermediate behaviour between the two other classes [22,24]. For the purpose of illustrating the importance of mycolate conformation in MOM inner leaflet function (see later), ketomycolates are restricted to W-

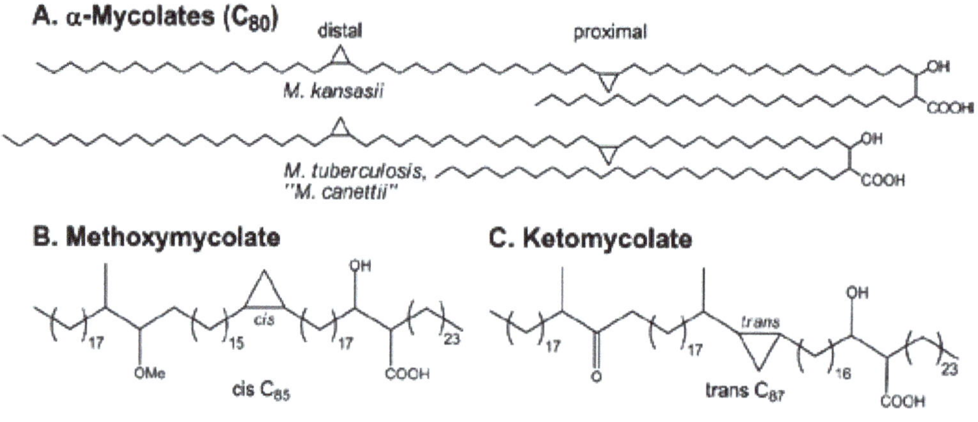

Figure 1. Representative structures of mycolic acids. **A.** α-Mycolates (C_{80}), comparing *M. kansasii* and *M. tuberculosis* complex. **B, C.** The main methoxy- and ketomycolates from *M. tuberculosis*.

conformations, methoxymycolates are shown with both semi-folded sZ and fully folded W-shapes [24] and α-mycolates have extended eU-conformations [24] (Figure 2).

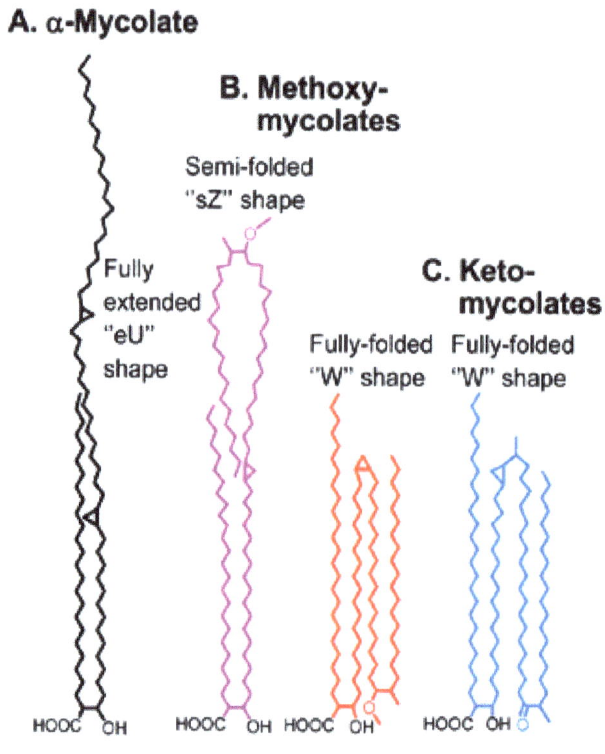

Figure 2. Two-dimensional representative conformations of *M. tuberculosis* mycolic acids. **A.** Extended α-mycolate. **B.** Two alternatives for methoxymycolates. **C.** Fully folded ketomycolate.

3. Esters of mycolic acids

The so-called "cord factors" are the best known mycolic acid esters in mycobacteria; they are principally trehalose dimycolates (TDMs) with trehalose monomycolates (TMMs) also being encountered (Figure 3). The proportions of TDMs and TMMs vary widely in mycobacteria so an integral structural role is not indicated, their main importance lying in the key role as intermediates in the transfer of mycolic acids on to arabinosyl units in the cell envelope [13]. Glucose monomycolates (GMMs) are common in mycobacteria, but in highly variable proportions [25]. Consistent proportions, however, are recorded for monomycoloyl glycerols (MMGs) (Figure 3) in the *Mycobacterium bovis* members of the *M. tuberculosis* complex [26,27], thereby suggesting some cell envelope structural involvement. Mycobacteria also produce very complex mixtures of di- and triacylglycerols, some of which contain non-hydroxylated fatty acids that correspond to the meromycolate portion of mycolic acids [28,29], the so-called "mycobacteric" acids [2]. Triacylglycerols have a storage role in "lipid bodies" [30] but they have also been suggested as contributors to the MOM outer leaflet [31]; the complex mixtures of di- and triacylglycerols must be fully unravelled before precise roles can be properly defined.

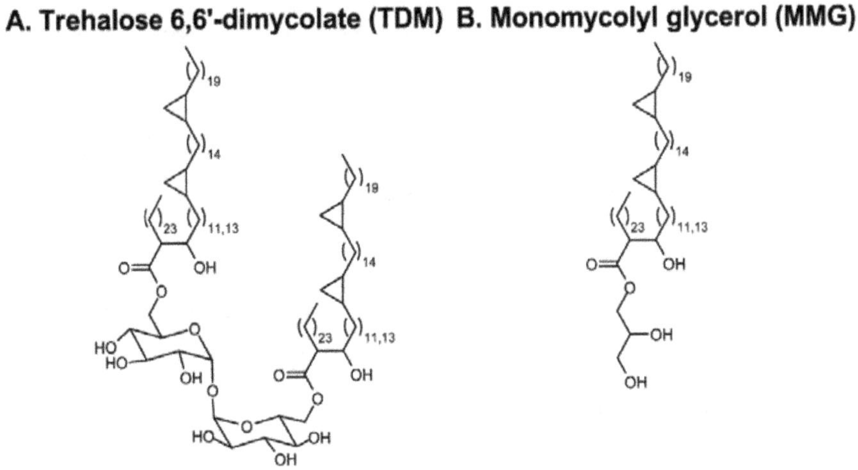

Figure 3. Mycolic acid esters. **A.** Trehalose dimycolate (TDM). **B.** Monomycoloyl glycerol (MMG).

4. Phthiocerol and phenolphthiocerol dimycocerosate families

The phthiocerol and phenolphthiocerol long-chain diols are esterified by multimethyl-branched "mycocerosic" acids whose chiral centres have ***R*** absolute configuration in members of the *M. tuberculosis* complex and *M. kansasii* (Figure 4) [32-35]. Phthiocerol dimycocerosates (PDIMs) are mainly based on long-chain diols, the phthiocerol As and phthiodiolones (Figure 4). Related families of the phenolphthiocerol dimycocerosates have characteristic antigenic oligosaccharides linked to the phenolic residue and these are commonly known as "phenolic glycolipids" (PGLs) (Figure 4) [33-36]. PDIMs are large (> 90 carbons) hydrophobic molecules that are considered to be "free lipid" constituents of the outer leaflet of the external MOM, interacting with the chains of the covalently bound MAs of the inner leaflet. The PDIMs from the *M. tuberculosis* complex are relatively large in comparison with those of other taxa. Other interesting cases are the so-called "Beijing" variants of *M. tuberculosis* [37] and *M. kansasii* [32, 33,35] where only restricted selections of members of the phthiocerol family are encountered.

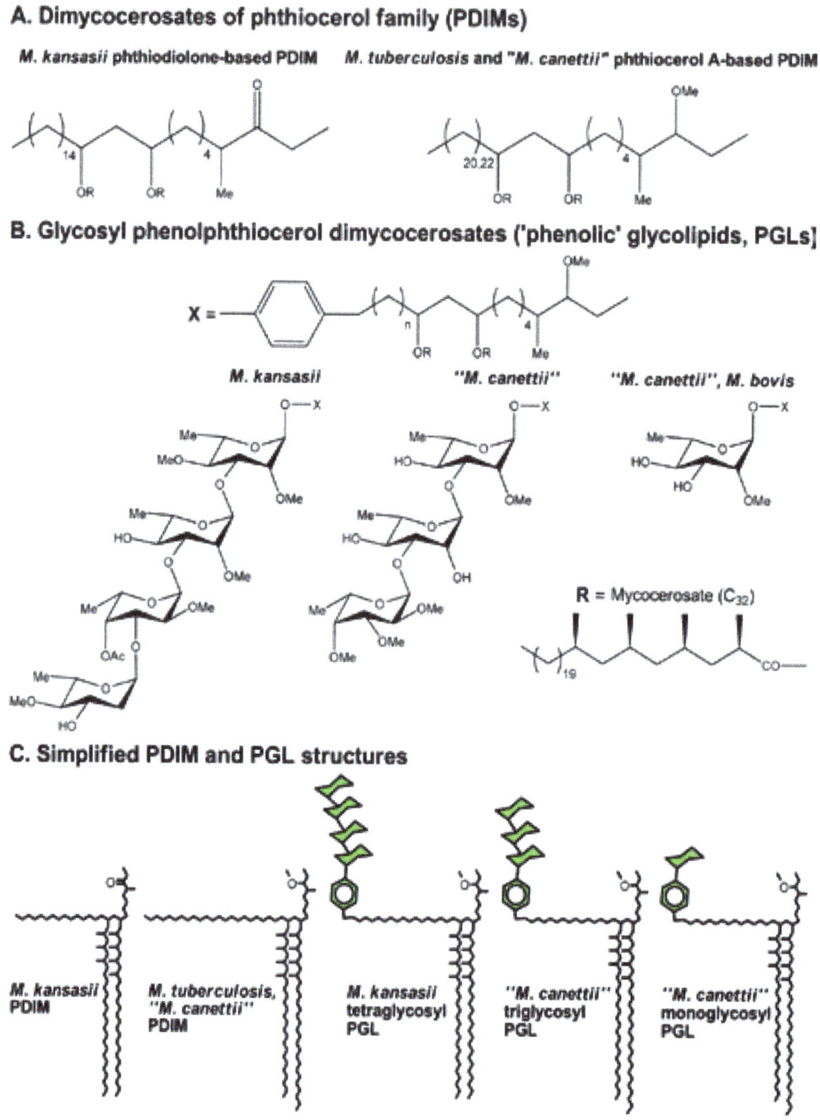

Figure 4. Representative structures of mycocerosate esters of phthiocerols and glycosyl phenophthiocerols. **A.** Phthiocerol family. **B.** Glycosyl phenophthiocerol (phenolic glycolipids). **C.** Simplified structures for illustrative use in Figures 10 and 11.

The oligosaccharide substituents of PGLs have demonstrable antigenicity [38] but the individual sugar units are relatively hydrophobic. Certain members of the *M. tuberculosis* complex, such as the rare smooth morphology tubercle bacilli termed "*Mycobacterium canettii*", have two PGL types with different oligosaccharides but *M. bovis,* for example, has only a single type (Figure 4). The PGLs from *M. kansasii* have close structural similarities to those from "*M. canettii*" (Figure 4), but not to those from *Mycobacterium marinum* [33-36]. The chiral centres in the multimethyl-branched fatty acid substituents in both the PGLs and PDIMs from *M. marinum* and *Mycobacterium ulcerans* are of *S* absolute configuration [33-36]. Significantly, the 1,3-diol units in the phthiocerol and phenolphthiocerol moieties (Figure 4) from *M. marinum* and *M. ulcerans* have *erythro* geometric configuration in contrast to the more common *threo* stereochemistry [33-36].

5. Acyl trehaloses

In addition to TDMs and TMMs, there are families of trehalose-based glycolipids acylated with multimethyl branched fatty acids with *S* absolute configuration of their chiral centres (Figure 5) [34,39,40]. The main fatty acids encountered are C_{24} mycosanoic, C_{27} mycolipenic, C_{27} mycolipanolic, C_{37} phthioceranic and C_{40} hydroxyphthioceranic acids (Figure 5). Diacyl trehaloses (DATs) are the simplest representatives, based on C_{24} mycosanoic and C_{27} mycolipanolic acids. The C_{27} mycolipenates are the characteristic acyl components of pentaacyl trehaloses (PATs) (Figure 5). The exceptionally long phthioceranic and hydroxyphthioceranic acids are the fatty acids found in a family of sulfated trehalose glycolipids (SGLs) (Figure 5) [3,41].

6. Lipooligosaccharides

A highly polar series of lipids, which include trehalose in their saccharide core, are termed lipooligosaccharides (LOSs) [42,43]. Such lipids are absent in many modern *M. tuberculosis* isolates but they are characteristic of "*M. canettii*" and *M. kansasii* (Figure 6). Lipooligosaccharides are associated with biofilms and motility [44]. Indeed, it has been shown that smooth variants of *M. kansasii,* containing LOSs, are rapidly cleared from the organs of infected animals, but rough variants, lacking all LOSs, produce chronic systemic infections [45].

7. Phosphatidylinositol mannosides and other polar lipids

The mycobacterial plasma membrane incorporates conventional polar lipids, such as phosphatidylethanolamine (PE), phosphatidylinositol (PI) and diphosphatidylglycerol (DPG) (Figure 7), which can interact together to form the basis of a typical membrane bilayer. However, most mycobacteria have a remarkably consistent family of four phosphatidylinosi-

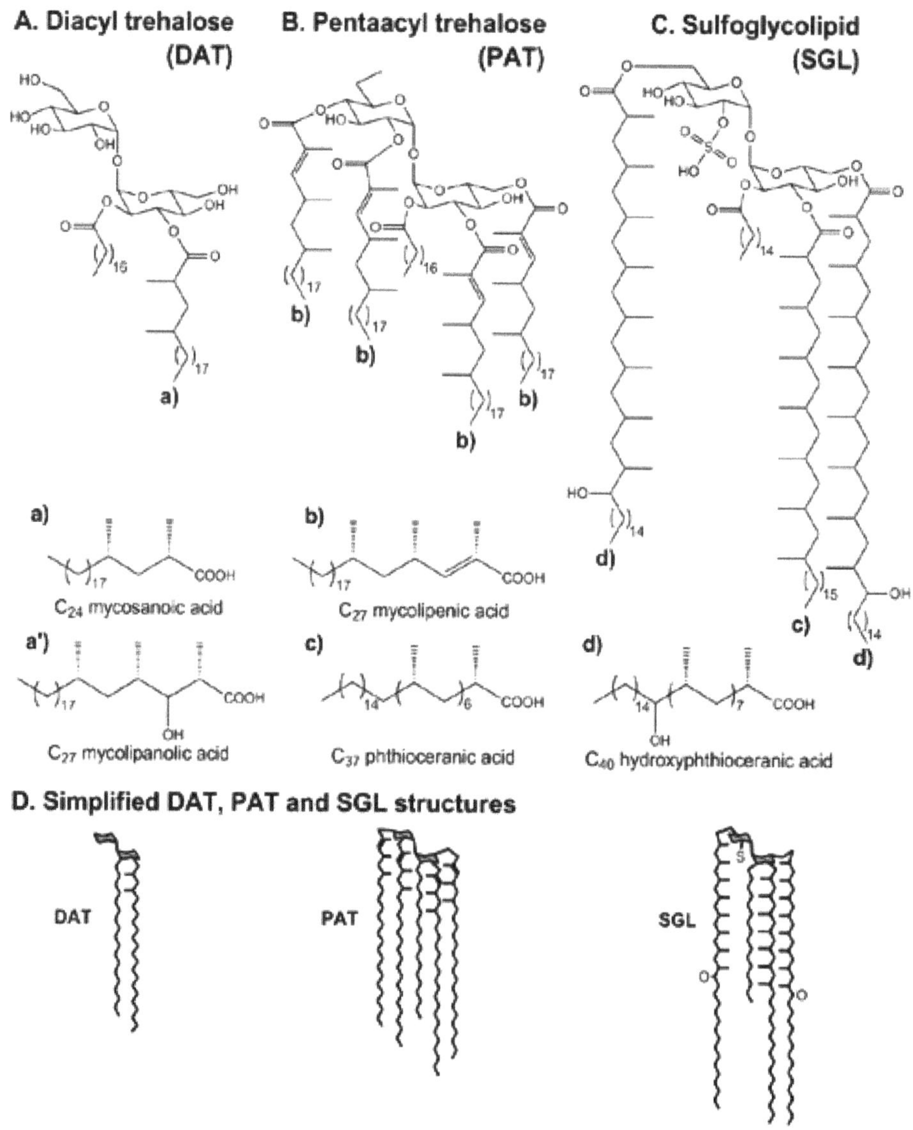

Figure 5. Acyl trehaloses. **A.** Diacyl trehalose (DAT). **B.** Pentaacyl trehalose (PAT). **C.** Sulfoglycolipid (SGL). **D.** Simplified structures for illustrative use in Figures 10 and 11.

tol mannosides (PIMs); these comprise mono- ($AcPIM_2$) and diacyl phosphatidylinositol dimannosides (Ac_2PIM_2) and mono- ($AcPIM_6$) and diacyl phosphatidylinositol hexamannosides (Ac_2PIM_6) (Figure 7) [46-49]. Recent research has provided evidence that PIM_2 and PIM_6 classes may be unevenly distributed over the two leaflets of the mycobacterial plasma membrane [31]. These findings will be interpreted, later, as showing that PIMs may act to reinforce the plasma membrane, perhaps adding a further level of selective permeability to the mycobacterial cell envelope.

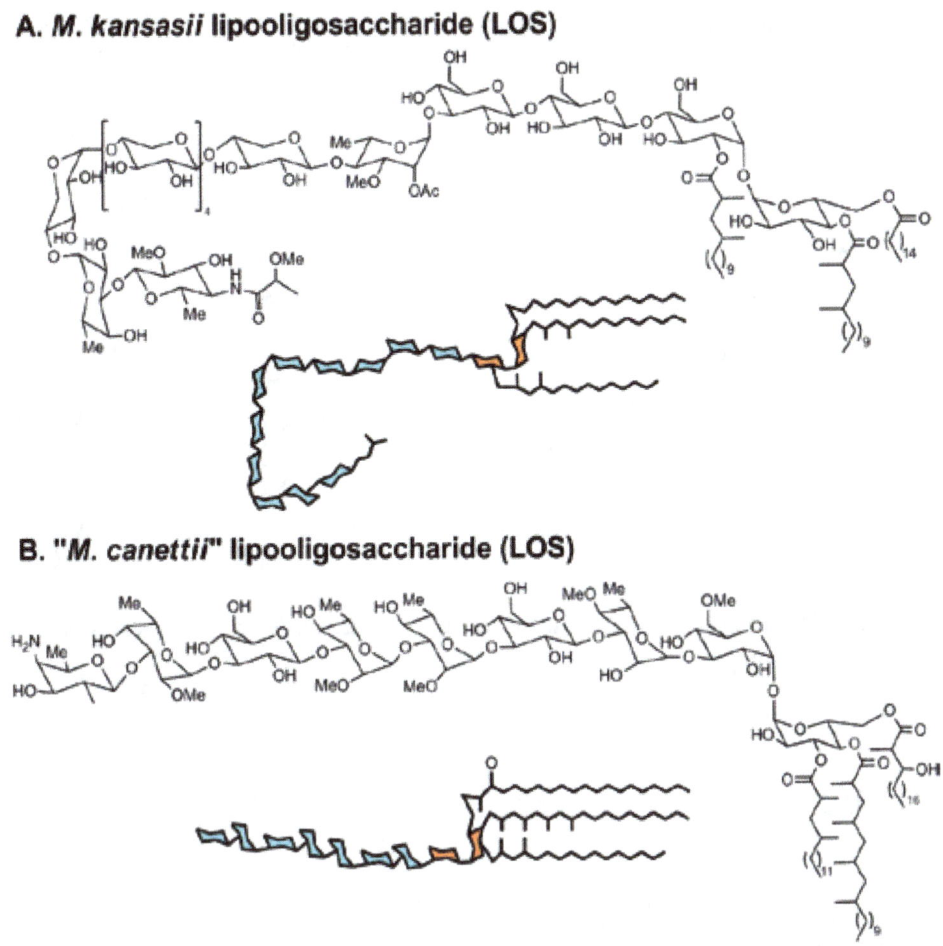

Figure 6. Lipooligosaccharides (LOSs). A. *M. kansasii*. B. *"M. canettii"*. Simplified structures are included.

8. Lipomannan and lipoarabinomannan

The basic structures of the PIMs polar lipid family (Figure 8) share the same manno-phosphatidylinositol (MPI) anchor with two classes of characteristic large lipoglycans, namely lipomannans (LMs) and lipoarabinomannans (LAMs) (Figure 8) [50-54].

9. Mycoloylarabinogalactan-peptidoglycan (mAGP)

The overall chemical structure of this complex macromolecule has been clarified during the past decade [55-58]. A specific linker unit covalently binds the proximal galactan portion of the arabinogalactan to peptidoglycan with the distal arabinose moieties providing anchorage for the 70 to 90 carbon long-chain mycolic acids (Figure 9) [19,55-58]. While chemical connec-

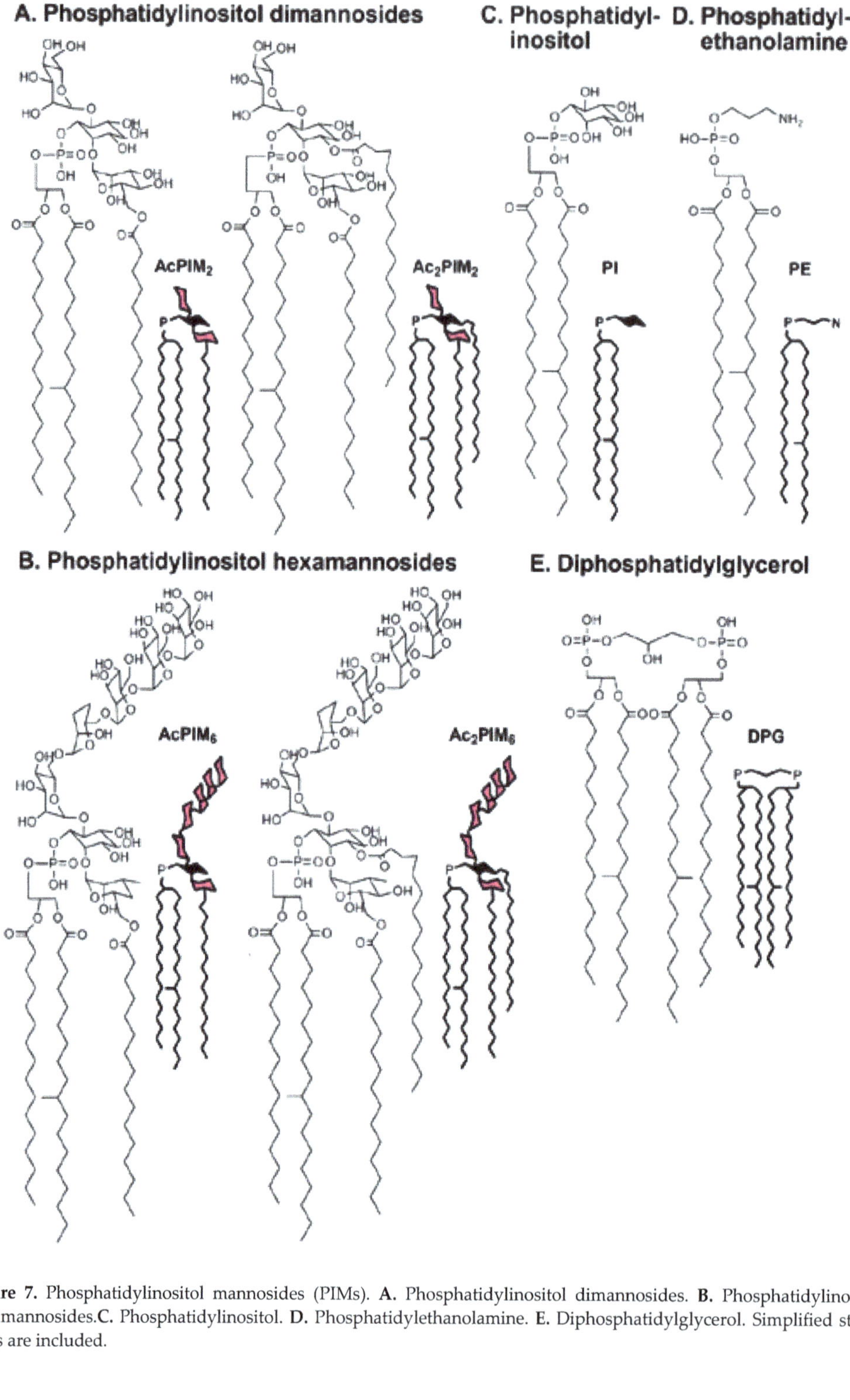

Figure 7. Phosphatidylinositol mannosides (PIMs). **A.** Phosphatidylinositol dimannosides. **B.** Phosphatidylinositol hexamannosides.**C.** Phosphatidylinositol. **D.** Phosphatidylethanolamine. **E.** Diphosphatidylglycerol. Simplified structures are included.

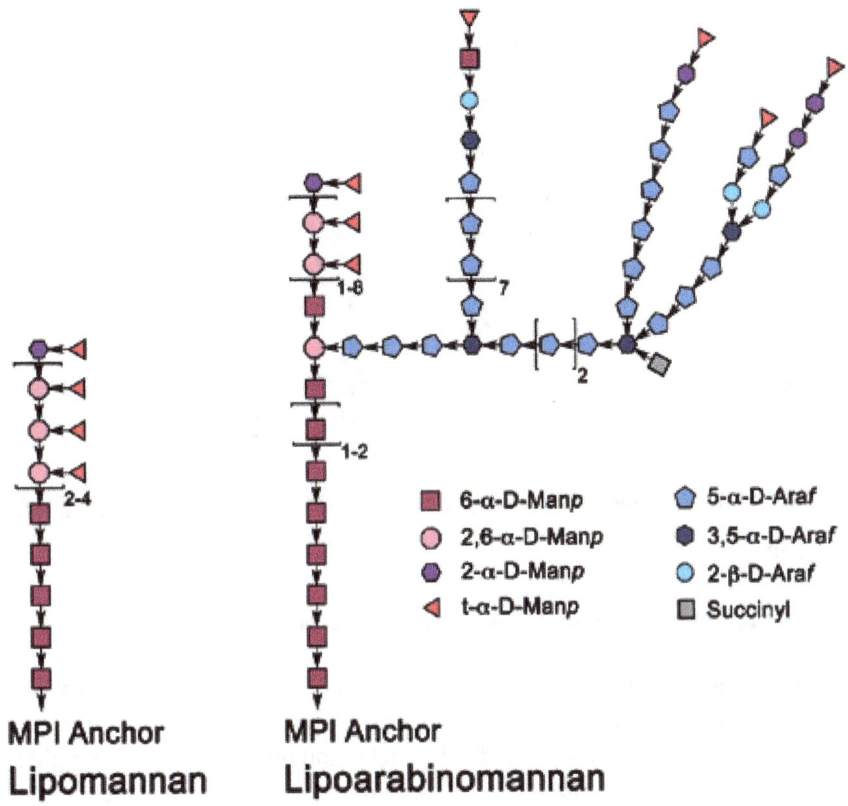

Figure 8. Essential structural topography of *M. tuberculosis* lipomannan and lipoarabinomannan. **MPI** is manno-phosphatidylinositol.

tivity is established, conformational preferences of the carbohydrate domains remain a matter of conjecture with diverse interpretations. It is becoming evident that versatile peptidoglycans can adopt different conformational arrangements, depending on the length of the polymeric disaccharide chains with helices being possible for shorter units [59]. It was shown that a synthetic peptidoglycan adopted a right-handed helical conformation [60]. A distinctive feature of mycobacterial peptidoglycan is the presence of a proportion of *N*-glycolyl muramic acid substituents, rather than the *N*-acetyl groups found in many other bacterial taxa [55-59]. The size and complexity of the mycoloylarabinogalactan- peptidoglycan, which is an extensive single macromolecule, provides a major challenge in perceiving how it can be coherently organised in three dimensions. This is not such a difficulty in many other bacterial taxa where no really major macromolecules are directly attached to peptidoglycan. It is now well established that the mycolic acids form a coherent inner leaflet of the MOM and this necessitates support from a well-integrated underlying platform.

The proposed mAGP arrangement (Figure 10) is based on a "scaffold" model [61,62], where peptide cross-linked helices are interspersed with helices of the galactan part of the arabinogalactan; the arabinan portion is then arranged to provide linkage points for mycolic acids. An

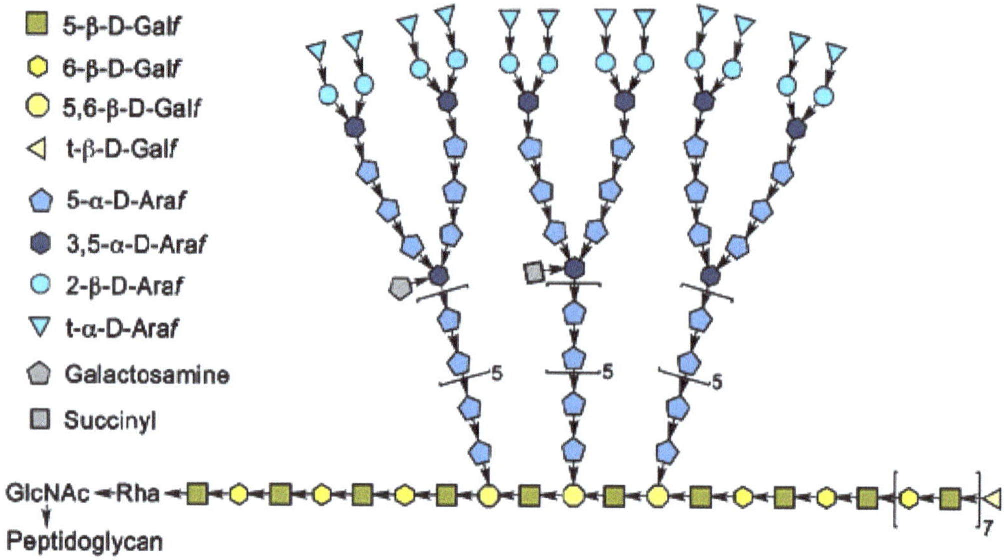

Figure 9. Essential structural topography of *M. tuberculosis* arabinogalactan-peptidoglycan.

attractive arrangement can be envisaged with the galactan extending to a level similar to that of the peptidoglycan helix to produce an essentially level "mosaic platform" as a stable anchorage for mycolic acids. While the helical galactan can provide a relatively rigid base unit, the arabinan may be more flexible so that the bound mycolic acids can jostle for position and occupy optimal locations. Indeed, arabinan flexibility may be an important factor in allowing hydrophobic interactions to govern the relative location of mycolic acid chains and associated free lipids. Calculations [63] indicate that the arabinofuranose polymer is reluctant to adopt a rigid compact helical conformation, thereby allowing a degree of flexibility.

10. Cell envelope organisation

The original model [4], with an inner and outer membrane, was based mainly on chemical principles, supported by freeze-etching results [64] that showed two clear distinct parallel cleavage planes in the mycobacterial cell envelope. The dual membrane proposal was confirmed by a confocal microscopy study that showed differential location of two fluorescent dyes of different lipophilicity [65]. The outer membrane was visualised directly by cryo-electron microscopy and the essential dimensions of the mycobacterial cell envelope were revealed [7-9]. An updated model for the cell envelope organisation for tubercle bacilli is proposed in Figure 10. Justification for the details of the proposal will build outwards from the plasma membrane.

The inner plasma membrane in mycobacteria has been traditionally regarded as conventional, even though a significant role was lacking for the unusual phosphatidylinositol mannosides

(PIMs) (Figure 7). A resolution of this conundrum has been indicated in a study [31], which showed strong evidence for locating Ac_2PIM_2 (Figure 7) as the sole polar component of the inner leaflet of the inner membrane. It was suggested that PIM_6 would be present in the outer leaflet of the inner membrane, projecting into the periplasm. It is not clear why there are two versions of PIM_2 and PIM_6, with either three or four fatty acid chains (Figure 7), but as a working hypothesis both PIM_2 lipids are placed in the inner leaflet and both PIM_6 lipids in the outer leaflet of the plasma membrane (Figure 10). As demonstrated by two-dimensional thin-layer chromatography [26], the proportions of the principal four PIM types are remarkably consistent, as is the proportion of PI. It is possible that equal proportions of PIMs with three and four fatty acid constituents are optimal for close packing in membranes; detailed physical studies on these lipids would be instructive. The proportions of PIM_2 exceed those of PIM_6 so if PIM_2 lipids are considered to predominate in the inner leaflet [31], then PI, PE and DPG (Figure 7) may complete the outer leaflet along with PIM_6. There is a distinct possibility that mycobacterial inner plasma membranes, rich in PIMs with three and four fatty acid chain anchors, have special physical properties that enhance its stability and perhaps governs permeability. Indeed, it has been suggested that this inner membrane may be "a bilayer environment of unusually low fluidity" [31] contributing to drug resistance. It was also noted [31] that the behaviour of PIM_2 liposomes had been found [66] to have behaviour suggestive of exceptional stability. It is now apparent that the inner mycobacterial plasma membrane is a highly specialised organelle, worthy of being distinguished with special nomenclature. Given the developing popularity of "MOM" for the mycobacterial outer membrane, a related simple suggestion might be "MIM" for the "mycobacterial inner membrane". It was found that disruption of PIM_2 production causes growth arrest [67,68] but the higher PIMs were dispensable [69], thereby indicating an important structural role for PIM_2. It has also been indicated that the acylation state of PIMs is also significant [70].

The outer leaflet of the MIM inner plasma membrane is also a suggested location for the PIM-related LM and LAM (Figure 10), but unequivocal evidence is elusive with alternative MOM location being a possibility. In a well-balanced objective analysis [71], it was concluded that LAM had at least an initial anchorage in MIM. However, in some cases [72,73], the undoubted presence of LAM at the cell surface required invoking specific lipoglycan transport mechanisms that need to be fully defined. At least a transient MIM location for LAM is supported by the presence of related lipoglycans in other actinomycetes, which do not have mycolic acids and an outer membrane, as summarised recently [72]. The basic fact that the lipid anchors of LM and LAM are identical to those in PIMs (Figures 7,8) suggests very strongly that all these components have a common anchorage in MIM. This should not rule out possible interactions with the hydrophobic MOM surface, but such lipophilic binding is predictably less specific and it is very difficult to envisage LM and LAM as important integral components of the MOM outer leaflet. The PIM-based lipid anchors appear to be all very similar for related LM and LAM lipoglycans across the genus *Mycobacterium* and related mycolata; however, enormous variations in the surface of the MOM in such taxa would militate strongly against any specific incorporation of LM and LAM into the MOM outer leaflet. Immunogold atomic force microscopy failed to detect cell surface LAM in *M. bovis* BCG, but LAM was revealed after treatment with drugs that attack cell envelope targets [74]. For *Corynebacterium glutamicum,* it was found

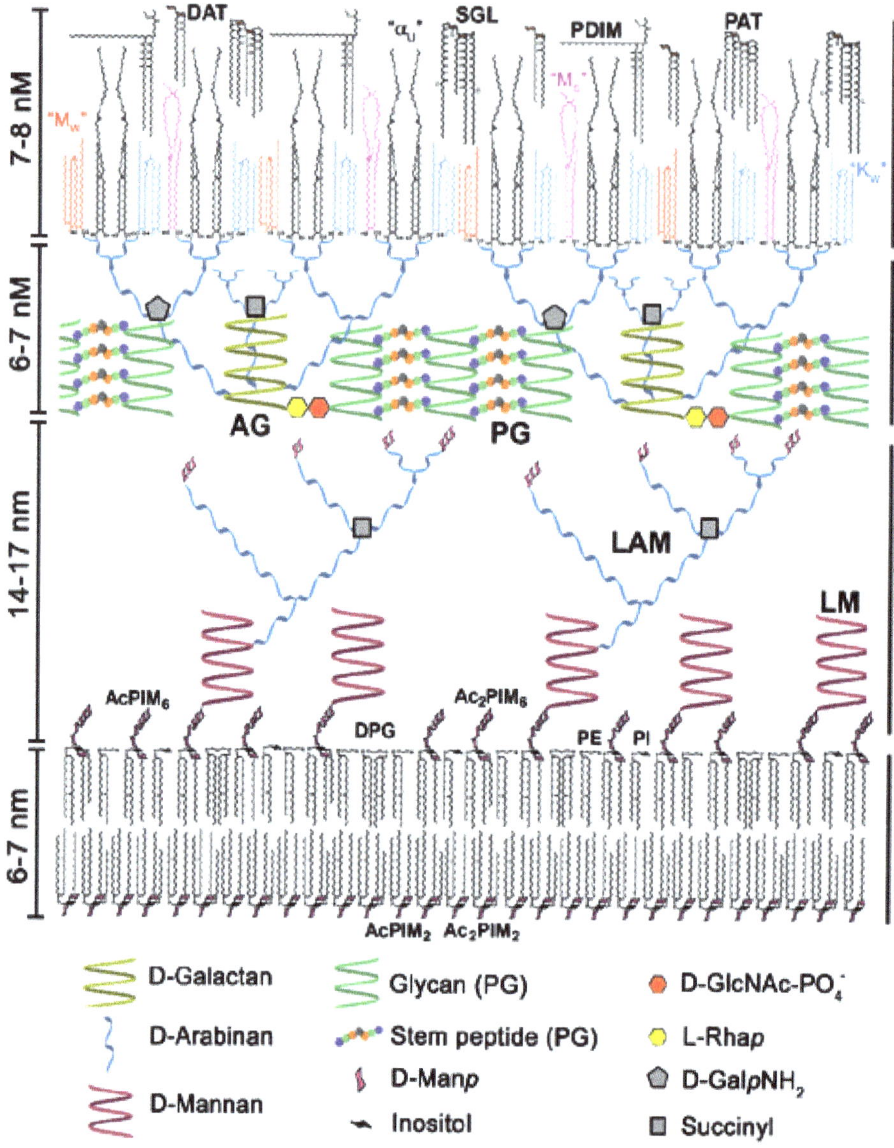

Figure 10. Two-dimensional representation of the location and interaction of structural components in the cell envelope of *M. tuberculosis.* MOM and MIM are "mycobacterial outer membrane" and "mycobacterial inner membrane", respectively. AGP is the arabinogalactan-peptidoglycan. Mycolic acid conformations (Figure 2) in the MOM are labelled "α_u" for α-mycolate for fully extended "eU" shape, "K_w" and "M_w" for fully folded keto- and methoxymycolate "W" shape, respectively, and "M_s" for semi-folded "sZ" shape. Correlating dimensions of all components are drawn to fit within the spatial constraints imposed by cryo-electron microscopy [8,9]. Dimensions of peptidoglycan (PG) helices are derived from synthetic material [60]. Helices of the mannan sections of lipomannan (LM) and lipoarabinomannan (LAM) and both the arabinan and galactan components of arabinogalactan (AG) were modelled using GLYCAM. Woods Group. (2005-2014) GLYCAM Web. Complex Carbohydrate Research Center, University of Georgia, Athens, GA. (http://www.glycam.com) [63]. Details of simplified lipid structures are in Figures 4-6.

that LM and LAM are embedded in the plasma membrane, along with the PIMs [75]. Overall, the importance of lipophilic anchors in external LM and LAM is diminished by the observation that their lipid-free glycan counterparts, mannan and arabinomannan, may be one destination of these components [72].

The extensive supposed "periplasmic space" (Figure 10) will, in fact, be an area of intense activity as all cellular components of the MOM whose synthesis is initiated in the cytoplasm, and continued through MIM, may be assembled and organised within [51-54]. The fact that many of these cell envelope components are relatively large may explain why such a relatively extensive compartment is needed. Cryo-electron microscopy studies [7-9,76] gave indications of some rather indistinct structural elements within the periplasm, labelled as layers L1 and L2 [7,76]. The internal L1 layer is most probably associated with "granular" material of protein origin, with the outer L2 layer corresponding to some of the peptidoglycan-arabinogalactan matrix [76]. It has been proposed that the maintenance of the relatively low-density periplasmic space could be facilitated by the presence of large polymeric material [9]. The helical mannan polysaccharide moiety in LM (Figure 10) may have such a role, but it could also act as a scaffold or template to compartmentalise various biochemical activities. In *M. smegmatis* it was shown that LAM was dramatically reduced as the bacteria approached stationary phase, but LM, mycolic acids and arabinogalactan were unchanged; this indicates that all these latter three components have important structural roles [73].

The accommodation and conformation of the mycoloyl arabinogalactan peptidoglycan macromolecular structure is a major challenge in the relatively limited space available (Figure 10). An informed choice has been made to use the "scaffold" approach of [61,62], with a helical peptidoglycan network interspersed with helical galactan units, as detailed in Figure 10. The relatively heavy peptidoglycan peptide cross-linking [52] may be a factor in favouring the scaffold arrangement in mycobacteria. This proposal echoes a previously advanced arrangement [52] that did not attempt to make precise spatial correlations and neglected to include the extensive periplasm. It would be interesting to explore the possibility that the *N*-glycolyl muramic acid substituents may have some influence on mycobacterial peptidoglycan conformation. The proposed coherent peptidoglycan – galactan "mosaic platform" layer (Figure 10) could provide a coherent anchorage for the arabinan moieties, some of which are esterified with mycolic acids. As noted previously, conformations of MAs vary with structural type and these are illustrated with W-conformations for keto-MAs, an extended U-conformation for α-MAs and equal numbers of W- and U-conformations for methoxy-MAs (Figure 2, 10). The MAs are comprised of approximately 50% α-MAs [17,18] as reflected in Figure 10. Such covalently bound MAs are instrumental in providing a stable MOM inner leaflet with potential for interaction with diverse free lipids to produce an effective outer membrane permeability barrier. Detailed spatial calculations attempted to simulate the accommodation of W-folded α-MAs into the MOM [77]; however, other MA conformations must be incorporated to provide a full picture. In a detailed quantitative study [31] of the cell envelope of *M. smegmatis* it was demonstrated that there were sufficient hydrocarbon chains in both inner and outer membranes to confirm the viability of the original dual membrane model [4].

A wide range of free lipid types are considered to form the outer leaflet of the outer mycomembrane of members of the *M. tuberculosis* complex. These range in polarity from the hydrophilic LOSs (Figure 6), through PGLs (Figure 4), DATs, SGLs and PATs (Figure 5), to the highly apolar hydrophobic PDIMs (Figure 4). All these unusual lipids have specialised fatty acid components, incorporating varying numbers of methyl branches located near to the carboxyl group (Figures 4-6). For the original chemical model of the mycobacterial cell envelope [4], it was conjectured that the presence of methyl branches might moderate the depth of insertion of the fatty acids into the MOM bilayer. This remains an attractive hypothesis, though detailed physical studies would be of value. The proximal multimethyl branches would favour a coiled conformation, leaving the distal straight-chain portion of such fatty acids to interact with mycolic acid chains. The straight-chain fatty acids in DATs, PATs (Figure 5) and LOSs (Figure 6) could possibly be layered parallel to the MOM surface providing elements of lateral stabilisation. In certain previous cell envelope models [9,78] there has been an unjustified tendency to include inverted TDMs as major components in the MOM outer leaflet. A proven role of TDMs is as an agent for the transfer of mycolic acids onto the arabinan matrix, presumably in the assembly of the inner leaflet of the MOM. It is more likely, therefore that TDMs would align themselves with the trehalose unit adjacent to the arabinan, as previously indicated [4]. Similarly, monomycoloyl glycerols (MMGs) (Figure 3) in *M. bovis* would be more readily accommodated with an internal glycerol unit. Such a location might possibly act to modify MOM fluidity in *M. bovis* whose mycolic acid composition has high proportions of *cis*-cyclopropyl keto-MAs, in comparison with the predominant *trans*-cyclopropyl keto-MAs in *M. tuberculosis* [17,18]. However, in related taxa, such as *Corynebacterium glutamicum*, it is probable that the structurally much simpler mycolic acids, and perhaps their trehalose esters, are able to participate as members of the outer leaflet of the outer membrane [8,78].

11. Evolutionary and pathogenicity aspects of cell envelope composition

It is of particular interest to attempt to obtain an understanding of the influence and importance of cell envelope composition in mycobacterial pathogenicity and evolution. A consensus is developing that an attractive evolutionary pathway can be envisaged from environmental *Mycobacterium kansasii*, through *"M. canettii"* to all the modern biotypes of the *M. tuberculosis* complex [79-83]. *M. kansasii* is the environmental organism that phenotypically resembles *M. tuberculosis* most closely and this relationship has been supported by genomic comparisons [79-81]. Cogent arguments have been advanced to associate the evolution of ancient tubercle bacilli, such as *"M. canettii"*, with bacteria similar to *M. kansasii*, including indications of horizontal gene transfer between these taxa [80,81]. Key genes acquired by horizontal gene transfer include those coding for mycobacterial lipids, transferases and proteins related to adaptation to anaerobic conditions [80,81]. *M. kansasii* continues to cause pulmonary disease in Silesian and South African miners, the bacterium being contracted from water in showers [81]. A detailed study has shown that the unusual smooth morphology *"M. canettii"* strains appear to form a pivotal role in the evolution of tuberculosis [84]. Although extant strains of

"M. canettii" still cause human tuberculosis, they differ significantly in infectivity and appear to be relatively ancestral [85,86]. Genomic studies indicate that the very diverse *"M. canettii"* isolates appear to coalesce into a form of bottleneck after which all the modern human and animal biotypes evolved in a relatively linear manner [83,84,87,88]. A plausible working hypothesis for the evolution of *M. tuberculosis sensu stricto* is outlined in Figure 11, highlighting the possible contribution of cell envelope lipid composition.

The most fundamental underlying difference between members of the *M. tuberculosis* complex, broadly including *"M. canettii"*, and *M. kansasii* and related environmental taxa is seen in the mycolic acids. The α-mycolic acids from *M. kansasii* have the regular spacing of the proximal and distal *cis*-cyclopropyl groups (Figure 1), common to a wide range of mycobacteria [17,18]. In clear contrast, α-mycolates from *"M. canettii"* and members of the *M. tuberculosis* complex have the chain between the hydroxyl group and the proximal cyclopropyl group shortened most significantly from 17 methylene groups in, for example, *M. kansasii* to 11 and 13 methylenes in members of the *M. tuberculosis* complex [4,17,18,79]. Additionally, the chains in 2-position and the terminal meromycolate chain are both relatively extended by two carbons. As noted above [20,22,24,79], *M. tuberculosis* α-mycolic acids extend more readily in molecular dynamics simulations with apparent interaction of the chain in 2-position with the chain between the two cyclopropyl groups, in a "fully extended shape" (Figure 2) [22] or "eU" conformation [24]. The methoxymycolates and ketomycolates of *"M. canettii"* and *M. tuberculosis* (Figure 1) conform to the general pattern of these components in related mycobacteria, such as *M. kansasii*, but, significantly, these oxygenated mycolates are slightly larger than any others [17,18]. The particular ability of α-mycolates to adopt extended flexible U-conformations is probably significant for interactions with free lipid components of the MOM outer leaflet. Indeed it is possible that the exceptionally long terminal chain in *M. tuberculosis* α-mycolic acids may penetrate right to the MOM outer leaflet to contribute to the hydrophobicity of the cell envelope surface. In this context, the balance of the three main types of mycolates is probably significant; the ratios of the α-, methoxy- and ketomycolates are, respectively, ~10:5:8 for *M. kansasii*, ~10:6:8 for *"M. canettii"* and ~10:5:5 for *M. tuberculosis* [17,18,79]. It is conceivable that having 50% α-mycolates may optimise hydrophobic interactions with the particular range of free lipids in the MOM outer leaflet in *M. tuberculosis.* In a detailed consideration [79], it was found possible to discern quite a range of distinct differences in the overall mycolic acid composition of these three taxa; the overall conclusion was an apparent simplification and tightening up of mycolate composition in modern *M. tuberculosis*.

There are also very significant changes in cell envelope MOM free lipid composition between all the taxa, shown in Figure 11. *M. kansasii* has characteristic polar LOSs (Figure 6), relatively polar PGLs (Figure 4) and PDIMs based only on phthiodiolones (Figure 4). These three lipid families appear to be the principal components of the outer leaflet of the MOM of *M. kansasii*, possibly contributing to a relatively polar cell surface compatible with a native hydrophilic environment. The PGLs of *M. kansasii* and *"M. canettii"* provide an appealing phenotypic link, with a loss of a single sugar to give a triglycosyl PGL and three sugar units to give a monoglycosyl PGL (Figures 4 and 11), as also highlighted previously [81]. However, some most significant new lipid structural principles are introduced in *"M. canettii"* (Figure 11). Two major classes of acyl trehalose glycolipids, the DATs and PATs (Figure 5), are encountered [86]. The relatively polar DATs are good antigens, which probably contribute to the cell surface properties of tubercle bacilli [38]. In contrast, the barely antigenic PATs are very non-polar and are likely to increase cell surface hydrophobicity quite significantly. The reduced 9-sugar oligosaccharide in the LOSs of *"M. canettii"*, compared with the 13-sugar oligosaccharide in *M. kansasii* might also result in reduced hydrophilicity. It is not known if all the diverse isolates of *"M. canettii"* have similar lipid profiles, but it certainly appears that the MOM free lipid composition of this taxon has some redundancy with perhaps an over-generous provision of lipid types (Figure 11). This redundancy might correlate with a high propensity for horizontal gene transfer, positively accumulating new mycobacterial lipid principles at the expense of a rather overblown excess of lipid biosynthesis. This might support a concept that *"M. canettii"* is a low pathogenicity intermediate taxon in evolutionary transit, rather than an efficient pathogen with a particular niche. In contrast, as will be detailed below, the modern *M. tuberculosis* complex has emerged out the ancestral melange as a group of efficient pathogens with a range of specialised hosts.

Aspects of the cell envelope lipid composition of *"M. canettii"* are essentially the same as for *M. tuberculosis sensu stricto*, including mycolic acid composition, but there are a number of key differences. Significantly, the LOSs and PGLs present in *"M. canettii"* are absent in *M. tuberculosis*, but the latter is uniquely characterised by the presence of SGLs [89]. As noted above, the highly polar LOSs are associated with hydrophilic interactions, such as motility and biofilm formation [44]. The PGLs are also relatively polar, but in addition to having a structural role in the outer leaflet of the MOM, particularly specific functions are elusive. SGLs behave on chromatography as quite polar lipids, presumably due to the presence of the sulfated trehalose unit. However, SGLs have very large nonpolar phthioceranic and hydroxyphthioceranic fatty acid acyl chains (Figure 5), which are likely to provide enhanced hydrophobicity. In two informative studies, it was shown that deficiencies in SGLs [90] and DATs and PATs [91] did not have decisive effects on replication and persistence. In bacterial disease, clear distinctions must be made between transmissibility and the pathogenic process once the infection has been established. It would appear that the very hydrophobic SGLs and PATs (Figure 5) may have primary value in the transmission process, perhaps accompanied by some secondary roles in pathogenicity.

Previous studies have shown an important link between hydrophobicity and aerosol performance in *Mycobacterium avium* [92]. Preliminary studies are under way to compare the hydrophobicity of *"M. canettii"* and *M. tuberculosis*. For cultures grown on solid media in the presence of Congo Red [93], the smooth colonies of *M. kansasii* and *"M. canettii"* resisted staining by the dye, but two different rough strains of *M. tuberculosis* absorbed so much dye that they almost merged into the background (Figure 12). In preliminary standard partitioning experiments between hexadecane and water [94], it was found that *M. tuberculosis* was approximately one fifth more hydrophobic than *"M. canettii"* (details not shown). These simple experiments indicate a distinct difference in hydrophobicity between one member of the smooth supposed ancestral "Cannetti" taxon and rough modern human tubercle bacilli. It follows, therefore, that *M. tuberculosis sensu stricto* may be specifically adapted for aerosol

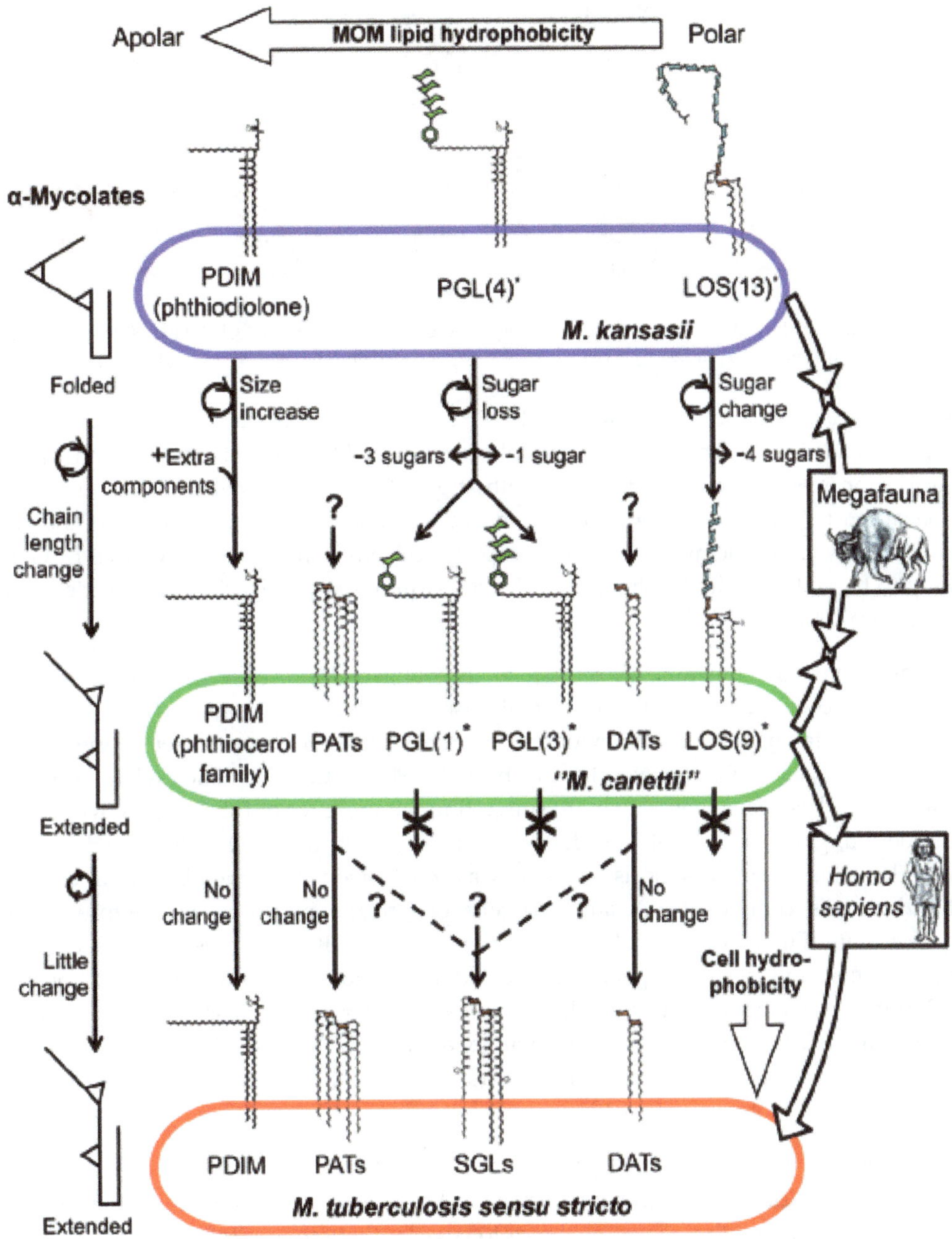

Figure 11. A generalised scenario for the significance of lipid composition in the evolution of *M. tuberculosis*. Details of the simplified lipid structures are in Figures 4-6. The numbers of sugars in particular LOSs and PGLs are shown in brackets with an asterisk, e.g. LOS (13)*.

transmission, whereas *"M. canettii"* is less favoured for this mode of transmission [85,86]. A link between cell envelope hydrophobicity and aerosol transmission is also probably signifi-

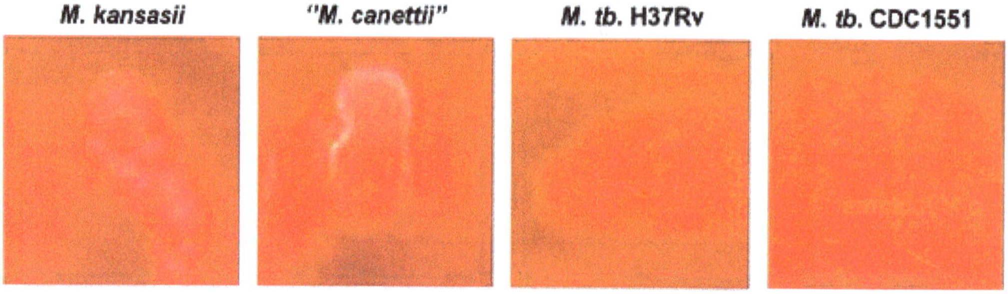

Figure 12. Differential uptake of Congo Red by *M. kansasii* ATCC12478, *"M. canettii"* CIPT 140010059 MNC1485, *M. tuberculosis* H37Rv and *M. tuberculosis* CDC1551. Strains were cultivated on 7H11 agar with 40μg/ml Congo Red.

cant in *Mycobacterium abscessus* infections [95,96]. Airway infections are often associated with rough variants that lack polar glycopeptidolipids and are likely to be more hydrophobic and aerosol transmissible than the usual smooth strains [95,96]. It was also shown that rough *Gordona* species were much more hydrophobic than smooth morphology variants of the same strain [97]. By use of chemical force microscopy the cell envelope surface of *M. bovis* BCG was found to be uniformly hydrophobic, but drugs disrupting mycolic acid synthesis destroyed this feature [74].

A jump from environmental *M. kansasii* to the obligate *M. tuberculosis* human pathogen requires the cooperation of suitable animal hosts, in which evolutionary changes can take place. The total dearth of any evidence for tuberculosis in *Homo sapiens,* prior to the Holocene, suggests zoonotic evolutionary hosts [79,98,99]. Characteristic skeletal lesions in a variety of Pleistocene megafauna are suggesting the presence of tuberculosis over a wide time period, going back to at least 120 ka BP [100,101]. In one well-documented example of a 17ka extinct bison, diagnosis by lesion was conclusively confirmed by amplification of *M. tuberculosis* complex DNA and recovery of pristine mycolipenate (Figure 5) and mycocerosate (Figure 4) tuberculosis lipid biomarkers [99,102,103]. The complex digestive organs in megafauna, such as bison and mastodons are potentially ideal vessels to facilitate evolutionary development, as the rich population of other microbial species present would be well situated to participate in horizontal gene transfer. There is substantial evidence for Pleistocene horizontal gene transfer in ancestral strains of the tubercle bacillus before linear evolution in the Holocene [80,81,104].

It is conceivable that, during the Pleistocene, thinly spread members of *Homo sapiens,* and also *Homo neanderthalensis,* may have contracted evolving ancestral tuberculosis from infected megafauna. However, there is no evidence to suggest that modern tuberculosis developed from ancestral strains solely in the human vehicles, mentioned above. Indeed, recent studies indicate that Neanderthals all became extinct before about 40ka BP [105], which precedes the perceived ~30 to 12ka BP evolutionary bottleneck in tubercle bacilli [84,87,106]. A feasible scenario, therefore, for the emergence of all the modern biotypes of the *M. tuberculosis* complex through the bottleneck would involve a complex web of interactions between *H. sapiens* and Pleistocene animal reservoirs until the dramatically ameliorated climatic conditions at the beginning of the Holocene allowed humans to form settlements and promulgate communal tuberculosis. The apparent ready spread of human *M. tuberculosis* in early Holocene settlements was probably a result of the ability of the tubercle bacillus to fly in aerosols. This could be a consequence of the dramatically enhanced hydrophobicity of *M. tuberculosis sensu stricto* as compared with the most likely ancestral strains, labelled *"M. canettii"*. It will not be easy to pinpoint a precise event when modern *M. tuberculosis* made its decisive debut on the human stage. As noted above, the digestive systems of Pleistocene megafauna were probably very efficient vessels for the evolution of tubercle bacilli and the change from the relatively hydrophilic *"M. canettii"*, in the digestive tract, to the hydrophobic *M. tuberculosis* that could be expelled from the lung. The enormous diversity of the extant surviving *"M. canettii"* taxon [84] probably points to an even greater range of smooth ancestral strains being passaged, recycled and adapted through animals and the environment. Indeed it probably reasonable to suggest that the great genetic diversity of smooth strains of the tubercle bacilli may be a result of their emergence over a wide time scale and geographical area.

12. Conclusion

The cell envelope of *M. tuberculosis* and related taxa is an assemblage of efficiently coordinated and closely interacting macromolecules and exquisitely designed lipid moieties. One of the most characteristic organelles is the "mycobacterial outer membrane" or "MOM", but recent studies have shown that the "mycobacterial inner membrane", or "MIM", may be comparable in importance (Figure 10). Indeed the MIM, if it has a very characteristic inner leaflet composed predominately of PIM_2 phospholipids, may be a formidable barrier protecting the cytoplasm (Figure 10). The MOM is composed of an outer leaflet of "free lipids", which interacts with a monolayer of mycolic acids covalently bound to the relatively flexible arabinan portion of an arabinogalactan that, in turn, is linked to peptidoglycan. Utilising the hypothesis of the "scaffold" model, the peptidoglycan and the galactan section of the arabinogalactan form helices perpendicular to the cell surface resulting in a stable type of "mosaic platform" from which the MOM can be linked *via* an arabinan cushion (Figure 10). The space between the MIM and peptidoglycan, usually termed the "periplasm", is envisaged as being the initial place for the linkage of the characteristic lipoglycans, namely "lipomannan" (LM) and "lipoarabinomannan" (LAM) (Figure 10). However, LAM certainly is transported to the external capsular regions, but LM may linger in the periplasm affording a degree of organisation and stability. Overall, it is important to note that the mycobacterial cell envelope is a dynamic three-dimensional organelle; the hypothetical arrangement pictured in Figure 10 can only be a two-dimensional snapshot illustrating likely locations and interactions.

Given the hypothesis that tubercle bacilli evolved from an environmental organism, such as *M. kansasii*, *via* a mammalian adapted semi-environmental ancestral taxon, such as *"M. canettii"*, parallel linked changes in the lipid components of the MOM can be discerned (Figure 11). A clear phenotypic link between *M. kansasii* and *"M. canettii"* is provided by clearly comparable "phenolic glycolipids" (PGLs) (Figure 4). The introduction of distinct mycolic acid

(Figure 1) and acyl trehalose (DATs, PATs, Figure 5) structures shows that "*M. canettii*" has an indisputable link with modern members of the *M. tuberculosis* complex (Figure 11). Refinement of the MOM lipid composition of "*M. canettii*", leads to the simplified MOM free lipids of *M. tuberculosis,* comprising PDIMs, DATs, PATs (Figures 4,5) and the very characteristic sulfoglycolipids (SGLs, Figure 5). The apparent enhanced hydrophobicity of the cell envelope of *M. tuberculosis sensu stricto* correlates well with the ability to be transmitted in aerosols. In broad evolutionary terms, a plausible scenario involves various Pleistocene megafauna passaging environmental mycobacteria, such as *M. kansasii,* until horizontal gene transfer resulted in the diverse family of smooth morphology strains labelled "*M. canettii*". Further evolutionary development, with possible human involvement for the first time, produced modern *M. tuberculosis* whose novel ability to fly in aerosols probably coincided with congregating settled humans multiplying together along with tubercle bacilli as new devastating companions.

Acknowledgements

The Leverhulme Trust Project Grant F/00 094/BL (OY-CL, DEM, GSB). GSB was supported by a Personal Research Chair from Mr. James Bardrick and the UK Medical Research Council. The UK Medical Research Council and the Medical Research Foundation provided support to AB.

Author details

David E. Minnikin[1*], Oona Y-C Lee[1], Houdini H.T. Wu[1], Vijayashankar Nataraj[1], Helen D. Donoghue[2], Malin Ridell[3], Motoko Watanabe[4], Luke Alderwick[1], Apoorva Bhatt[1] and Gurdyal S. Besra[1]

*Address all correspondence to: d.e.minnikin@bham.ac.uk

1 Institute of Microbiology and Infection, School of Biosciences, University of Birmingham, Birmingham, UK

2 Centre for Clinical Microbiology, Division of Infection and Immunity, University College London, London, UK

3 Department of Microbiology and Immunology, Institute of Biomedicine, University of Gothenburg, Gothenburg, Sweden

4 School of Pharmacy, Tokyo University of Pharmacy and Life Sciences, Tokyo, Japan

References

[1] Anderson RJ. Structural peculiarities of acid-fast bacterial lipids. Chemical Reviews 1941;29: 225-243.

[2] Asselineau J. The Bacterial Lipids. Paris: Hermann; 1966.

[3] Goren MB, Brennan PJ. Mycobacterial lipids: Chemistry and biologic activities. In: Tuberculosis. Youmans G.P. (ed.) Philadelphia USA: W.B. Saunders Company; 1979. p63-193.

[4] Minnikin, DE. Lipids: Complex lipids, their chemistry, biosynthesis and role. In: Ratledge C, Stanford J. (eds.) The Biology of Mycobacteria. London, UK:, Academic Press; 1982. p95-184.

[5] Daffé M, Draper P. The Envelope Layers of Mycobacteria with Reference to their Pathogenicity. Advances in Microbial Physiology 1998;39: 131-203.

[6] Brennan PJ, Nikaido H. The Envelope of Mycobacteria. Annual Reviews of Biochemistry 1995; 64: 29-63.

[7] Hoffmann C, Leis A, Niederweis M., Plitzko JM, Engelhardt H. Disclosure of the mycobacterial outer membrane: Cryo-electron tomography and vitreous sections reveal the lipid bilayer structure. PNAS 2008;105: 3963-3967.

[8] Zuber B, Chami M, Houssin C, Dubochet J, Griffiths G, Daffé M. Direct visualization of the outer membrane of mycobacteria and corynebacteria in their native state. Journal of Bacteriology 2008;190: 5672-5680.

[9] Daffé M, Zuber B. The Fascinating Coat Surrounding Mycobacteria. In: Remaut H., Fronzes R. (eds.) Bacterial Membranes: Structural and Molecular Biology. Linton, Cambridge UK: Caister Academic Press; 2014. p179-192.

[10] Daffé M, Etienne G. The capsule of *Mycobacterium tuberculosis* and its implications for pathogenicity. Tubercle and Lung Disease 1999:79: 153–169.

[11] Draper P, Daffé M. The Cell Envelope of *Mycobacterium tuberculosis* with Special Reference to the Capsule and Outer Permeability Barrier. In: Cole ST, Eisenach KD, McMurray DN, Jacobs WR. (eds.) Tuberculosis and the Tubercle Bacillus. Washington, DC: American Society for Microbiology; 2005. p287-305.

[12] Niederweis M. Mycobacterial Porins. In: Daffé M., Reyrat, J-M. (eds.) The Mycobacterial Cell Envelope. Washington, DC: American Society for Microbiology; 2008. p153-165.

[13] Kremer L, Besra GS. A Waxy Tale, by *Mycobacterium tuberculosis*. In: Cole ST, Eisenach KD, McMurray DN, Jacobs WR. (eds.) Tuberculosis and the Tubercle Bacillus. Washington, DC: American Society for Microbiology; 2005. p287-305.

[14] Verschoor JA, Baird MS, Grooten J. Towards understanding the functional diversity of cell wall mycolic acids of *Mycobacterium tuberculosis*. Progress in Lipid Research 2012;51: 325–339.

[15] Marrakchi H, Bardou F, Laneélle M, Daffé M. A comprehensive overview of mycolic acid structure and biosynthesis. In: Daffé M, Reyrat JM. (eds). The Mycobacterial Cell Envelope. Washington, DC: American Society for Microbiology; 2008. p41–62.

[16] Marrakchi H, Lanéelle M-A, Daffé M. Mycolic Acids: Structures, Biosynthesis, and Beyond. Chemistry & Biology 2014;21: 67- 85.

[17] Watanabe M, Aoyagi Y, Ridell M, Minnikin DE. Separation and characterization of individual mycolic acids in representative mycobacteria. Microbiology 2001;147: 1825–1837.

[18] Watanabe M., Aoyagi Y, Mitome H, Fujita T, Naoki H, Ridell M, Minnikin DE. Location of functional groups in mycobacterial meromycolate chains; the recognition of new structural principles in mycolic acids. Microbiology 2002;148: 1881-1902.

[19] McNeil M, Daffé M, Brennan PJ. Location of the Mycolyl Ester Substituents in the Cell Walls of Mycobacteria. Journal of Biological Chemistry 1991;266: 13217-13223.

[20] Villeneuve M., Kawai M, Kanashima H, Watanabe M, Minnikin DE, Nakahara H. Temperature dependence of the Langmuir monolayer packing of mycolic acids from *Mycobacterium tuberculosis*. Biochimica et Biophysica Acta Biomembranes 2005;1715: 71–80.

[21] Villeneuve M, Kawai M, Watanabe M, Aoyagi Y, Hitotsuyanagi Y, Takeya K, Gouda H, Hirono S, Minnikin DE, Nakahara H. Conformational behavior of oxygenated mycobacterial mycolic acids from *Mycobacterium bovis* BCG. Biochimica et Biophysica Acta Biomembranes 2007;1768: 1717–1726.

[22] Villeneuve M, Kawai M, Watanabe M, Aoyagi Y, Hitotsuyanagi Y, Takeya K, Gouda H, Hirono S, Minnikin DE, Nakahara H. Differential conformational behaviors of alpha-mycolic acids in Langmuir monolayers and computer simulations. Chemistry and Physics of Lipids 2010;163: 569–579.

[23] Villeneuve M, Kawai M, Horiuchi K, Watanabe M, Aoyagi Y, Hitotsuyanagi Y, Takeya K, Gouda H, Hirono S, Minnikin DE. Conformational folding of mycobacterial methoxy and ketomycolic acids facilitated by α-methyl *trans*-cyclopropane groups rather than *cis*-cyclopropane units. Microbiology 2013;159: 2405–2415.

[24] Groenewald W, Baird MS, Verschoor JA, Minnikin DE, Croft AK. Differential spontaneous folding of mycolic acids from *Mycobacterium tuberculosis*. Chemistry and Physics of Lipids 2014;180: 15–22.

[25] Moody DB, Reinhold BB, Guy MR, Beckman EM, Frederique DE, Furlong ST, Ye S, Reinhold VN, Sieling PA, Modlin RL, Besra GS, Porcelli SA. Structural requirements

for glycolipid antigen recognition by CD1b-restricted T cells. Science 1997;278: 283-286.

[26] Dobson G, Minnikin DE, Minnikin SM, Parlett JH, Goodfellow M, Ridell M, Magnusson M. Systematic analyses of complex mycobacterial lipids. In: Goodfellow M, Minnikin DE. (eds.) Chemical Methods in Bacterial Systematics. London, UK: Academic Press; 1985. p237- 265.

[27] Andersen CS, Agger EM, Rosenkrands I, Gomes JM, Bhowruth V, Gibson KJ, Petersen RV, Minnikin DE, Besra GS, Andersen P. A Simple Mycobacterial Monomycoloylated Glycerol Lipid has Potent Immunostimulatory Activity. Journal of Immunology 2009; 182: 424-432.

[28] Kremer L, de Chastellier C, Dobson G, Gibson KJ, Bifani P, Balor S, Gorvel J-P, Locht C, Minnikin DE, Besra GS. Identification and structural characterization of an unusual mycobacterial monomeromycoloyldiacylglycerol. Molecular Microbiology 2005;57: 1113–1126.

[29] Rafidinarivo E, Lanéelle M-A, Montrozier H, Valero-Guillén P, Astola J, Luquin M, Promé J-C, Daffé M. Trafficking pathways of mycolic acids: structures, origin, mechanism of formation, and storage form of mycobacteric acids. Journal of Lipid Research 2009;50: 477–490.

[30] Garton NJ, Christensen H, Minnikin DE, Adegbola RA, Barer MR. Intracellular lipophilic inclusions of mycobacteria *in vitro* and in sputum. Microbiology 2002;148: 2951–2958.

[31] Bansal-Mutalik R, Nikaido H. Mycobacterial outer membrane is a lipid bilayer and the inner membrane is unusually rich in diacyl phosphatidylinositol dimannosides. PNAS 2014;111: 4958-4963.

[32] Minnikin DE, Dobson G, Goodfellow M, Magnusson M, Ridell M. Distribution of Some Mycobacterial Waxes Based on the Phthiocerol Family. Journal of General Microbiology 1985;131: 1375-1381.

[33] Daffé M, Lanéelle M-A. Distribution of Phthiocerol Diester, Phenolic Mycosides and Related Compounds in Mycobacteria. Journal of General Microbiology 1988;134: 2049-2055.

[34] Minnikin DE, Kremer L, Dover LG, Besra GS. The methyl-branched fortifications of *Mycobacterium tuberculosis*. Chemistry and Biology 2002; 9: 545-553.

[35] Onwueme KC, Cheryl J, Vos CJ, Zurita J, Ferreras JA, Quadri LEN. The dimycocerosate ester polyketide virulence factors of mycobacteria. Progress in Lipid Research 2005;44: 259–302.

[36] Guilhot C, Chalut C, Daffé M. Biosynthesis and Roles of Phenolic Glycolipids and Related Molecules in *Mycobacterium tuberculosis*. In: Daffé M, Reyrat J-M. (eds.) The

Mycobacterial Cell Envelope. Washington, DC: American Society for Microbiology; 2008. p273-289.

[37] Huet SG, Constant C, Malaga W, Lanéelle M-A, Kremer K, van Soolingen D, Daffé M, Guilhot C. A lipid profile typifies the Beijing strains of *Mycobacterium tuberculosis*. Identification of a mutation responsible for a modification of the structures of phthiocerol dimycocerosates and phenolic glycolipids. Journal of Biological Chemistry 2009;284: 27101–27113.

[38] Ridell M, Wallerström G, Minnikin DE, Bolton RC, Magnusson M. A comparative serological study of antigenic glycolipids from *Mycobacterium tuberculosis*. Tubercle and Lung Disease 1992;73: 101-105.

[39] Jackson M, Stadthagen G, Gicquel B. Long-chain multiple methyl-branched fatty acid-containing lipids of *Mycobacterium tuberculosis*: Biosynthesis, transport, regulation and biological activities. Tuberculosis 2007;87: 78–86.

[40] Daffé M, Lacave C, Lanéelle M-A, Gillois M, Lanéelle G. Polyphthienoyl trehalose, glycolipids specific for virulent strains of the tubercle bacillus. European Journal of Biochemistry 1988;172: 579-584.

[41] Bertozzi CR, Schelle MW. Sulfated Metabolites from *M. tuberculosis*: Sulfolipid-1 and Beyond. In: Daffé M, Reyrat J-M. (eds.) The Mycobacterial Cell Envelope. Washington, DC: American Society for Microbiology; 2008. p291-304.

[42] Daffé M, McNeil M, Brennan PJ. Novel Type-Specific Lipooligosaccharides from *Mycobacterium tuberculosis*. Biochemistry 1991;30: 378-388.

[43] Gilleron M, Puzo G. Lipooligosaccharidic antigens from *Mycobacterium kansasii* and *Mycobacterium gastri*. Glycoconjugate Journal 1995;12: 298-308.

[44] Ren H, Dover LG, Islam ST, Alexander DC, Chen JM, Besra GS, Liu J. Identification of the lipooligosaccharide biosynthetic gene cluster from *Mycobacterium marinum*. Molecular Microbiology 2007;63: 1345-1359.

[45] Belisle JT, Brennan PJ. Chemical basis of rough and smooth variation in mycobacteria. Journal of Bacteriology 1989;171: 3465-3470.

[46] Gilleron M, Quesniaux VFJ, Puzo G. Acylation State of the Phosphatidylinositol Hexamannosides from *Mycobacterium bovis* Bacillus Calmette Guérin and *Mycobacterium tuberculosis* H37Rv and Its Implication in Toll-like Receptor Response. Journal of Biological Chemistry 2003; 278: 29880-29889.

[47] Gilleron M, Ronet C, Mempel M, Monsarrat B, Gachelin G, Puzo G. Acylation state of the phosphatidylinositol mannosides from *Mycobacterium bovis* bacillus Calmette Guérin and ability to induce granuloma and recruit natural killer T cells. Journal of Biological Chemistry 2001;276: 34896-34904.

[48] Guerin ME, Kordulάková J, Alzari PM, Brennan PJ, Jackson M. Molecular Basis of Phosphatidyl-myo-inositol Mannoside Biosynthesis and Regulation in Mycobacteria. Journal of Biological Chemistry 2010;285: 33577-33583.

[49] Morita YS, Fukuda T, Sena CBC, Yamaryo-Botte Y, McConville MJ, Kinoshita T. Inositol lipid metabolism in mycobacteria: Biosynthesis and regulatory mechanisms. Biochimica et Biophysica Acta 2011;1810: 630–641.

[50] Nigou J, Gilleron M, Puzo G. Lipoarabinomannans: from structure to biosynthesis. Biochimie 2003;85: 153-166.

[51] Mishra AK, Driessen NN, Appelmelk BJ, Besra GS. Lipoarabinomannan and related glycoconjugates: structure, biogenesis and role in *Mycobacterium tuberculosis* physiology and host-pathogen interaction. FEMS Microbiology Reviews 2011;35: 1126–1157.

[52] Kaur D, Guerin ME, Škovierová H, Brennan PJ, Jackson M. Biogenesis of the cell wall and other glycoconjugates of *Mycobacterium tuberculosis*. Advances in Applied Microbiology 2009;69: 23-78.

[53] Jankute M, Grover S, Rana AK, Besra GS. Arabinogalactan and lipoarabinomannan biosynthesis: structure, biogenesis and their potential as drug targets. Future Microbiology 2012;7: 129-147.

[54] Jankute M, Grover S, Birch HL, Besra GS. Genetics of Mycobacterial Arabinogalactan and Lipoarabinomannan Assembly. In: Hatfull GF, Jacobs WR. (eds.) Molecular Genetics of Mycobacteria, 2nd Edition. Washington, DC: American Society for Microbiology; 2014. p535-557.

[55] Barry CE, Crick DC, McNeil MR. Targeting the formation of the cell wall core of *M. tuberculosis*. Infectious Disorders and Drug Targets 2007;7: 182-202.

[56] Crick DC, Brennan PJ. Biosynthesis of the Arabinogalactan-Peptidoglycan Complex of *Mycobacterium tuberculosis*. In: Daffé M., Reyrat, J-M. (eds.) The Mycobacterial Cell Envelope. Washington, DC: American Society for Microbiology; 2008. p25-40.

[57] Crick DC, Chatterjee D, Scherman MS, McNeil MR. Structure and Biosynthesis of the Mycobacterial Cell Wall. Comprehensive Natural Products II: Chemistry and Biology 2010;6: 381–406. DOI: 10.1016/B978-008045382-8.00173-8.

[58] Daffé M. The Global Architecture of the Mycobacterial Cell Envelope. In: Daffé M., Reyrat, J-M. (eds.) The Mycobacterial Cell Envelope. Washington, DC: American Society for Microbiology; 2008. p3-11.

[59] Turner RD, Vollmer W, Foster SJ. Different walls for rods and balls: the diversity of peptidoglycan. Molecular Microbiology 2014;91: 862-874.

[60] Meroueh SO, Bencze KZ, Hesek D, Lee M, Fisher JD, Timothy L. Stemmler TL, Mobashery S. Three-dimensional structure of the bacterial cell wall peptidoglycan. PNAS 2006;103: 4404–4409.

[61] Dmitriev BA, Ehlers S, Rietschel ET, Brennan PJ. Molecular mechanics of the mycobacterial cell wall: from horizontal layers to vertical scaffolds. International Journal of Medical Microbiology 2000;290: 251-258.

[62] Dmitriev B, Toukach F, Ehlers S. Towards a comprehensive view of the bacterial cell wall. Trends in Microbiology 2005;13: 569-574.

[63] Kirschner KN, Yongye AB, Tschampel SM, Daniels CR, Foley BL, Woods RJ. GLYCAM06: A Generalizable Biomolecular Force Field. Carbohydrates. Journal of Computational Chemistry 2008;29: 622-655.

[64] Barksdale L, Kim K-S. *Mycobacterium*. Bacteriological Reviews 1977; 41: 217–372.

[65] Christensen H, Garton NJ, Horobin RW, Minnikin DE, Barer MR. Lipid domains of mycobacteria studied with fluorescent molecular probes. Molecular Microbiology 1999;31: 1561–1572.

[66] Sprott GD, Dicaire CJ, Gurnani K, Sad S, Krishnan L. Activation of Dendritic Cells by Liposomes Prepared from Phosphatidylinositol Mannosides from *Mycobacterium bovis* Bacillus Calmette-Guérin and Adjuvant Activity *in vivo*. Infection and Immunity 2004;72: 5235–5246.

[67] Kordulákovà J, Gilleron M, Mikusova K, Puzo G, Brennan PJ, Gicquel B, Jackson, M. Definition of the First Mannosylation Step in Phosphatidylinositol Mannoside Synthesis. Journal of Biological Chemistry 2002;277: 31335–31344.

[68] Guerin ME, Kaur D, Somashekar BS, Gibbs S, Gest P, Chatterjee D, Brennan PJ, Jackson M. New insights into the early steps of phosphatidylinositol mannoside biosynthesis in mycobacteria: PimB' is an essential enzyme of *Mycobacterium smegmatis*. Journal of Biological Chemistry 2009;284: 25687–25696.

[69] Driessen NN, Ummels R, Maaskant JJ, Gurcha SS, Besra GS, Ainge GD, Larsen DS, Painter GF, Vandenbroucke-Grauls CM, Geurtsen J, Appelmelk BJ. Role of phosphatidylinositol mannosides in the interaction between mycobacteria and DC-SIGN. Infection and Immunity 2009;77: 4538–4547.

[70] Kordulákovà J, Gilleron M, Puzo G, Brennan PJ, Gicquel B, Mikusovà K, Jackson M. Identification of the required acyltransferase step in the biosynthesis of the phosphatidylinositol mannosides of *Mycobacterium* species. Journal of Biological Chemistry 2003;278: 36285–36295.

[71] Gilleron M, Jackson M, Nigou J, Puzo G. Structure, Biosynthesis and Activities of the Phosphatidyl-*myo*-Inositol-based Lipoglycans. In: Daffé M, Reyrat, J-M. (eds.) The Mycobacterial Cell Envelope. Washington, DC: American Society for Microbiology; 2008. p75-105.

[72] Pitarque S, Larrouy-Maumus G, Payré B, Jackson M, Puzo G, Nigou J. The immunomodulatory lipoglycans, lipoarabinomannan and lipomannan, are exposed at the mycobacterial cell surface. Tuberculosis 2008;88: 560-565.

[73] Dhiman RK, Dinadayala P, Ryan GJ, Lenaerts AJ, Schenkel AR, Crick DC. Lipoarabinomannan Localization and Abundance during Growth of *Mycobacterium smegmatis*. Journal of Bacteriology 2011;193: 5802-5809.

[74] Alsteens D, Verbelen C, Dague E, Raze D, Baulard AR, Dufrêne YF. Organization of the mycobacterial cell wall: a nanoscale view. Pflugers Arch- European Journal of Physiology 2008;456: 117-125.

[75] Marchand CH, Salmeron C, Bou Raad R, Méniche X, Chami M, Masi M, Blanot D, Daffé M, Tropis M, Huc E, Le Maréchal P, Decottignies P, Bayan N. Biochemical Disclosure of the Mycolate Outer Membrane of *Corynebacterium glutamicum*. Journal of Bacteriology 2012;194: 587-597.

[76] Sani M, Houben ENG, Geurtsen J, Pierson J, de Punder K, van Zon M, Wever B, Piersma SR, Jiménez CR, Daffé M, Appelmelk BJ, Bitter W, van der Wel1 N, Peters PJ. Direct Visualization by Cryo-EM of the Mycobacterial Capsular Layer: A Labile Structure Containing ESX-1-Secreted Proteins. PLoS Pathogens 2010;6: e1000794.

[77] Bhamidi S, Scherman MS, Jones V, Crick DC, Belisle JT, Brennan PJ, McNeil MR. Detailed structural and quantitative analysis reveals the spatial organization of the cell walls of *in vivo* grown *Mycobacterium leprae* and *in vitro* grown *M. tuberculosis*. Journal of Biological Chemistry 2011;286: 23168-23177.

[78] Dover LG, Cerdeño-Tárraga AM, Pallen MJ, Parkhill J, Besra GS. Comparative cell wall core biosynthesis in the mycolated pathogens, *Mycobacterium tuberculosis* and *Corynebacterium diphtheriae*. FEMS Microbiology Reviews 2004:28: 225–250.

[79] Minnikin DE, Lee OY-C, Wu HHT, Besra GS, Bhatt A, Nataraj V, Rothschild BM, Spigelman M, Donoghue HD. Ancient mycobacterial lipids: Key reference biomarkers in charting the evolution of tuberculosis. Tuberculosis 2015;95: S133-S139.

[80] Veyrier F, Pletzer D, Turenne C, Behr MA. Phylogenetic detection of horizontal gene transfer during the step-wise genesis of *Mycobacterium tuberculosis*. BMC Evolutionary Biology 2009;9: 196.

[81] Veyrier FJ, Dufort A, Behr MA. The rise and fall of the *Mycobacterium tuberculosis* genome. Trends in Microbiology 2011;19: 156-161.

[82] Bottai D, Stinear TP, Supply P, Brosch R. Mycobacterial Pathogenomics and Evolution. In: Hatfull GF, Jacobs WR. (eds.) Molecular Genetics of Mycobacteria, 2nd Edition. Washington, DC: American Society for Microbiology; 2014. p27-47.

[83] Smith NH, Hewinson RG, Kremer K, Brosch R, Gordon SV. Myths and misconceptions: the origin and evolution of *Mycobacterium tuberculosis*. Nature Reviews in Microbiology 2009;7: 537-544.

[84] Supply P, Marceau M, Mangenot S, Roche D, Rouanet C, Khanna V, Majlessi L, Criscuolo A, Tap J, Pawlik A, Fiette L, Orgeur M, Fabre M, Parmentier C, Frigui W, Simeone R, Boritsch EC, Debrie AS, Willery E, Walker D, Quail MA, Ma L, Bouchier C,

Salvignol G, Sayes F, Cascioferro A, Seemann T, Barbe V, Locht C, Gutierrez MC, Leclerc C, Bentley SD, Stinear TP, Brisse S, Médigue C, Parkhill J, Cruveiller S, Brosch R. Genomic analysis of smooth tubercle bacilli provides insights into ancestry and pathoadaptation of *Mycobacterium tuberculosis*. Nature Genetics 2013;45: 172-179.

[85] Fabre M, Hauck Y, Soler C, Koeck J-L, van Ingen J, van Soolingen D, Vergnaud G, Pourcel C. Molecular characteristics of *"Mycobacterium canettii"* the smooth *Mycobacterium tuberculosis* bacilli. Infection, Genetics and Evolution 2010;10: 1165–1173.

[86] Koeck J-L, Fabre M, Simon F, Daffé M, Garnotel E, Matan AB, Gérôme P, Bernatas JJ, Buisson Y, Pourcel C. Clinical characteristics of the smooth tubercle bacilli *'Mycobacterium canettii'* infection suggest the existence of an environmental reservoir. Clinical Microbiology and Infection 2011;17: 1013–1019.

[87] Gutierrez MC, Brisse S, Brosch R, Fabre M, Omaïs B, Marmiesse M, Supply P, Vincent V. Ancient origin and gene mosaicism of the progenitor of *Mycobacterium tuberculosis*. PLoS Pathogens 2005;1(1): e5.

[88] Gordon SV, Bottai D, Simeone R, Stinear TP, Brosch R. Pathogenicity in the tubercle bacillus: molecular and evolutionary determinants. BioEssays 2009;31: 378–388.

[89] Soto CY, Cama M, Gibert I, Luquin M. Application of an easy and reliable method for sulfolipid-I detection in the study of its distribution in *Mycobacterium tuberculosis* strains. FEMS Microbiology Letters 2000;187: 103-107.

[90] Rousseau C, Turner OC, Rush E, Bordat Y, Sirakova TD, Kolattukudy PE, Ritter S, Orme IM, Gicquel B, Jackson M. Sulfolipid Deficiency Does Not Affect the Virulence of *Mycobacterium tuberculosis* H37Rv in Mice and Guinea Pigs. Infection and Immunity 2003; 71: 4684–4690.

[91] Rousseau C, Neyrolles O, Bordat Y, Giroux S, Sirakova TD, Prevost M-C, Kolattukudy PE, Gicquel B, Jackson M. Deficiency in mycolipenate- and mycosanoate-derived acyltrehaloses enhances early interactions of *Mycobacterium tuberculosis* with host cells. Cellular Microbiology 2003;5: 405–415.

[92] Falkinham JO. Mycobacterial Aerosols and Respiratory Disease. Emerging Infectious Diseases 2003;9: 763-767.

[93] Cangelosi GA, Palermo CO, Laurent J-P, Hamlin AM, Brabant WH. Colony morphotypes on Congo red agar segregate along species and drug susceptibility lines in the *Mycobacterium avium-intracellulare* complex. Microbiology 1999;145: 1317-1324.

[94] Stokes RW, Norris-Jones R, Brooks DE, Beveridge TJ, Doxsee D, Thorson LM. The Glycan-Rich Outer Layer of the Cell Wall of *Mycobacterium tuberculosis* Acts as an Antiphagocytic Capsule Limiting the Association of the Bacterium with Macrophages. Infection and Immunity 2004;72: 5676–5686.

[95] Jönsson B, Gilljam M, Lindblad A, Ridell M, Wold AE, Welinder-Olsson C. Molecular epidemiology of *Mycobacterium abscessus*, with focus on cystic fibrosis. Journal Clinical Microbiology 2007;45: 1497–1504.

[96] Jönsson B, Ridell M, Wold AE. Phagocytosis and cytokine response to rough and smooth colony variants of *Mycobacterium abscessus* by human peripheral blood mononuclear cells. APMIS 2013;121: 45–55.

[97] Bendinger B, Rijnaarts HHM, Altendorf K, Zehnder AJB. Physicochemical Cell Surface and Adhesive Properties of Coryneform Bacteria Related to the Presence and Chain Length of Mycolic Acids. Applied and Environmental Microbiology 1993;59: 3973-3977.

[98] Hershkovitz I, Donoghue HD, Minnikin DE, Besra GS, Lee OY-C, Gernaey AM, Galili E, Eshed V, Greenblatt CL, Lemma E, Kahila Bar-Gal G, Spigelman M. Detection and molecular characterization of 9000-year-old *Mycobacterium tuberculosis* from a Neolithic settlement in the Eastern Mediterranean. PLoS ONE 2008;3: e3426.

[99] Lee OY-C, Wu HHT, Donoghue HD, Spigelman, M, Greenblatt CL, Bull ID, Rothschild, BM, Martin, LD, Minnikin, DE, Besra, GS. *Mycobacterium tuberculosis* Complex Lipid Virulence Factors Preserved in the 17,000-Year-Old Skeleton of an Extinct Bison, *Bison antiquus*. PLoS ONE 2012;7: e41923.

[100] Rothschild BM, Martin LD. Did ice-age bovids spread tuberculosis? Naturwissenschaften 2006;93: 565-569.

[101] Rothschild BM, Laub R. Hyperdisease in the late Pleistocene: validation of an early 20th century hypothesis. Naturwissenschaften 2006;93: 557–564.

[102] Minnikin DE, Lee OY-C, Wu HHT, Besra GS, Donoghue HD. Molecular biomarkers for ancient tuberculosis. In: Cardona P-J. (ed.) Understanding Tuberculosis – Deciphering the Secret Life of the Bacilli. Rijeka, Croatia.: InTech -Open Access Publisher. 2012. p. 1-36. http://www.intechopen.com/books/understanding tuberculosis-deciphering-the-secret-life-of-the-bacilli

[103] Rothschild BM, Martin LD, Lev G, Bercovier H, Bar-Gal GK, Greenblatt C, Donoghue H, Spigelman M, Brittain D. *Mycobacterium tuberculosis* complex DNA from an extinct bison dated 17,000 years BP. Clinical and Infectious Diseases 2001;33: 305–311.

[104] Jang J, Becq J, Gicquel B, Deschavanne P, Neyrolles O. Horizontally acquired genomic islands in the tubercle bacilli. Trends in Microbiology 2008;16: 303-308.

[105] Higham T, Douka K, Wood R, Ramsey CB, Brock F, Basell L, Camps M, Arrizabalaga A, Baena J, Barroso-Ruíz C, Bergman C, Boitard C, Boscato P, Caparrós M, Conard NJ, Draily C, Froment A, Galván B, Gambassini P, Garcia-Moreno A, Grimaldi S, Haesaerts P, Holt B, Iriarte-Chiapusso MJ, Jelinek A, Jordá Pardo JF, Maíllo-Fernández JM, Marom A, Maroto J, Menéndez M, Metz L, Morin E, Moroni A, Negrino F, Panagopoulou E, Peresani M, Pirson S, de la Rasilla M, Riel-Salvatore J, Ronchitelli A, Santamaria D, Semal P, Slimak L, Soler J, Soler N, Villaluenga A, Pinhasi R, Jacobi

R. The timing and spatiotemporal patterning of Neanderthal disappearance. Nature 2014;512: 306-309.

[106] Djelouadji Z, Raoult D, Drancourt M. Palaeogenomics of *Mycobacterium tuberculosis*: epidemic bursts with a degrading genome. Lancet Infectious Diseases 2011;11: 641–650.

10

Regulation of the Immune Response by *Mycobacterium tuberculosis* Beijing Genotype

Marcia Campillo-Navarro, Isabel Wong-Baeza,
Jeanet Serafín-López, Rogelio Hernández-Pando,
Sergio Estrada-Parra, Iris Estrada-García and
Rommel Chacón-Salinas

1. Introduction

Tuberculosis (TB) is an old infectious disease that has affected humans for millennia [1]. This disease is caused by infection with bacilli belonging to the *Mycobacterium tuberculosis* (Mtb) complex and is responsible for 1.3 million deaths around the world, making TB the second leading cause of death by infectious disease caused by a single pathogen. In addition to this high number of deaths, a large proportion of individuals present latent TB infection (LTBI): it is estimated that at least one third of the human population could have LTBI [2]. Why more than 90% of the individuals infected with Mtb do not develop the active form of the disease is unclear, although the immune status of the individual seems to play a crucial role for Mtb containment [3]. This is evident in individuals with Human Immunodeficiency Virus co-infection, who are more prone to develop active TB: a quarter of TB deaths occur in individuals co-infected with HIV [2].

However, other factors are associated with TB development, such as the host environment and the genetic diversity of Mtb. This genetic diversity has been organized into genotypes and lineages, according to the genetic profiles obtained by techniques such as IS6110 fingerprinting, spoligotyping and mycobacterial interspersed repetitive units-variable number of tandem repeats (MIRU-VNTR). Interestingly, these genotypes show a differential distribution around the world and exhibit different levels of virulence [4]. One of the genotypes that has attracted more attention in recent years is the Beijing family, because it is highly prevalent among TB patients, it favours the spread of multidrug-resistant tuberculosis, and it has been suggested that BCG vaccination confers poor protection against it [5].

It is not clear why the Beijing genotype prevails in infected individuals. One factor that could be responsible for this phenomenon is the interaction that Mtb Beijing establishes with the immune response. In this chapter, we analyze and discuss current knowledge regarding the cellular and molecular mechanisms of the immune response to Mtb, and how these mechanisms are affected by the Beijing genotype in relation to human infections.

2. Immune response to *Mycobacterium tuberculosis*

Mtb can enter the body through several routes, but the most usual one is through the airways [6]. This process is initiated by the release of small saliva droplets containing Mtb bacilli that are expelled by active TB patients [7]. Some droplets are small enough to cross the mucociliary barrier and reach the alveoli, where they interact with the first cellular element of the immune response, the alveolar macrophage [8]. Macrophages are armed with a vast array of innate immune receptors that allow direct recognition of Mtb; these receptors include Toll-like receptors (TLR), Nod-like receptors (NLR), C-type lectin receptors (CLR) and scavenger receptors [9]. After recognition, macrophages ingest bacilli by phagocytosis, but they are unable to kill them due to the evolutionary mechanisms acquired by Mtb that actively inhibit phagosome maturation and protect Mtb from destruction by toxic compounds, such as reactive nitrogen and oxygen intermediates and hydrolytic enzymes from lysosomes; these mechanisms allow intracellular Mtb survival and proliferation [10, 11].

In addition to this intracellular proliferation, Mtb also induces a strong inflammatory response, characterized by macrophage production of cytokines like TNF-α, IL-1β and IL-6, which promote the recruitment of more macrophages from the blood [12]. The recruited macrophages are able to ingest bacilli but, like alveolar macrophages, they are unable to eliminate the ingested Mtb. The continuous recruitment of macrophages during these early stages provides a constant supply of cells susceptible to infection, as well as an increase of inflammatory signals that induces the recruitment of more susceptible cells from the blood, without causing significant tissue damage. At the same time, lung resident dendritic cells (DCs) engulf bacilli or their derived products; the inflammatory environment promotes DCs migration from the lungs to the draining lymph nodes, where they activate Mtb antigen-specific naïve T cells and induce a strong T cell response characterized by proliferation and activation of Mtb antigen-specific CD4+and CD8+T cells [13]. These T cells travel through the blood and are recruited to the infection site by the ongoing inflammatory process.

Upon recognition of the infected macrophages, T cells produce significant amounts of TNF-α and IFN-γ, the cytokines that characterize a Th1 response. TNF-α and IFN-γ increase the microbicidal mechanisms of the infected macrophages, which eventually leads to the intracellular killing of Mtb. Macrophage activation can be limited by the secretion of IL-4, IL-10 and TGF-β produced by Th2 and T regulatory (Treg) cells [14-16]. The Th1 response, however, does not lead to a complete elimination of Mtb, but to the formation of an organized cellular structure, the granuloma, where live mycobacteria persist in a dormant state known as latent infection [17]. The structure of the granuloma varies, but usually its center is formed by caseum, a structure that contains abundant remains of dead cells and forms a hypoxic, acidic and lipid-rich environment that limits extracellular Mtb proliferation. The caseum is limited by highly activated macrophages (multinucleated Langhans cells and foamy macrophages) surrounded by CD4+and CD8+T cells [18]. While the host immune response is unaffected, the granuloma structure is preserved and Mtb is contained within; however, the alteration of crucial elements of the immune response, such as the decrease of CD4+T cells during HIV infection or the blockade of TNF-α by therapeutic antibodies, causes disorganization of the granuloma structure, caseum liquefaction and oxygen access, which promotes Mtb extracellular proliferation and dissemination into the airways, from where Mtb can reach susceptible hosts [19-21] (Figure 1).

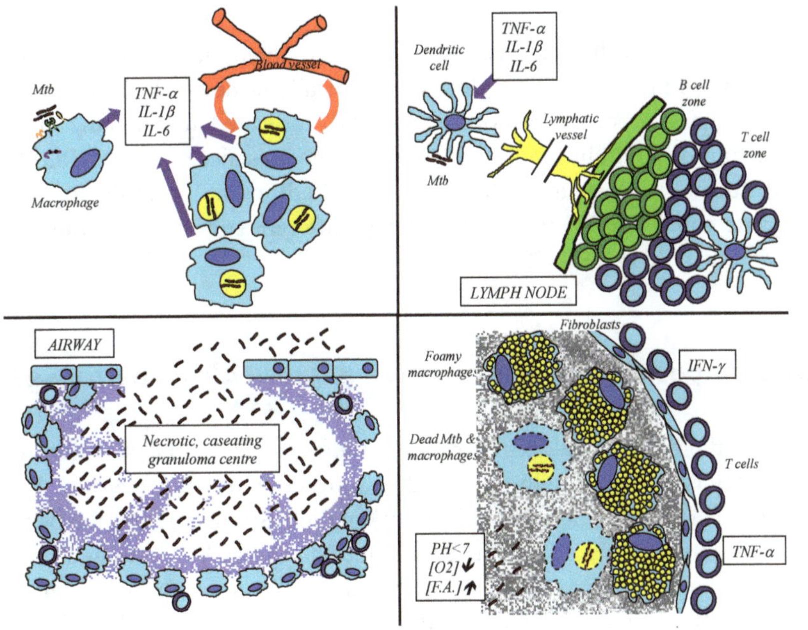

Figure 1. Development of the immune response to *Mycobacterium tuberculosis*. The main four stages of the immune response to *Mycobacterium tuberculosis* (Mtb) are depicted. Macrophages are the first component of the cellular immune response that is encountered by Mtb (top left); they are used by Mtb to replicate and to induce an inflammatory response that allows the recruitment of more macrophages susceptible to infection. Dendritic cells (top right) carry Mtb antigens from the infection site to the draining lymph nodes, to activate antigen-specific T cells. The mycobacterial granuloma (bottom right) plays a fundamental role in Mtb containment. Alterations in the dynamic equilibrium of the granuloma (bottom left) promote disorganization and access of extracellular Mtb to oxygen, which allows its replication and dissemination through the airways.

3. *Mycobacterium tuberculosis* Beijing genotype

Because Mtb strains present over 99 % of similarity at their nucleotide sequence level and have identical sequences of their 16S RNAs [22, 23], for several years it was thought that they were genetically homogeneous and lacked genetic diversity. However, the development and use of different genetic tools for the study of Mtb revealed greater diversity. Studies that analyzed repetitive DNA elements in Mtb led to the discovery of high polymorphism in several strains. The study of restriction fragment length polymorphism (RFLP) in IS6110 allowed van Soolingen *et al* to identify a group of strains, isolated in Beijing, Mongolia, South Korea and Thailand, which shared a unique RFLP pattern. Since the majority of these strains came from Beijing, they became known as the "Beijing family". Further genetic characterization showed that all these strains shared an identical spoligotyping of the direct repeat (DR) region, and similar patterns of polymorphic GC-rich sequence (PGRS) as well as an IS1081 restriction fragments [24]. Mtb strains with these genetic characteristics were later found outside the Southeast Asian region, in Russia, Spain, the United States, Cuba, Peru, Colombia, Iran, Israel and South Africa [5, 25].

Beijing strains were classified as "typical", if they presented one or more IS6110 insertions in the noise transfer function (NTF) region, or "atypical", if they lacked this insertion [26, 27]. Analysis of large sequence polymorphisms (LSP) indicated that Beijing strains could be divided into four different lineages, depending on the presence of RD105, RD142, RD150 and RD181 [28]. Further studies, using PCR to analyze 40 different loci in Beijing strains, showed that this group could also be divided into seven different sub-lineages, thus revealing great genetic diversity in this group [29].

4. Clinical importance of *Mycobacterium tuberculosis* Beijing genotype

In addition to the high prevalence of Beijing strains in the Southeast Asian region, Beijing strains have been associated with outbreaks in different parts of the world. The strains that were responsible for a TB outbreak in New York in the 1990's were from the Beijing genotype, and they were more frequent in patients co-infected with HIV, reaching a mortality rate of more than 80%. Interestingly, strains from this outbreak had multidrug resistance to isoniazid, rifampicin, streptomycin, ethambutol, ethionamide, rifabutin and kanamycin, favouring treatment failure [30-32]. Later studies showed the global emergence of this genotype in different parts of the world [25, 33, 34].

Several epidemiological studies have documented the hyper-virulence of the Beijing genotype. For example, patients infected with Beijing strains have increased rates of treatment failure and relapse [35-39]. In line with these studies, Kong *et al* showed that patients infected with Beijing strains developed more extra-thoracic TB than patients infected with other genotypes [40]. Other studies demonstrated that individuals infected with strains from the Beijing genotype were more likely to progress to active TB [41, 42] and had increased drug resistance [43, 44]. Furthermore, patients infected with these strains were younger than patients infected with other genotypes [45], and they developed febrile responses in earlier stages of treatment [46]. Moreover, infection with Beijing strains was associated with HIV co-infection [47] and BCG vaccination [48]. However, others have been unable to find an association between infection with Beijing strains and the aforementioned clinical manifestations of the disease [38, 45, 49-54].

Few studies focused on the immune response have been conducted in patients infected with Beijing strains. Sun *et al* found that the sera of patients infected with Beijing and non-Beijing strains had similar levels of IFN-γ and IL-18, while peripheral blood mononuclear cells (PBMCs) expressed similar mRNA levels for IFN-γ, IL-2, IL-18. However, patients infected with Beijing strains had decreased levels of IL-4 [55]. In contrast with these results, Rakotosamimanana *et al* observed that PBMCs from patients infected with the "modern" Mtb strains from Beijing and Central Asia produced less IFN-γ in response to ESAT-6 than PBMCs from patients infected with other genotypes [56]. These results suggest that Mtb Beijing genotype could induce an altered immune response that could favor infection by these strains.

5. Effects of *Mycobacterium tuberculosis* Beijing genotype on the immune response: *in vivo* models

The first evidence of the hyper-virulence of the Mtb Beijing genotype came from studies with different mouse models of infection. Manca *et al* showed that the Beijing strain HN878, isolated from cases from an outbreak in Texas, led to higher bacterial loads in the lungs and to accelerated death in immune-competent mice, compared to a non-Beijing strain. Moreover, the lymph node and spleen cells from HN878-infected mice showed decreased proliferation and IFN-γ production after *in vitro* re-stimulation, suggesting a defective induction of a Th1 response because of the early induction of type I IFN by HN878 [57, 58]. Later studies showed that the decrease in the Th1 response was associated with the induction of Treg cells in mice and also in guinea pigs, an animal model that resembles human tuberculosis [59, 60]. Intracisternal infection of rabbits with Mtb leads to the development of tuberculous meningitis. In this model of infection, the Beijing strains HN878 and W4 led to higher bacterial loads in the cerebrospinal fluid and brain, increased dissemination to the lungs and liver, earlier leukocytosis, increased levels of TNF-α during the later stages of the infection, and severe clinical manifestations, compared to the low-virulence strain CDC1551 [61].

López *et al* reported that three Beijing strains, representing the predominant genotypes in Asia, were hyper-virulent in a mouse model of progressive pulmonary tuberculosis, compared to other genotypes (Somali, Haarlem, Canetti and H37Rv). This hyper-virulence was reflected as an increased number of bacteria in the lungs and a rapid death of the mice infected with the Beijing strains. The mice infected with the Beijing strains had altered immune responses: they expressed TNF-α and iNOS in their lungs during the early stages of the disease, but had a defective production of iNOS and IFN-γ during the later stages of the infection [62]. Further studies associated this phenomenon with a decrease in Th1 cells caused by apoptosis and with a defective cytotoxicity, indicative of a deficient CD8+T cell response [63, 64]. A more recent report with the Beijing strain K1, isolated in Korea, showed that this strain is hyper-virulent, and the lungs of infected mice had a decreased production of Th1 and Th2 cytokines [65]. The hyper-virulence of the Beijing strains was also observed when they were compared to East African-Indian strains in mice [66].

However, Dormans *et al* showed that hyper-virulence is not associated with all the Beijing strains. He observed that strain 9402008, isolated from Asia, caused little lung pathology, bacterial load and mortality in mice [67]. Furthermore, Aguilar *et al* showed that Beijing strains isolated in South Africa, which presented low transmissibility in humans, were less virulent than the Beijing strains that were highly transmissible [68]. The highly transmissible Beijing strains caused an early induction of TNF-α and delayed IL-4 production, as well as defective induction of IFN-γ and iNOS in the lungs during the later stages of the disease, compared to the low-virulence Beijing strains [68]. This difference in virulence among Beijing strains was also observed in a mouse model of infection with seven Beijing strains isolated in Vietnam [69], and in guinea pigs infected with ten Beijing strains isolated in the USA. Interestingly, the lungs of these guinea pigs also showed differential patterns of T cell infiltration and cytokine production: virulent strains induced less IFN-γ during the later stages of the infection, compared to low-virulence strains [70]. A more recent study showed that heterogeneity in virulence was also observed in mice infected with Beijing strains isolated from Brazil and Mozambique [71].

From these *in vivo* experiments, it is clear that hyper-virulence is not a unique characteristic that applies to all the strains from the Beijing genotype. However, all the hyper-virulent strains from the Beijing group share a common characteristic: they are able to interfere with the Th1 response that is crucial for infection containment, favoring the dissemination of bacilli in the lung and an increased pathology.

6. Effects of *Mycobacterium tuberculosis* Beijing genotype on the immune response: *in vitro* models

6.1. Macrophages

Several studies have analyzed the ability of the Beijing strains to replicate inside macrophages and to induce cytokine production by these cells. One of the first studies that showed a differential response of macrophages to the Beijing strains was performed in human macrophages. The Beijing strain 210, isolated in the USA, grew faster in human macrophages than other Mtb strains tested, but there were no differences among the strains regarding the induction of TNF-α, IL-6, IL-10 or IL-12 [72]. A faster intracellular replication of the bacilli in human macrophages was also observed with four different Beijing strains [73]. In contrast with these results, Manca *et al* showed that human monocytes infected with the Beijing strain HN878 produced increased mRNA levels for IL-4, IL-11, IL-13, type I IFN, TRAIL and VEGF, compared to monocytes infected with the low-virulence strain CDC1551 [74], and our group reported that the hyper-virulent Beijing strain 9501000 induced higher expression of IL-1β,

TNF-α and IL-12 in mouse bone marrow-derived macrophages (mBMDM), in comparison to a low-virulence strain of the Canetti genotype [75].

Theus *et al* used fifteen different strains of the Beijing genotype and infected IFN-γ-activated THP-1 cells (a human monocyte-like cell line); interestingly, they observed a spectrum of growth and TNF-α induction among these Beijing strains [76]. Tanveer *et al* observed that ten Beijing strains induced similar levels of TNF-α in PMA-stimulated THP-1 cells than Central Asian strains, but lower levels of TNF-α than H37Rv [77]. A low production of TNF-α, IL-6, IL-10 and CXCL1 was also observed in monocyte-derived human macrophages infected with nine different Beijing strains, compared to macrophages infected with H37Rv [78]. In line with this study, Reiling *et al* reported that human macrophages stimulated with four Beijing strains produced lower levels of TNF-α, IL-1β, IL-6, IL-12 and CCL5 than Haarlem strains [66], and Portevin *et al* extended this observation to "modern" Mtb lineages, including Beijing genotype strains [79]. However, Krishnan *et al* observed that seven Beijing strains induced higher IL-1β and TNF-α production than Euro-American strains, but there was considerable heterogeneity in the amount of cytokines induced by each Beijing strain [69]. Heterogeneity in the amount of IL-1β produced was also observed in mBMDM infected with seven Beijing strains [80].

Altogether, these results point to a heterogenic response of macrophages to different isolates of the Beijing genotype. Besides the obvious differences in the biological systems used in the studies summarized in the previous paragraphs, which could explain the differing results, experiments that have used the same *in vitro* model show that the induction of heterogenic cytokine responses is a common characteristic of the Beijing genotype. Two patterns are observed: one is characterized by low induction of pro-inflammatory cytokines, which is associated with a poor regulation of intracellular bacterial replication. The second pattern is characterized by a higher production of pro-inflammatory cytokines, and *in vivo* evidence indicates that, during the early stages of an infection with these strains, there is an inflammatory response of equal or higher magnitude than the inflammatory response induced by other genotypes. This, however, raises a question: how could high levels of pro-inflammatory cytokines be favorable to the pathogen? The paradox may be explained by the function that these cytokines play during Mtb infection. For instance, macrophage-produced TNF-α is associated with macrophage self-activation and control of the intracellular replication of Mtb during the early stages of the infection but, according to a mouse model of infection, it is the T cell-produced TNF-α that is essential for mycobacterial containment during the chronic infection [81]. The recruitment of macrophages with low anti-mycobacterial capacity during the early stages actually favors infection dissemination [82], so the induction of an inflammatory environment that allows the recruitment of such cells could be actively pursued by some virulent Mtb strains.

6.2. Dendritic cells

Although DCs play a crucial role for the mounting of T cell responses to Mtb, few studies have analyzed how Beijing strains affect DC functions. The first studies on this subject analyzed cytokine production by DCs. Wang *et al* observed that human derived DCs stimulated with

Beijing strains produced low levels of TNF-α, IL-6 and CCL3, compared to DCs stimulated with H37Rv [78]. Portevin *et al* observed that human DCs stimulated with "modern" Mtb lineages, which include Beijing genotype strains, produced less pro-inflammatory cytokines than DCs stimulated with "ancient" Mtb lineages [79], while Krishnan *et al* did not observe any difference in cytokine production by mouse bone marrow derived DCs (mBMDDCs) stimulated with Beijing strains, H37Rv or other genotypes [69]. Recently, our group reported that a hyper-virulent Beijing strain failed to activate mBMDDCs (assessed by MHC class II expression) but did not affect the induction of CCR7 expression, which is essential to drive DC migration from the tissues to the lymph nodes. Moreover, these DCs had higher levels of PDL-1 and IL-10 than DCs stimulated with low-virulence strains. Interestingly, the phenotypic changes correlated with alterations in DC function, as revealed by their inability to induce a Th1 response [83]; a phenomenon usually observed during *in vivo* infections with hyper-virulent Beijing strains.

6.3. Human peripheral blood mononuclear cells

Human PBMCs consist mainly of monocytes, T cells, B cells and NK cells. Assays where PBMCs are stimulated with pathogens or their antigens can be used to evince T cell-mediated immune responses [84]. In one of the first studies that used PBMCs to assess granuloma formation *in vitro*, the authors analyzed two Beijing strains and did not observe a difference in the number or size of the granulomas induced by these strains, compared to the granulomas induced by Haarlem, Latin American-Mediterranean or East African-Indian strains [78]. Our group reported that the PBMCs from healthy BCG-vaccinated individuals stimulated with Beijing strains presented CD4+and CD8+T cell proliferation responses similar to those induced by the less virulent Canetti and H37Rv strains, and that the Beijing strains induced higher production of IL-10 and IL-12, but similar levels of IFN-γ [85]. Recently, van Laarhoven *et al* analyzed the effect of fourteen Beijing strains on cytokine production by PBMCs from non-BCG-vaccinated healthy individuals; "modern" Beijing strains induced lower levels of IL-1β, IFN-γ and IL-22 than "ancient" Beijing strains [86]. In contrast, Portevin *et al* did not observe a difference in cytokine production by PBMCs stimulated with several Beijing strains [79]. One explanation for the different response of PBMC's, beyond the genetic diversity of Beijing strains, is the immune status of the donors: only one study analyzed the response of BCG vaccinated individuals, and BCG vaccination has been associated with increased susceptibility to infection with Beijing strains [48].

The studies described above show that Beijing strains modulate the response of different cell populations that participate during the immune response to this pathogen. However, most of these studies are focused on macrophages, leaving aside other cell populations that are known to participate in the immune response to mycobacteria, such as pneumocytes, neutrophils, mast cells, NK, NKT cells, γδ T cells, B cells, etc. Studying how these cells respond to Beijing strains will help to understand the mechanism used by this Mtb genotype to override the immune response.

7. Components of *Mycobacterium tuberculosis* Beijing genotype that modulate the immune response

7.1. Lipids

Several Mtb components are associated with evasion of the immune response. Among them, lipids have been widely studied, mainly because of the atypical structure of the mycobacterial cell wall and the predominance of some types of lipids in this cell wall. Lipid extracts from the Beijing strain HN878 induced higher expression of IL-13, G-CSF and VEGF in human macrophages, compared to the expression induced by lipids from the CDC1551 strain [74]. The cell wall lipids from hyper-virulent Beijing strain 9501000 also induced higher expression of TNF-α and IL-10 than the cell wall lipids from H37Rv and Canetti genotype [87].

Reed *et al* showed that three hyper-virulent Beijing strains expressed a phenolic glycolipid (PGL) that was not expressed by the lower-virulence strains H37Rv and CDC1551. When the HN878 strain lost the expression of this PGL, its hyper-virulence in mice and rabbits was diminished, and the cytokine pattern that it induced in macrophages became similar to that induced by H37Rv [88]. Later studies showed that 102 Beijing strains had unaltered *pks15/1*, the open reading frame (ORF) coding for the enzyme responsible for PGL production [28]. However, the presence of intact *pks15/1* is not exclusive of the Beijing genotype [89], and some Beijing strains that express this ORF do not produce PGL [90]. In addition, a study reported that induction of PGL production by non-Beijing strains did not increase their virulence [91]. Regarding other lipids, Reed *et al* observed that 36 Beijing strains, but not Indo-Oceanic or Euro-American strains, uniformly expressed triacylglycerides [90]. Huet *et al* showed that Beijing strains presented a pattern of phthiocerol dimycoceroserates (PDIM) different to that of other Mtb strains; this difference was associated with the mutation $Rv2952^{G526A}$ in the Beijing strains, but it was not associated with the virulence of these Beijing strains [92]. Another study reported that total lipids extracts from Beijing strains induced higher TNF-α production by mBMDM than total lipids extracts from Euro-American strains. These Beijing strains had a characteristic pattern of PDIM, which was different to that of other Mtb strains [69].

These studies indicate that lipids from Mtb Beijing play an important role in the regulation of macrophage activation and in the induction of cytokine production. However, further studies are needed to clarify how these lipids impact other arms of the immune response that are crucial for infection containment, such as DCs and T cells specific for Mtb lipid antigens [93]. Another potential role for the lipids of the Beijing strains could be as carbon and energy reservoirs, which would be valuable in the harsh conditions that the bacilli find inside macrophages or in the anoxic granulomas [90].

7.2. Proteins

One of the first studies that analyzed proteins identified that a Beijing strain, but not Canetti or H37Rv strains, expressed mRNA for PE_PGRS Rv3652 [94]. Wu *et al* observed that the Beijing strain 210 had higher SigA mRNA levels than H37Rv, and that blockade of SigA expression attenuated bacterial growth in human macrophages and in the lungs of infected mice, a phenomenon that was associated with increased Mtb susceptibility to reactive oxygen intermediates [95]. Later studies showed that SigA induced up-regulation of Eis, which in turn promoted TNF-α and IL-10 production by macrophages [96, 97].

Pheiffer *et al,* using proteomic techniques, found that a Beijing strain expressed higher levels of α-crystallin and lower levels of Hsp65, PstS1 and 47kDa protein than H37Rv [98]. Interestingly, Reed *et al* found that Beijing strains constitutively expressed high mRNA levels of genes in the DosR regulon, including *dosR*, Rv3130c, *hspX*, *fdxA* and *narX*; the levels of these mRNAs were up to 50 times higher than the levels found in non-Beijing strains [90]. Usually, Mtb induces the expression of the DosR regulon under two conditions: 1) in the lungs of infected mice and in artificial granulomas [99], and 2) inside macrophages that are activated with IFN-γ [100]. In consequence, the authors hypothesized that a constitutive high expression of the genes in the DosR regulon would allow a fast adaptation of Mtb to this harsh conditions leading to Mtb survival. The mechanisms that maintain this high expression of the DosR regulon are unknown, but mutations in DosT sensor kinase and chromosomal duplication have been implicated in this phenomenon [101, 102].

Rindi *et al* found that Beijing strains expressed high levels of PPE44, a member of the Mtb PPE proteins that are related with antigenic variation [103]. Another approach, using proteomic analysis among several Beijing strains with different virulence, showed that the virulent strains over-expressed 53 proteins involved in regulation, cell wall synthesis and cell processes [104]. Recent reports indicate that the virulent Beijing strain K1 expressed higher levels of ESAT-6, HSP-X and CFP-10 than strains from other genotypes, and it also expressed InsB, a protein which shares homology with ESAT-6 [105, 106].

Altogether, these results indicate that Beijing strains express a different set of proteins that could participate in many stages of the infection. First, they could modify the innate immune response through a differential engagement of pattern recognition receptors (PRRs), inducing a response that would favors infection [107]. Second, they could facilitate a rapid adaptation of the bacilli to the adverse conditions found during infection (hypoxic, or rich in reactive nitrogen and oxygen intermediates, for example) [90]. Third, the regulation of the expression of proteins that are recognized by the adaptive immune response could facilitate immune evasion and fostering survival of the bacteria [98].

7.3. Other molecules

Carbohydrates from Beijing strains have been poorly analyzed. Usually, carbohydrates are associated with lipids or proteins, and they are abundant on bacterial cell walls. Carbohydrates play a crucial role in the recognition of microbes by innate immune cells through PRRs, and consequently, they could modulate the whole immune response to the bacilli [108, 109].

As we have seen, the immune response is crucial role for infection containment, but other non-immune factors contribute to Mtb virulence, and a conjunction of all these factors defines the outcome of the infection. Metabolomic studies of hyper-virulent and hypo-virulent Beijing strains have reported a difference in the presence of different metabolites, including amino acids, carbohydrates and lipids [110]. How this difference impacts bacterial phenotype needs further clarification.

8. Evolution as a driving force in the success of *Mycobacterium tuberculosis* Beijing genotype

The studies cited above highlight a great variation in the responses to infection with Beijing strains, both *in vivo* and *in vitro*. One explanation for this variation could be the genetic diversity of the Beijing strains, but some studies have been unable to correlate the different responses with the genetic diversity of the Beijing genotype [111, 112]. So, how can we understand this variation? Evolution has played a fundamental role in shaping the actual scenario of TB on earth. Humans have co-existed with Mtb since our appearance as a species on this planet, and Mtb accompanied humans since the first migrations from Africa to other parts of the world [1, 113]. These migrations and settlings allowed a co-evolution of each human population with its pathogens, including Mtb, and this is reflected in the distribution of Mtb diversity: six different Mtb lineages are stably associated with specific human populations, according to their geographic distribution [4]. Mtb lineages are so well adapted to their hosts that even in cosmopolitan areas, where diverse human populations from different geographic origins coexist, a specific Mtb lineage preferentially infects individuals from a specific geographic origin (sympatric transmission) [114]. Allopatric human transmission of Mtb occurs, but infection of individuals from one geographic origin with Mtb from a different lineage is usually associated with other factors, such as HIV co-infection. Patients with allopatric infections have increased pulmonary impairment, compared to patients with sympatric infections [114, 115].

Mtb Beijing genotype belongs to the East-Asian lineage, and it is strongly associated with hosts from this geographic area. When Mtb Beijing genotype is introduced to new areas, where it is uncommon, it preferentially infects hosts that also come from its original geographic area. Studies in Italy and Sweden indicate that infection with Mtb Beijing genotype is uncommon among natives and more frequent among migrants from areas commonly infected by this genotype, which suggests a poor adaptation of Mtb Beijing genotype to the native hosts [116, 117]. In fact, the genetic diversification of Mtb Beijing genotype has been associated with adaptation to particular human populations [118].

Which host factors predispose to infection with Mtb Beijing genotype? Some studies indicate that infection with Beijing strains occurs preferentially in hosts that have particular polymorphisms in immune response genes. In Vietnamese patients, infection with Beijing strains was associated with the presence of the TLR-2 allele T597C [119], and recent reports indicate that TLR-2 polymorphisms are differentially distributed in human populations according to their geographic localization and ethnicity [120]. Whether these polymorphisms affect the immune response to Beijing strains still needs to be analyzed, but differential activation of TLR-2 and TLR-4 by Mtb strains from different genotypes has an impact on the immune response to the bacilli [121].

Crevel *et al* found that, in Indonesian patients, the polymorphism D453N G and an insertion in the 3'untranslated region (UTR) of the *slc11a1* gene (formerly known as *nramp1*) were strongly associated with Beijing strains infection [122]; polymorphisms in this gene (which codes for an iron transporter in macrophages) have been associated with TB susceptibility [123]. Salie *et al* documented an association between MHC class I alleles and infection with Beijing strains in South Africans, where the allele B*07:05 increased the odds of infection with Beijing strains, while the allele B*35:01 had the opposite effect. Interestingly, B*07:05 is a frequent allele in East Asian populations [124]. MHC class I molecules are essential for antigen presentation to CD8+T cells, which are needed for the containment of Mtb infection [125]. These studies provide evidence of a co-evolution between Beijing strains and their hosts.

9. Conclusion

Mtb Beijing genotype has attracted attention because of its high prevalence among TB patients, but despite multiple studies, the causes of this success remain obscure. An interesting aspect of Mtb Beijing genotype infection is the diversity of the immune responses that are induced in humans and in experimental models (*in vivo* and *in vitro*). It is possible that this diversity results from the adaptation of Mtb Beijing genotype to the genetic background of its hosts and to other evolutionary pressures, such as drug treatment, BCG vaccination and HIV co-infection. These factors, and others still unknown, will shape the strategies used by Beijing strains to override the immune response and to establish successful infections in the host.

Acknowledgements

This work was supported by SIP, IPN and Conacyt (157100 CB-2010-01).

Author details

Marcia Campillo-Navarro[1], Isabel Wong-Baeza[1], Jeanet Serafín-López[1],
Rogelio Hernández-Pando[2], Sergio Estrada-Parra[1], Iris Estrada-García[1] and
Rommel Chacón-Salinas[1*]

*Address all correspondence to: rommelchacons@yahoo.com.mx

1 Department of Immunology, National School of Biological Sciences, ENCB-IPN, Mexico

2 Department of Experimental Pathology, National Institute of Medical Sciences and Nutrition Salvador-Zubirán, Mexico

References

[1] Comas I, Coscolla M, Luo T, Borrell S, Holt KE, Kato-Maeda M, et al. Out-of-Africa migration and Neolithic coexpansion of Mycobacterium tuberculosis with modern humans. Nature Genetics. 2013;45(10):1176-82.

[2] WHO. Global Tuberculosis Report 2013. Geneva: WHO, 2013.

[3] Raviglione MC, Snider DE, Jr., Kochi A. Global epidemiology of tuberculosis. Morbidity and mortality of a worldwide epidemic. JAMA : the Journal of the American Medical Association. 1995;273(3):220-6.

[4] Gagneux S, DeRiemer K, Van T, Kato-Maeda M, de Jong BC, Narayanan S, et al. Variable host-pathogen compatibility in Mycobacterium tuberculosis. Proceedings of the National Academy of Sciences of the United States of America. 2006;103(8):2869-73.

[5] Glynn JR, Whiteley J, Bifani PJ, Kremer K, van Soolingen D. Worldwide occurrence of Beijing/W strains of Mycobacterium tuberculosis: a systematic review. Emerging Infectious Diseases. 2002;8(8):843-9.

[6] Smith I. Mycobacterium tuberculosis pathogenesis and molecular determinants of virulence. Clinical Microbiology Reviews. 2003;16(3):463-96.

[7] Fennelly KP, Martyny JW, Fulton KE, Orme IM, Cave DM, Heifets LB. Cough-generated aerosols of Mycobacterium tuberculosis: a new method to study infectiousness. American Journal of Respiratory and Critical Care Medicine. 2004;169(5):604-9.

[8] Engele M, Stossel E, Castiglione K, Schwerdtner N, Wagner M, Bolcskei P, et al. Induction of TNF in human alveolar macrophages as a potential evasion mechanism of virulent Mycobacterium tuberculosis. Journal of Immunology. 2002;168(3):1328-37.

[9] Schafer G, Jacobs M, Wilkinson RJ, Brown GD. Non-opsonic recognition of Mycobacterium tuberculosis by phagocytes. Journal of Innate Immunity. 2009;1(3):231-43.

[10] Armstrong JA, Hart PD. Response of cultured macrophages to Mycobacterium tuberculosis, with observations on fusion of lysosomes with phagosomes. The Journal of Experimental Medicine. 1971;134(3 Pt 1):713-40.

[11] Via LE, Deretic D, Ulmer RJ, Hibler NS, Huber LA, Deretic V. Arrest of mycobacterial phagosome maturation is caused by a block in vesicle fusion between stages controlled by rab5 and rab7. The Journal of Biological Chemistry. 1997;272(20):13326-31.

[12] Tsao TC, Hong J, Huang C, Yang P, Liao SK, Chang KS. Increased TNF-alpha, IL-1 beta and IL-6 levels in the bronchoalveolar lavage fluid with the upregulation of their mRNA in macrophages lavaged from patients with active pulmonary tuberculosis. Tubercle and lung disease : the Official Journal of the International Union against Tuberculosis and Lung Disease. 1999;79(5):279-85.

[13] Tian T, Woodworth J, Skold M, Behar SM. In vivo depletion of CD11c+ cells delays the CD4+ T cell response to Mycobacterium tuberculosis and exacerbates the outcome of infection. Journal of Immunology. 2005;175(5):3268-72.

[14] Seah GT, Scott GM, Rook GA. Type 2 cytokine gene activation and its relationship to extent of disease in patients with tuberculosis. The Journal of Infectious Diseases. 2000;181(1):385-9.

[15] Boussiotis VA, Tsai EY, Yunis EJ, Thim S, Delgado JC, Dascher CC, et al. IL-10-producing T cells suppress immune responses in anergic tuberculosis patients. The Journal of Clinical Investigation. 2000;105(9):1317-25.

[16] Bonecini-Almeida MG, Ho JL, Boechat N, Huard RC, Chitale S, Doo H, et al. Down-modulation of lung immune responses by interleukin-10 and transforming growth factor beta (TGF-beta) and analysis of TGF-beta receptors I and II in active tuberculosis. Infection and Immunity. 2004;72(5):2628-34.

[17] Silva Miranda M, Breiman A, Allain S, Deknuydt F, Altare F. The tuberculous granuloma: an unsuccessful host defence mechanism providing a safety shelter for the bacteria? Clinical & Developmental Immunology. 2012;2012:139127.

[18] Tsai MC, Chakravarty S, Zhu G, Xu J, Tanaka K, Koch C, et al. Characterization of the tuberculous granuloma in murine and human lungs: cellular composition and relative tissue oxygen tension. Cellular Microbiology. 2006;8(2):218-32.

[19] Jones BE, Young SM, Antoniskis D, Davidson PT, Kramer F, Barnes PF. Relationship of the manifestations of tuberculosis to CD4 cell counts in patients with human immunodeficiency virus infection. The American Review of Respiratory Disease. 1993;148(5):1292-7.

[20] de Noronha AL, Bafica A, Nogueira L, Barral A, Barral-Netto M. Lung granulomas from Mycobacterium tuberculosis/HIV-1 co-infected patients display decreased in situ TNF production. Pathology, Research and Practice. 2008;204(3):155-61.

[21] Chakravarty SD, Zhu G, Tsai MC, Mohan VP, Marino S, Kirschner DE, et al. Tumor necrosis factor blockade in chronic murine tuberculosis enhances granulomatous inflammation and disorganizes granulomas in the lungs. Infection and Immunity. 2008;76(3):916-26.

[22] Boddinghaus B, Rogall T, Flohr T, Blocker H, Bottger EC. Detection and identification of mycobacteria by amplification of rRNA. Journal of Clinical Microbiology. 1990;28(8):1751-9.

[23] Sreevatsan S, Pan X, Stockbauer KE, Connell ND, Kreiswirth BN, Whittam TS, Musser JM. Restricted structural gene polymorphism in the Mycobacterium tuberculosis complex indicates evolutionarily recent global dissemination. Proceedings of the National Academy of Sciences of the United States of America. 1997;94(18):9869-74.

[24] van Soolingen D, Qian L, de Haas PE, Douglas JT, Traore H, Portaels F, et al. Predominance of a single genotype of Mycobacterium tuberculosis in countries of east Asia. Journal of Clinical Microbiology. 1995;33(12):3234-8.

[25] Bifani PJ, Mathema B, Kurepina NE, Kreiswirth BN. Global dissemination of the Mycobacterium tuberculosis W-Beijing family strains. Trends in Microbiology. 2002;10(1):45-52.

[26] Kurepina NE, Sreevatsan S, Plikaytis BB, Bifani PJ, Connell ND, Donnelly RJ, et al. Characterization of the phylogenetic distribution and chromosomal insertion sites of five IS6110 elements in Mycobacterium tuberculosis: non-random integration in the dnaA-dnaN region. Tubercle and Lung Disease : the Official Journal of the International Union against Tuberculosis and Lung Disease. 1998;79(1):31-42.

[27] Mokrousov I, Narvskaya O, Otten T, Vyazovaya A, Limeschenko E, Steklova L, Vyshnevskyi B. Phylogenetic reconstruction within Mycobacterium tuberculosis Beijing genotype in northwestern Russia. Research in Microbiology. 2002;153(10):629-37.

[28] Tsolaki AG, Gagneux S, Pym AS, Goguet de la Salmoniere YO, Kreiswirth BN, Van Soolingen D, Small PM. Genomic deletions classify the Beijing/W strains as a distinct genetic lineage of Mycobacterium tuberculosis. Journal of Clinical Microbiology. 2005;43(7):3185-91.

[29] Hanekom M, van der Spuy GD, Streicher E, Ndabambi SL, McEvoy CR, Kidd M, et al. A recently evolved sublineage of the Mycobacterium tuberculosis Beijing strain family is associated with an increased ability to spread and cause disease. Journal of Clinical Microbiology. 2007;45(5):1483-90.

[30] Agerton TB, Valway SE, Blinkhorn RJ, Shilkret KL, Reves R, Schluter WW, et al. Spread of strain W, a highly drug-resistant strain of Mycobacterium tuberculosis, across the United States. Clinical Infectious Diseases. 1999;29(1):85-92.

[31] Bifani PJ, Plikaytis BB, Kapur V, Stockbauer K, Pan X, Lutfey ML, et al. Origin and interstate spread of a New York City multidrug-resistant Mycobacterium tuberculosis clone family. JAMA : the Journal of the American Medical Association. 1996;275(6):452-7.

[32] Frieden TR, Sherman LF, Maw KL, Fujiwara PI, Crawford JT, Nivin B, et al. A multi-institutional outbreak of highly drug-resistant tuberculosis: epidemiology and clinical outcomes. JAMA : the Journal of the American Medical Association. 1996;276(15): 1229-35.

[33] Johnson R, Warren R, Strauss OJ, Jordaan AM, Falmer AA, Beyers N, et al. An outbreak of drug-resistant tuberculosis caused by a Beijing strain in the western Cape, South Africa. The International Journal of Tuberculosis and Lung Disease : the official journal of the International Union against Tuberculosis and Lung Disease. 2006;10(12):1412-4.

[34] Affolabi D, Faihun F, Sanoussi N, Anyo G, Shamputa IC, Rigouts L, et al. Possible outbreak of streptomycin-resistant Mycobacterium tuberculosis Beijing in Benin. Emerging Infectious Diseases. 2009;15(7):1123-5.

[35] Parwati I, Alisjahbana B, Apriani L, Soetikno RD, Ottenhoff TH, van der Zanden AG, et al. Mycobacterium tuberculosis Beijing genotype is an independent risk factor for tuberculosis treatment failure in Indonesia. The Journal of Infectious Diseases. 2010;201(4):553-7.

[36] Burman WJ, Bliven EE, Cowan L, Bozeman L, Nahid P, Diem L, et al. Relapse associated with active disease caused by Beijing strain of Mycobacterium tuberculosis. Emerging Infectious Diseases. 2009;15(7):1061-7.

[37] Lan NT, Lien HT, Tung le B, Borgdorff MW, Kremer K, van Soolingen D. Mycobacterium tuberculosis Beijing genotype and risk for treatment failure and relapse, Vietnam. Emerging Infectious Diseases. 2003;9(12):1633-5.

[38] Sun YJ, Lee AS, Wong SY, Paton NI. Association of Mycobacterium tuberculosis Beijing genotype with tuberculosis relapse in Singapore. Epidemiology and infection. 2006;134(2):329-32.

[39] Huyen MN, Buu TN, Tiemersma E, Lan NT, Dung NH, Kremer K, et al. Tuberculosis relapse in Vietnam is significantly associated with Mycobacterium tuberculosis Beijing genotype infections. The Journal of Infectious Diseases. 2013;207(10):1516-24.

[40] Kong Y, Cave MD, Zhang L, Foxman B, Marrs CF, Bates JH, Yang ZH. Association between Mycobacterium tuberculosis Beijing/W lineage strain infection and extrathoracic tuberculosis: Insights from epidemiologic and clinical characterization of the three principal genetic groups of M. tuberculosis clinical isolates. Journal of Clinical Microbiology. 2007;45(2):409-14.

[41] de Jong BC, Hill PC, Aiken A, Awine T, Antonio M, Adetifa IM, et al. Progression to active tuberculosis, but not transmission, varies by Mycobacterium tuberculosis lineage in The Gambia. The Journal of Infectious Diseases. 2008;198(7):1037-43.

[42] Pang Y, Song Y, Xia H, Zhou Y, Zhao B, Zhao Y. Risk factors and clinical phenotypes of Beijing genotype strains in tuberculosis patients in China. BMC infectious diseases. 2012;12:354.

[43] Thwaites G, Caws M, Chau TT, D'Sa A, Lan NT, Huyen MN, et al. Relationship between Mycobacterium tuberculosis genotype and the clinical phenotype of pulmonary and meningeal tuberculosis. Journal of Clinical Microbiology. 2008;46(4):1363-8.

[44] Drobniewski F, Balabanova Y, Nikolayevsky V, Ruddy M, Kuznetzov S, Zakharova S, et al. Drug-resistant tuberculosis, clinical virulence, and the dominance of the Beijing strain family in Russia. JAMA : the Journal of the American Medical Association. 2005;293(22):2726-31.

[45] Anh DD, Borgdorff MW, Van LN, Lan NT, van Gorkom T, Kremer K, van Soolingen D. Mycobacterium tuberculosis Beijing genotype emerging in Vietnam. Emerging Infectious Diseases. 2000;6(3):302-5.

[46] van Crevel R, Nelwan RH, de Lenne W, Veeraragu Y, van der Zanden AG, Amin Z, et al. Mycobacterium tuberculosis Beijing genotype strains associated with febrile response to treatment. Emerging Infectious Diseases. 2001;7(5):880-3.

[47] Middelkoop K, Bekker LG, Mathema B, Shashkina E, Kurepina N, Whitelaw A, et al. Molecular epidemiology of Mycobacterium tuberculosis in a South African community with high HIV prevalence. The Journal of Infectious Diseases. 2009;200(8):1207-11.

[48] Kremer K, van-der-Werf MJ, Au BK, Anh DD, Kam KM, van-Doorn HR, et al. Vaccine-induced immunity circumvented by typical Mycobacterium tuberculosis Beijing strains. Emerging Infectious Diseases. 2009;15(2):335-9.

[49] Chan MY, Borgdorff M, Yip CW, de Haas PE, Wong WS, Kam KM, Van Soolingen D. Seventy percent of the Mycobacterium tuberculosis isolates in Hong Kong represent the Beijing genotype. Epidemiology and Infection. 2001;127(1):169-71.

[50] Palittapongarnpim P, Luangsook P, Tansuphaswadikul S, Chuchottaworn C, Prachaktam R, Sathapatayavongs B. Restriction fragment length polymorphism study of Mycobacterium tuberculosis in Thailand using IS6110 as probe. The International Journal of Tuberculosis and Lung Disease : the official journal of the International Union against Tuberculosis and Lung Disease. 1997;1(4):370-6.

[51] Prodinger WM, Bunyaratvej P, Prachaktam R, Pavlic M. Mycobacterium tuberculosis isolates of Beijing genotype in Thailand. Emerging Infectious Diseases. 2001;7(3): 483-4.

[52] Feng JY, Su WJ, Tsai CC, Chang SC. Clinical impact of Mycobacterium tuberculosis W-Beijing genotype strain infection on aged patients in Taiwan. Journal of Clinical Microbiology. 2008;46(9):3127-9.

[53] Glynn JR, Crampin AC, Traore H, Yates MD, Mwaungulu FD, Ngwira BM, et al. Mycobacterium tuberculosis Beijing genotype, northern Malawi. Emerging Infectious Diseases. 2005;11(1):150-3.

[54] Hasan Z, Tanveer M, Kanji A, Hasan Q, Ghebremichael S, Hasan R. Spoligotyping of Mycobacterium tuberculosis isolates from Pakistan reveals predominance of Central Asian Strain 1 and Beijing isolates. Journal of Clinical Microbiology. 2006;44(5): 1763-8.

[55] Sun YJ, Lim TK, Ong AK, Ho BC, Seah GT, Paton NI. Tuberculosis associated with Mycobacterium tuberculosis Beijing and non-Beijing genotypes: a clinical and immunological comparison. BMC Infectious Diseases. 2006;6:105.

[56] Rakotosamimanana N, Raharimanga V, Andriamandimby SF, Soares JL, Doherty TM, Ratsitorahina M, et al. Variation in gamma interferon responses to different in-

fecting strains of Mycobacterium tuberculosis in acid-fast bacillus smear-positive patients and household contacts in Antananarivo, Madagascar. Clinical and Vaccine Immunology. 2010;17(7):1094-103.

[57] Manca C, Tsenova L, Bergtold A, Freeman S, Tovey M, Musser JM, et al. Virulence of a Mycobacterium tuberculosis clinical isolate in mice is determined by failure to induce Th1 type immunity and is associated with induction of IFN-alpha /beta. Proceedings of the National Academy of Sciences of the United States of America. 2001;98(10):5752-7.

[58] Manca C, Tsenova L, Barry CE, 3rd, Bergtold A, Freeman S, Haslett PA, et al. Mycobacterium tuberculosis CDC1551 induces a more vigorous host response in vivo and in vitro, but is not more virulent than other clinical isolates. Journal of Immunology. 1999;162(11):6740-6.

[59] Ordway D, Henao-Tamayo M, Harton M, Palanisamy G, Troudt J, Shanley C, et al. The hypervirulent Mycobacterium tuberculosis strain HN878 induces a potent TH1 response followed by rapid down-regulation. Journal of Immunology. 2007;179(1): 522-31.

[60] Shang S, Harton M, Tamayo MH, Shanley C, Palanisamy GS, Caraway M, et al. Increased Foxp3 expression in guinea pigs infected with W-Beijing strains of M. tuberculosis. Tuberculosis. 2011;91(5):378-85.

[61] Tsenova L, Ellison E, Harbacheuski R, Moreira AL, Kurepina N, Reed MB, et al. Virulence of selected Mycobacterium tuberculosis clinical isolates in the rabbit model of meningitis is dependent on phenolic glycolipid produced by the bacilli. The Journal of Infectious Diseases. 2005;192(1):98-106.

[62] Lopez B, Aguilar D, Orozco H, Burger M, Espitia C, Ritacco V, et al. A marked difference in pathogenesis and immune response induced by different Mycobacterium tuberculosis genotypes. Clinical and Experimental Immunology. 2003;133(1):30-7.

[63] Rios-Barrera VA, Campos-Pena V, Aguilar-Leon D, Lascurain LR, Meraz-Rios MA, Moreno J, et al. Macrophage and T lymphocyte apoptosis during experimental pulmonary tuberculosis: their relationship to mycobacterial virulence. European Journal of Immunology. 2006;36(2):345-53.

[64] Quintero-Macias L, Silva-Sanchez A, Valderrabano-Ortiz E, Munguia-Fuentes R, Aguilar-Leon D, Hernandez-Pando R, Flores-Romo L. Reduced in vivo cytotoxicity and increased Mycobacterial burden are associated with virulent Mycobacterium tuberculosis strains during lung infection. Immunological Investigations. 2012;41(1): 51-60.

[65] Jeon BY, Kwak J, Hahn MY, Eum SY, Yang J, Kim SC, Cho SN. In vivo characteristics of Korean Beijing Mycobacterium tuberculosis strain K1 in an aerosol challenge model and in the Cornell latent tuberculosis model. Journal of Medical Microbiology. 2012;61(Pt 10):1373-9.

[66] Reiling N, Homolka S, Walter K, Brandenburg J, Niwinski L, Ernst M, et al. Clade-specific virulence patterns of Mycobacterium tuberculosis complex strains in human primary macrophages and aerogenically infected mice. mBio. 2013;4(4).

[67] Dormans J, Burger M, Aguilar D, Hernandez-Pando R, Kremer K, Roholl P, et al. Correlation of virulence, lung pathology, bacterial load and delayed type hypersensitivity responses after infection with different Mycobacterium tuberculosis genotypes in a BALB/c mouse model. Clinical and Experimental Immunology. 2004;137(3): 460-8.

[68] Aguilar D, Hanekom M, Mata D, Gey van Pittius NC, van Helden PD, Warren RM, Hernandez-Pando R. Mycobacterium tuberculosis strains with the Beijing genotype demonstrate variability in virulence associated with transmission. Tuberculosis. 2010;90(5):319-25.

[69] Krishnan N, Malaga W, Constant P, Caws M, Tran TH, Salmons J, et al. Mycobacterium tuberculosis lineage influences innate immune response and virulence and is associated with distinct cell envelope lipid profiles. PloS One. 2011;6(9):e23870.

[70] Kato-Maeda M, Shanley CA, Ackart D, Jarlsberg LG, Shang S, Obregon-Henao A, et al. Beijing sublineages of Mycobacterium tuberculosis differ in pathogenicity in the guinea pig. Clinical and Vaccine Immunology. 2012;19(8):1227-37.

[71] Ribeiro SC, Gomes LL, Amaral EP, Andrade MR, Almeida FM, Rezende AL, et al. Mycobacterium tuberculosis strains of the modern sublineage of the Beijing family are more likely to display increased virulence than strains of the ancient sublineage. Journal of Clinical Microbiology. 2014;52(7):2615-24.

[72] Zhang M, Gong J, Yang Z, Samten B, Cave MD, Barnes PF. Enhanced capacity of a widespread strain of Mycobacterium tuberculosis to grow in human macrophages. The Journal of Infectious Diseases. 1999;179(5):1213-7.

[73] Li Q, Whalen CC, Albert JM, Larkin R, Zukowski L, Cave MD, Silver RF. Differences in rate and variability of intracellular growth of a panel of Mycobacterium tuberculosis clinical isolates within a human monocyte model. Infection and Immunity. 2002;70(11):6489-93.

[74] Manca C, Reed MB, Freeman S, Mathema B, Kreiswirth B, Barry CE, 3rd, Kaplan G. Differential monocyte activation underlies strain-specific Mycobacterium tuberculosis pathogenesis. Infection and Immunity. 2004;72(9):5511-4.

[75] Chacon-Salinas R, Serafin-Lopez J, Ramos-Payan R, Mendez-Aragon P, Hernandez-Pando R, Van Soolingen D, et al. Differential pattern of cytokine expression by macrophages infected in vitro with different Mycobacterium tuberculosis genotypes. Clinical and Experimental Immunology. 2005;140(3):443-9.

[76] Theus S, Eisenach K, Fomukong N, Silver RF, Cave MD. Beijing family Mycobacterium tuberculosis strains differ in their intracellular growth in THP-1 macrophages.

The International Journal of Tuberculosis and Lung Disease : the official journal of the International Union against Tuberculosis and Lung Disease. 2007;11(10):1087-93.

[77] Tanveer M, Hasan Z, Kanji A, Hussain R, Hasan R. Reduced TNF-alpha and IFN-gamma responses to Central Asian strain 1 and Beijing isolates of Mycobacterium tuberculosis in comparison with H37Rv strain. Transactions of the Royal Society of Tropical Medicine and Hygiene. 2009;103(6):581-7.

[78] Wang C, Peyron P, Mestre O, Kaplan G, van Soolingen D, Gao Q, et al. Innate immune response to Mycobacterium tuberculosis Beijing and other genotypes. PloS One. 2010;5(10):e13594.

[79] Portevin D, Gagneux S, Comas I, Young D. Human macrophage responses to clinical isolates from the Mycobacterium tuberculosis complex discriminate between ancient and modern lineages. PLoS Pathogens. 2011;7(3):e1001307.

[80] Krishnan N, Robertson BD, Thwaites G. Pathways of IL-1beta secretion by macrophages infected with clinical Mycobacterium tuberculosis strains. Tuberculosis. 2013;93(5):538-47.

[81] Allie N, Grivennikov SI, Keeton R, Hsu NJ, Bourigault ML, Court N, et al. Prominent role for T cell-derived tumour necrosis factor for sustained control of Mycobacterium tuberculosis infection. Scientific reports. 2013;3:1809.

[82] Cambier CJ, Takaki KK, Larson RP, Hernandez RE, Tobin DM, Urdahl KB, et al. Mycobacteria manipulate macrophage recruitment through coordinated use of membrane lipids. Nature. 2014;505(7482):218-22.

[83] Reyes-Martinez JE, Nieto-Patlan E, Nieto-Patlan A, Gonzaga-Bernachi J, Santos-Mendoza T, Serafin-Lopez J, et al. Differential activation of dendritic cells by Mycobacterium tuberculosis Beijing genotype. Immunological Investigations. 2014;43(5):436-46.

[84] Muul LM, Heine G, Silvin C, James SP, Candotti F, Radbruch A, Worm M. Measurement of proliferative responses of cultured lymphocytes. Current Protocols in Immunology / edited by John E Coligan [et al] . 2011;Chapter 7:Unit7 10.

[85] Rivera-Ordaz A, Gonzaga-Bernachi J, Serafin-Lopez J, Hernandez-Pando R, Van Soolingen D, Estrada-Parra S, et al. Mycobacterium tuberculosis Beijing genotype induces differential cytokine production by peripheral blood mononuclear cells of healthy BCG vaccinated individuals. Immunological Investigations. 2012;41(2):144-56.

[86] van Laarhoven A, Mandemakers JJ, Kleinnijenhuis J, Enaimi M, Lachmandas E, Joosten LA, et al. Low induction of proinflammatory cytokines parallels evolutionary success of modern strains within the Mycobacterium tuberculosis Beijing genotype. Infection and Immunity. 2013;81(10):3750-6.

[87] Rocha-Ramirez LM, Estrada-Garcia I, Lopez-Marin LM, Segura-Salinas E, Mendez-Aragon P, Van Soolingen D, et al. Mycobacterium tuberculosis lipids regulate cyto-

kines, TLR-2/4 and MHC class II expression in human macrophages. Tuberculosis. 2008;88(3):212-20.

[88] Reed MB, Domenech P, Manca C, Su H, Barczak AK, Kreiswirth BN, et al. A glycolipid of hypervirulent tuberculosis strains that inhibits the innate immune response. Nature. 2004;431(7004):84-7.

[89] Chaiprasert A, Yorsangsukkamol J, Prammananan T, Palittapongarnpim P, Leechawengwong M, Dhiraputra C. Intact pks15/1 in non-W-Beijing Mycobacterium tuberculosis isolates. Emerging Infectious Diseases. 2006;12(5):772-4.

[90] Reed MB, Gagneux S, Deriemer K, Small PM, Barry CE, 3rd. The W-Beijing lineage of Mycobacterium tuberculosis overproduces triglycerides and has the DosR dormancy regulon constitutively upregulated. Journal of Bacteriology. 2007;189(7):2583-9.

[91] Sinsimer D, Huet G, Manca C, Tsenova L, Koo MS, Kurepina N, et al. The phenolic glycolipid of Mycobacterium tuberculosis differentially modulates the early host cytokine response but does not in itself confer hypervirulence. Infection and Immunity. 2008;76(7):3027-36.

[92] Huet G, Constant P, Malaga W, Laneelle MA, Kremer K, van Soolingen D, et al. A lipid profile typifies the Beijing strains of Mycobacterium tuberculosis: identification of a mutation responsible for a modification of the structures of phthiocerol dimycocerosates and phenolic glycolipids. The Journal of Biological Chemistry. 2009;284(40): 27101-13.

[93] Neyrolles O, Guilhot C. Recent advances in deciphering the contribution of Mycobacterium tuberculosis lipids to pathogenesis. Tuberculosis. 2011;91(3):187-95.

[94] Flores J, Espitia C. Differential expression of PE and PE_PGRS genes in Mycobacterium tuberculosis strains. Gene. 2003;318:75-81.

[95] Wu S, Howard ST, Lakey DL, Kipnis A, Samten B, Safi H, et al. The principal sigma factor sigA mediates enhanced growth of Mycobacterium tuberculosis in vivo. Molecular Microbiology. 2004;51(6):1551-62.

[96] Samuel LP, Song CH, Wei J, Roberts EA, Dahl JL, Barry CE, 3rd, et al. Expression, production and release of the Eis protein by Mycobacterium tuberculosis during infection of macrophages and its effect on cytokine secretion. Microbiology. 2007;153(Pt 2):529-40.

[97] Wu S, Barnes PF, Samten B, Pang X, Rodrigue S, Ghanny S, et al. Activation of the eis gene in a W-Beijing strain of Mycobacterium tuberculosis correlates with increased SigA levels and enhanced intracellular growth. Microbiology. 2009;155(Pt 4):1272-81.

[98] Pheiffer C, Betts JC, Flynn HR, Lukey PT, van Helden P. Protein expression by a Beijing strain differs from that of another clinical isolate and Mycobacterium tuberculosis H37Rv. Microbiology. 2005;151(Pt 4):1139-50.

[99] Karakousis PC, Yoshimatsu T, Lamichhane G, Woolwine SC, Nuermberger EL, Grosset J, Bishai WR. Dormancy phenotype displayed by extracellular Mycobacterium tuberculosis within artificial granulomas in mice. The Journal of Experimental Medicine. 2004;200(5):647-57.

[100] Schnappinger D, Ehrt S, Voskuil MI, Liu Y, Mangan JA, Monahan IM, et al. Transcriptional Adaptation of Mycobacterium tuberculosis within Macrophages: Insights into the Phagosomal Environment. The Journal of Experimental Medicine. 2003;198(5):693-704.

[101] Fallow A, Domenech P, Reed MB. Strains of the East Asian (W/Beijing) lineage of Mycobacterium tuberculosis are DosS/DosT-DosR two-component regulatory system natural mutants. Journal of Bacteriology. 2010;192(8):2228-38.

[102] Domenech P, Kolly GS, Leon-Solis L, Fallow A, Reed MB. Massive gene duplication event among clinical isolates of the Mycobacterium tuberculosis W/Beijing family. Journal of Bacteriology. 2010;192(18):4562-70.

[103] Rindi L, Peroni I, Lari N, Bonanni D, Tortoli E, Garzelli C. Variation of the expression of Mycobacterium tuberculosis ppe44 gene among clinical isolates. FEMS Immunology and Medical Microbiology. 2007;51(2):381-7.

[104] de Souza GA, Fortuin S, Aguilar D, Pando RH, McEvoy CR, van Helden PD, et al. Using a label-free proteomics method to identify differentially abundant proteins in closely related hypo- and hypervirulent clinical Mycobacterium tuberculosis Beijing isolates. Molecular & Cellular Proteomics. 2010;9(11):2414-23.

[105] Park PJ, Kim AR, Salch YP, Song T, Shin SJ, Han SJ, Cho SN. Characterization of a novel antigen of Mycobacterium tuberculosis K strain and its use in immunodiagnosis of tuberculosis. Journal of Microbiology. 2014.

[106] Shin AR, Shin SJ, Lee KS, Eom SH, Lee SS, Lee BS, et al. Improved sensitivity of diagnosis of tuberculosis in patients in Korea via a cocktail enzyme-linked immunosorbent assay containing the abundantly expressed antigens of the K strain of Mycobacterium tuberculosis. Clinical and Vaccine Immunology. 2008;15(12):1788-95.

[107] Pathak SK, Basu S, Basu KK, Banerjee A, Pathak S, Bhattacharyya A, et al. Direct extracellular interaction between the early secreted antigen ESAT-6 of Mycobacterium tuberculosis and TLR2 inhibits TLR signaling in macrophages. Nature Immunology. 2007;8(6):610-8.

[108] Appelmelk BJ, van Die I, van Vliet SJ, Vandenbroucke-Grauls CM, Geijtenbeek TB, van Kooyk Y. Cutting edge: carbohydrate profiling identifies new pathogens that interact with dendritic cell-specific ICAM-3-grabbing nonintegrin on dendritic cells. Journal of Immunology. 2003;170(4):1635-9.

[109] Torrelles JB, Schlesinger LS. Diversity in Mycobacterium tuberculosis mannosylated cell wall determinants impacts adaptation to the host. Tuberculosis (Edinb). 2010;90(2):84-93.

[110] Meissner-Roloff RJ, Koekemoer G, Warren RM, Loots DT. A metabolomics investigation of a hyper- and hypo-virulent phenotype of Beijing lineage M. tuberculosis. Metabolomics. 2012;8(6):1194-203.

[111] Wu K, Dong D, Fang H, Levillain F, Jin W, Mei J, et al. An interferon-related signature in the transcriptional core response of human macrophages to Mycobacterium tuberculosis infection. PLoS One. 2012;7(6):e38367.

[112] Hanekom M, Gey van Pittius NC, McEvoy C, Victor TC, Van Helden PD, Warren RM. Mycobacterium tuberculosis Beijing genotype: a template for success. Tuberculosis (Edinb). 2011;91(6):510-23.

[113] Hershberg R, Lipatov M, Small PM, Sheffer H, Niemann S, Homolka S, et al. High functional diversity in Mycobacterium tuberculosis driven by genetic drift and human demography. PLoS Biology. 2008;6(12):e311.

[114] Gagneux S. Host-pathogen coevolution in human tuberculosis. Philosophical Transactions of the Royal Society of London Series B, Biological sciences. 2012;367(1590): 850-9.

[115] Pasipanodya JG, Moonan PK, Vecino E, Miller TL, Fernandez M, Slocum P, et al. Allopatric tuberculosis host-pathogen relationships are associated with greater pulmonary impairment. Infection, Genetics and Evolution. 2013;16:433-40.

[116] Ghebremichael S, Groenheit R, Pennhag A, Koivula T, Andersson E, Bruchfeld J, et al. Drug resistant Mycobacterium tuberculosis of the Beijing genotype does not spread in Sweden. PloS One. 2010;5(5):e10893.

[117] Zanini F, Carugati M, Schiroli C, Lapadula G, Lombardi A, Codecasa L, et al. Mycobacterium tuberculosis Beijing family: analysis of the epidemiological and clinical factors associated with an emerging lineage in the urban area of Milan. Infection, Genetics and Evolution. 2014;25:14-9.

[118] Hanekom M, van der Spuy GD, Gey van Pittius NC, McEvoy CR, Ndabambi SL, Victor TC, et al. Evidence that the spread of Mycobacterium tuberculosis strains with the Beijing genotype is human population dependent. Journal of Clinical Microbiology. 2007;45(7):2263-6.

[119] Caws M, Thwaites G, Dunstan S, Hawn TR, Lan NT, Thuong NT, et al. The influence of host and bacterial genotype on the development of disseminated disease with Mycobacterium tuberculosis. PLoS Pathogens. 2008;4(3):e1000034.

[120] Ioana M, Ferwerda B, Plantinga TS, Stappers M, Oosting M, McCall M, et al. Different patterns of Toll-like receptor 2 polymorphisms in populations of various ethnic and geographic origins. Infection and Immunity. 2012;80(5):1917-22.

[121] Carmona J, Cruz A, Moreira-Teixeira L, Sousa C, Sousa J, Osorio NS, et al. Strains Are Differentially Recognized by TLRs with an Impact on the Immune Response. PLoS One. 2013;8(6):e67277.

[122] van Crevel R, Parwati I, Sahiratmadja E, Marzuki S, Ottenhoff TH, Netea MG, et al. Infection with Mycobacterium tuberculosis Beijing genotype strains is associated with polymorphisms in SLC11A1/NRAMP1 in Indonesian patients with tuberculosis. The Journal of Infectious Diseases. 2009;200(11):1671-4.

[123] Blackwell JM, Goswami T, Evans CA, Sibthorpe D, Papo N, White JK, et al. SLC11A1 (formerly NRAMP1) and disease resistance. Cellular Microbiolology. 2001;3(12): 773-84.

[124] Salie M, van der Merwe L, Moller M, Daya M, van der Spuy GD, van Helden PD, et al. Associations between human leukocyte antigen class I variants and the Mycobacterium tuberculosis subtypes causing disease. The Journal of Infectious Diseases. 2014;209(2):216-23.

[125] Lewinsohn DA, Heinzel AS, Gardner JM, Zhu L, Alderson MR, Lewinsohn DM. Mycobacterium tuberculosis-specific CD8+ T cells preferentially recognize heavily infected cells. American Journal of Respiratory and Critical Care Medicine. 2003;168(11):1346-52.

Permissions

All chapters in this book were first published by InTech Open; hereby published with permission under the Creative Commons Attribution License or equivalent. Every chapter published in this book has been scrutinized by our experts. Their significance has been extensively debated. The topics covered herein carry significant findings which will fuel the growth of the discipline. They may even be implemented as practical applications or may be referred to as a beginning point for another development.

The contributors of this book come from diverse backgrounds, making this book a truly international effort. This book will bring forth new frontiers with its revolutionizing research information and detailed analysis of the nascent developments around the world.

We would like to thank all the contributing authors for lending their expertise to make the book truly unique. They have played a crucial role in the development of this book. Without their invaluable contributions this book wouldn't have been possible. They have made vital efforts to compile up to date information on the varied aspects of this subject to make this book a valuable addition to the collection of many professionals and students.

This book was conceptualized with the vision of imparting up-to-date information and advanced data in this field. To ensure the same, a matchless editorial board was set up. Every individual on the board went through rigorous rounds of assessment to prove their worth. After which they invested a large part of their time researching and compiling the most relevant data for our readers.

The editorial board has been involved in producing this book since its inception. They have spent rigorous hours researching and exploring the diverse topics which have resulted in the successful publishing of this book. They have passed on their knowledge of decades through this book. To expedite this challenging task, the publisher supported the team at every step. A small team of assistant editors was also appointed to further simplify the editing procedure and attain best results for the readers.

Apart from the editorial board, the designing team has also invested a significant amount of their time in understanding the subject and creating the most relevant covers. They scrutinized every image to scout for the most suitable representation of the subject and create an appropriate cover for the book.

The publishing team has been an ardent support to the editorial, designing and production team. Their endless efforts to recruit the best for this project, has resulted in the accomplishment of this book. They are a veteran in the field of academics and their pool of knowledge is as vast as their experience in printing. Their expertise and guidance has proved useful at every step. Their uncompromising quality standards have made this book an exceptional effort. Their encouragement from time to time has been an inspiration for everyone.

The publisher and the editorial board hope that this book will prove to be a valuable piece of knowledge for researchers, students, practitioners and scholars across the globe.

List of Contributors

Elizabeth M. MacDonald and Angelo A. Izzo
Mycobacteria Research Laboratories, Department of Microbiology, Immunology and Pathology, Colorado State University, Fort Collins, CO, USA

Carlos Adam Conte Junior
Department of Food Technology, Faculty of Veterinary, Fluminense Federal University, Niterói, Rio de Janeiro, Brazil

Vânia M. Flosi Paschoalin
Faculty of Veterinary Medicine, Universidad Nacional Mayor de San Marcos, San Borja, Lima, Peru

César Aquiles Lázaro de la Torre
Department of Food Technology, Faculty of Veterinary, Fluminense Federal University, Niterói, Rio de Janeiro, Brazil
Faculty of Veterinary Medicine, Universidad Nacional Mayor de San Marcos, San Borja, Lima, Peru

Eduardo Eustáquio de Souza Figueiredo
Department of Food and Nutrition, Federal University of Mato Grosso, Cuiabá/MT, Brazil
Faculty of Nutrition and Food Science and Technology, Federal University of Mato Grosso, Cuiabá/MT, Brazil

Walter Lilenbaum
Department of Microbiology, Fluminense Federal University, Niterói, Rio de Janeiro, Brazil
Biomedical Institute, Fluminense Federal University, Niterói - RJ, Brazil

H. J. Sánchez-Pérez
Health Department, The College of the Southern Border (El Colegio de la Frontera Sur, Ecosur), San Cristobal de Las Casas, Chiapas, Mexico
Prometeo researcher, Loja National University, Loja, Ecuador
Research Groups for Africa and Latin Americas (GRAAL), Barcelona, Spain

Anaximandro Gómez-Velasco
Health Department, The College of the Southern Border (El Colegio de la Frontera Sur, Ecosur), San Cristobal de Las Casas, Chiapas, Mexico Research Groups for Africa and Latin Americas (GRAAL), Barcelona, Spain
Postdoctoral Research Fellow, Mexican National Council for Science and Technology (CONACyT), Mexico

G. Leal
Health Care Department, Health and Society Area, Autonomous Metropolitan University, Xochimilco Campus, Mexico, Distrito Federal., Mexico

A. Bencomo-Alerm
Mycobacteriology Laboratory, Health Jurisdiction II, Chiapas Institute of Health, San Cristobal de Las Casas, Chiapas, Mexico

N. Romero-Sandova
Research Groups for Africa and Latin Americas (GRAAL), Barcelona, Spain
School of Medicine, Faculty of Medicine, Health and Life Sciences, International University of Ecuador, Quito, Ecuador

M. Martín-Mateo
Research Groups for Africa and Latin Americas (GRAAL), Barcelona, Spain
School of Medicine, Faculty of Medicine, Health and Life Sciences, International University of Ecuador, Quito, Ecuador
Faculty of Medicine, Autonomous University of Barcelona, Bellaterra, Barcelona, Spain

Marisol Ocampo C.
Head of the Tuberculosis Department, Fundación Instituto de Inmunología de Colombia, FIDIC, Carrera, and Bogotá, Colombia
School of Medicine and Health Sciences, Universidad del Rosario, Bogotá, Colombia

Ricardo César Tavares Carvalho, Leone Vinícius Furlanetto and Vânia Margaret Flosi Paschoalin
Institute of Chemistry, Federal University of Rio de Janeiro, Rio de Janeiro - RJ, Brazil

Rafael da Silva Duarte
Institute of Microbiology, Federal University of Rio de Janeiro, Rio de Janeiro - RJ, Brazil

Luciano Nakazato
Laboratory of Molecular Biology, Faculty of Veterinary Medicine, Federal University of Mato Grosso, Cuiabá/MT, Brazil

M. Orozco-Uribe, L. Donis-Maturano, J. Calderón-Amador and L. Flores-Romo
Department of Cell Biology, CINVESTAVIPN, Zacatenco, México City, Mexico

R. Chacón-Salinas, J. Castañeda-Casimiro, S. Estrada-Parra and I. Estrada-García
Department of Immunology, ENCB-IPN, México City, Mexico

Paula Cristina Alves Leitão
Faculty of Medical Sciences, Universidade de Pernambuco, Brazil

Luiz Alberto Alves Mota
Faculty of Medical Sciences, Universidade de Pernambuco, Brazil
Hospital Universitário Oswaldo Cruz, Brazil
Rede Nordeste de Biotecnologia (RENORBIO), Brazil

Ana Maria dos Anjos Carneiro-Leão
Department of Animal Morphology and Physiology - Universidade Federal Rural de Pernambuco, Brazil, Brazil

Magda Lorena Orduz and Wellman Ribón
Universidad Industrial de Santander, Bucaramanga, Colombia

David E. Minnikin, Oona Y-C Lee, Houdini H. T. Wu, Vijayashankar Nataraj, Luke Alderwick, Apoorva Bhatt and Gurdyal S. Besra
Institute of Microbiology and Infection, School of Biosciences, University of Birmingham, Birmingham, UK

Helen D. Donoghue
Centre for Clinical Microbiology, Division of Infection and Immunity, University College London, London, UK

Malin Ridell
Department of Microbiology and Immunology, Institute of Biomedicine, University of Gothenburg, Gothenburg, Sweden

Motoko Watanabe
School of Pharmacy, Tokyo University of Pharmacy and Life Sciences, Tokyo, Japan

Marcia Campillo-Navarro, Isabel Wong-Baeza, Jeanet Serafín-López, Sergio Estrada-Parra, Iris Estrada-García and Rommel Chacón-Salinas
Department of Immunology, National School of Biological Sciences, ENCB-IPN, Mexico

Rogelio Hernández-Pando
Department of Experimental Pathology, National Institute of Medical Sciences and Nutrition Salvador-Zubirán, Mexico

Index

www.ingramcontent.com/pod-product-compliance
Lightning Source LLC
LaVergne TN
LVHW062236200926
848484LV00006B/1552